MEDICAL LIBRARY

DUNCAN MacMILLAN HOUSE

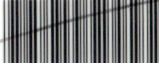

Although the long-term patterns of problem-behaviour that form personality disorders are part of the major classifications of disease, they have a generally unrecognized importance in clinical practice. These disorders are the origins of many medical consultations and social ills, perhaps associated with self-harm, suicide, neglect of children, criminality, alcohol and drug abuse, HIV transmission and 'accidents'. In a comprehensive summary and evaluation of the clinical literature, this book seeks to dispel the myth that personality disorder is simply a category for those problem individuals for whom nothing can be done.

With detailed coverage of recognition, assessment and management, Drs Dowson and Grounds provide a co-ordinated empirically-based account of those aspects of personality disorders that are of relevance to psychiatrists and allied disciplines, including clinical psychologists, social workers, criminologists, specialist nurses and primary care physicians. It describes how many individuals with personality disorders can be helped by health care services.

PERSONALITY DISORDERS:
RECOGNITION AND CLINICAL MANAGEMENT

PERSONALITY DISORDERS: RECOGNITION AND CLINICAL MANAGEMENT

JONATHAN H. DOWSON, MA, MB, BChir, MD (Cantab); DPM, PhD (Edin); FRCPsych

ADRIAN T. GROUNDS, BMedSci, BM, BS, DM (Nottingham); MRCPsych
University of Cambridge, UK

CAMBRIDGE
UNIVERSITY PRESS

Published by the Press Syndicate of the University of Cambridge
The Pitt Building, Trumpington Street, Cambridge CB2 1RP
40 West 20th Street, New York, NY 10011-4211, USA
10 Stamford Road, Oakleigh, Melbourne 3166, Australia

First published 1995

Printed in Great Britain at the University Press, Cambridge

A catalogue record for this book is available from the British Library

Library of Congress cataloguing in publication data

Dowson, Jonathan H.
Personality disorders : recognition and clinical management /
Jonathan H. Dowson, Adrian T. Grounds.
    p. cm.
Includes bibliographical references and index.
ISBN 0 521 45049 7 (hc)
1. Personality disorders.   I. Grounds, Adrian.   II. Title.
[DNLM: 1. Personality Disorders – diagnosis.   2. Personality
Disorders – therapy.   WM 190 D752p 1995]
RC554.D69 1995
616.85'8–dc20
DNLM/DLC
for Library of Congress   94-40749 CIP

ISBN 0 521 45049 7 hardback

Contents

Acknowledgement

We are most grateful to Mrs Anne Robson who prepared the original manuscripts.

Part One

Recognition

1

Personality disorders: basic concepts and clinical overview

J.H. DOWSON

Psychiatric disorders

'Personality disorders' consist of maladaptive patterns of motivated behaviour that are usually evident for at least several years. They form one of the main categories of psychiatric disorders.

Psychiatric disorders are usually defined in terms of signs and symptoms. 'Signs' are phenomena related to biological functioning and, in this context, consist of behaviour, while psychiatric 'symptoms' refer to the patient's complaints of adverse experiences. These include 'mental' phenomena, involving what has been called conscious awareness. The term 'patient' usually refers to someone who is being seen by a medical practitioner (or other health-care worker) in a professional context.

Behaviour can be defined as what an individual says or does, but only if it is associated with conscious awareness, so that an involuntary movement such as a tremor would not qualify. Also, behaviour includes what is not said or done; for example, patients with phobias may avoid a range of situations. The various mental phenomena which underlie motivated behaviour can be described by such terms as thoughts, ideas, memories, moods, attitudes and feelings, while the concept of conscious awareness can be extended to include the 'unconscious' or 'subconscious'; this involves higher mental activity that can influence conscious mental phenomena, although the person is not aware (or not fully aware) of these processes. For instance, a person may 'unconsciously' avoid keeping a series of appointments with his/her doctor because of a fear of having a serious illness diagnosed, even though the individual does not seem aware of the reason.

'Problem-behaviour in clinical practice' is a simple operational definition of psychiatric disorder, and can refer to problems from the patient's perspective as well as to difficulties that the patient causes for others. But this does not clarify which individuals with 'problem-behaviour' should

3

receive psychiatric and other medical services. Unfortunately, there is no satisfactory answer to this and there are two main attributes of a patient's problem-behaviour that are generally considered to require medical intervention. First, if there is an identifiable (or suspected) abnormal biological factor affecting the patient's behaviour (e.g. alcohol intoxication or a brain tumour) or, second, if medical care and treatment appears to be helpful, even if the concept of illness, disease or disorder would not usually be applied. The latter situation could occur if an individual has been involved in a serious traffic accident involving the death of several family members, and becomes suicidal. He/she may then be considered to need a period of care, restraint and sedation in a psychiatric hospital, even though the signs and symptoms appear as an understandable reaction to events.

Every branch of medicine involves the accumulation of knowledge, and the classification of relevant disorders (or 'diagnoses') is an essential part of this process. Classifications of psychiatric disorders can be based on groups of signs and symptoms, on causal factors, or on a rather untidy combination of both these approaches, which is apparent when the four main generally-accepted classes of psychiatric disorder are considered. The first, 'organic disorders', is based on the presence of causal factors, and consists of disorders that are due (at least in part) to an identifiable biological abnormality, such as the changes in brain structure in Alzheimer's disease. However, the remaining classes are mainly based on signs and symptoms; the second, the 'functional psychoses', includes schizophrenia and manic-depressive disorder, while the third, the 'neuroses', contains an heterogeneous group of syndromes, such as anxiety disorders and some types of depression. The fourth and final category is 'personality disorders', which, in contrast to all the previous categories, consists of repeated maladaptive patterns of behaviour which are usually present, in some degree, throughout adult life.

Why are personality disorders important?

While the repeated patterns of problem-behaviour that form personality disorders (PDs) are part of the major classifications of disease, they have a generally unrecognized importance in medical practice, although they provide the basis for numerous medical consultations. Also, PDs are often the origins of various social phenomena with serious consequences to society or to public health, such as homelessness (Scott, 1993), alcoholism, drug abuse, neglect of children, criminality, HIV transmission, 'accidents' and driving offences. Tiihonen & Eronen (1993), in a study of all subjects who had committed homicide in Finland over a specified period, found that males with antisocial PD were about 20 times more likely to commit homicide than males in the general population, and that homicide in this group was usually associated with alcohol dependence. Of 13 homicide recidivists in Finnish prisons or high-security hospitals, 11 had PD combined with severe alcoholism (Tiihonen & Hakola, 1994). In both primary care and hospital services, PDs appear to be associated with a high rate of consultations for physical symptoms without a clear diagnosis, and with many instances of self-harm. There is evidence that PDs can be causal factors (with varying degrees of specificity) for other psychiatric diagnoses such as some syndromes involving anxiety, depression and substance abuse, while PDs often complicate the diagnosis, management and outcome of co-occurring medical and psychiatric conditions. For example, an hypomanic illness may be mistakenly diagnosed as an antisocial PD, or exacerbate relatively mild maladaptive personality features. Also, if patients with an eating disorder have an associated PD, this often affects the severity and response to treatment, and co-occurring PDs have been shown to adversely affect the outcome of a range of non-PD psychiatric disorders (Reich & Vasile, 1993).

Patients with PDs are often mishandled in medical practice, because of a lack of knowledge of PD syndromes and a generally 'negative' attitude that can be evoked in their doctors. This is understandable, as the patient's behaviour in relation to a PD often involves difficult-to-manage behaviour such as excessive dependence on others, repeated complaints, problems in sustaining relationships and difficulties in many aspects of social functioning. Also, many health care workers believe that PDs are nothing to do with biology and medicine, despite the increasing evidence from twin and family studies that genetic as well as environmental factors are important for the development of many aspects of personality and PDs. A further reason is another erroneous belief that 'nothing can be done', but, in reality, many patients with PDs can be helped considerably by health care services.

Personality

Response/habit/trait/temperament

The concept of personality involves behavioural consistencies (Zuckerman, 1991), but describing 'behaviour' provides many pitfalls, even for the wary. An observed action (e.g. avoidance) may be given a label, such as 'defensive behaviour', which may make an assumption of a motive without sufficient evidence, while similar and related behaviours may be given several different designations. Also, different behaviours may receive the same label.

A specified 'response' in a specified situation can be considered as the basic unit of behaviour, for instance, a laboratory animal pressing a lever to obtain food in response to an auditory stimulus. But even this example is not a simple model, as the delay in, or duration of, the response may vary, and be accompanied by variable additional behaviour that is not measured.

A 'habit' involves some consistency of behaviour over a period of time, and as the human environment is not analogous to the relatively controlled conditions of a laboratory animal, and will always show some variation, the concept of a habit implies that there is some consistency of response in different situations. It must be remembered that although a habit consists of behaviour, this can be considered as being derived from higher mental activity.

A 'trait' has been considered as the basic unit of personality or PD, and consists of a specified group of related habits; for example, going to parties can be a habit contributing to the trait of sociability. Consistency of behaviour in different situations is more likely to be found in relation to a trait than to a habit, and the degree of a behaviour related to a trait is usually distributed approximately normally in the population.

An even broader concept combines traits to form basic dimensions of personality, or 'temperaments', which have been defined as 'inherited personality traits present in early childhood' (Buss & Plomin, 1986), and as 'the relatively stable features of the organism, primarily biologically determined ...' (Strelau, 1983). But, because of continuous interactions between the individual and the environment, modification of broad patterns of behaviour over time would be expected.

The hypothesis that there is a major genetic contribution to temperament implies that there may be associated biological markers, and that behaviour related to temperaments may have counterparts in non-human animals. Behaviour in non-human animals can be categorized as 'emotionality', 'sociability' and 'antisocial tendencies' (for example, involving intraspecies aggression) can be identified in non-human mammals, and Rutter (1987) considered that these have human counterparts, which probably have 'fairly direct' neurobiological correlates. Patterns of emotionality, sociability and activity (the latter can be associated with antisocial tendencies) can appear early in childhood and show a degree of stability, although the nature of the related behaviours may change during childhood and adult life. Other temperaments that have been postulated include impulsivity, tough-mindedness, constraint, the three factors of extraversion, neuroticism and psychoticism (which resemble sociability, emotionality, and antisocial tendencies, respectively; Eysenck, 1982), and a five factor model with extraversion (versus introversion), neuroticism (versus stability), agreeableness, conscientiousness and culture (i.e. openness to experience). Cloninger (1986) has argued for three main temperaments, i.e. harm avoidance, novelty seeking and reward dependence, each associated with specific neurotransmitter activity, and this model has been extended to include seven dimensions, by the addition of persistence, self-directedness, cooperativeness and self-transcendence (Cloninger, Svrakic & Przybeck, 1993). The latter dimension relates to how the individual identifies him/herself as autonomous, an integral part of humanity or an integral part of the universe as a whole.

Definitions and concepts

The concept of personality has been defined as 'the sum total of a person's actions and reactions' (Walton, 1973) and the 'enduring qualities of an individual shown in his/her ways of behaving in a wide variety of circumstances' (Gelder, Gath & Mayou, 1983). Hall & Lindsey (1978) considered that the organization and integration of behaviours was an important aspect of the concept, and they defined personality as 'that which gives order and congruence to all the different kinds of behaviour in which the individual engages'. Thus, although most definitions and assessments of personality focus on overt behaviour, the underlying higher mental activity, involving motivational, attitudinal and emotional elements, is an integral part of the personality concept. Rutter (1987) considered that it is the inclusion of patterns of thought and feelings, together with the meaningful patterns of behaviour that reflect motivation, which distinguishes the concept of personality from temperament.

Allport (1937) described the 'dynamic organisation' of personality, which refers to mental processes that are in a constant state of interaction, with the potential for change. These phenomena involve attitudes to self, patterns of relating to others and planning for the future. Also, psychoanalytic theory has focussed on the 'dynamic' (i.e. involving movement) aspects of higher mental activity and the meanings of experiences. These approaches recognized that symptoms such as anxiety are often found in the context of a personality abnormality that has been termed the 'neurotic character' (Alexander, 1930). Dynamic aspects of mental functioning include 'defence mechanisms', such as 'denial', which are the various observable methods by which an individual may keep certain thoughts at the 'back of the mind' and out of conscious awareness. However, the suggestion that the use of different psychological defence mechanisms can be used to classify personality has been considered to be unproven (Rutter, 1987).

Consistency

A 'trait' (i.e. a group of related habits) is considered to be the basic unit of personality, and a 'summary of consistencies of behaviour or an average of states over time, which will reflect the individual's characteristics, the situation and the individual-situation interaction' (Zuckerman, 1991). (A 'state' denotes behaviour at a given moment.) Some consistency has been demonstrated for sociability in children (Kagan & Moss, 1962) and for various traits in adults, in particular extraversion-sociability.

In relation to the consistency of temperaments, Rutter (1987) has pointed out that differences between children can be measured with reasonable reliability in relation to activity level and sociability, and that such assessments can have clinically significant implications; for example, measures of temperaments in children have been correlated with subsequent emotional disturbance in different contexts. (Reliability is the extent to which a test would give consistent results on being applied more than once to the same people under standard conditions.)

Behaviour reflects interactions between traits, temperaments and the environment, and data from several measuring instruments, as well as from several situations, may be needed for useful personality assessment. Also, the relationships between different behaviours may reflect a consistent pattern. Consistency of behaviour can be influenced by the degree of specificity of the environment and, in studies on monkeys, autonomic reactivity was reasonably consistent only when evaluated in stressful situations (Suomi, 1983). (This example has a direct parallel with clinical practice, as some patients can show consistent but episodic maladaptive behaviour, but only in the context of a life-crisis.) Another variable affecting consistency of behaviour is the effect of 'developmental' changes (i.e. changes related to increasing age), as a trait can give rise to different expressions of related behaviour at different ages; for example, a low level of activity may initially lead to the seeking of maternal closeness but later to an avoidance of new situations (Kagan, Reznick & Snidman, 1986; Rutter, 1987). Also, passivity and lack of physical adventurousness in childhood have been shown to predict adult non-competitiveness and certain characteristics of sexual behaviour (Kagan & Moss, 1962; Ryder, 1967).

Approaches

Personality has been evaluated from three main perspectives. The first focusses on the individual's social interactions, in particular early parent–child, peer, and close confiding relationships (Wolkind & Rutter, 1985; Hinde & Stevenson-Hinde, 1986); for example, Hodges & Tizard (1989) reported that early institutional care was associated with certain patterns of social interaction in later childhood. The second approach is cognitive, involving examination of consistent patterns of thoughts, feelings and attitudes about self and environment, for instance low self-esteem, which has been claimed to be an important causal factor for some depressive disorders (Brown & Harris, 1978; Peterson & Seligman, 1984). In the third approach, personality traits (such as empathy, suspiciousness, and sensation-seeking), can be variously defined and classified.

Personality disorders

Historical developments

Early concepts of PD were developed in the 19th century (Berrios, 1993), for example, Prichard (1835) defined 'moral insanity' as

a form of mental derangement in whom the moral and active principles of the mind are strongly perverted or depraved, the power of self-government is lost or greatly impaired, and the individual is found incapable, not of talking or reasoning on any subject proposed to him, but of conducting himself with decency and propriety in the business of life.

Subsequently, Maudsley (1868) described a similar but narrower category for someone with 'no capacity for true moral feeling . . .', and Koch (1891) used the term 'psychopathic inferiority' to denote those with clearly abnormal behaviour in the presence of a normal mental state. Kraepelin (1905) described 'morbid mental states in which the peculiar disposition of the personality must be considered the real foundation of the malady', while Schneider (1923) termed all PDs as 'psychopathic', and described ten different types. This broad category of 'psychopathic personality' contrasts with subsequent narrower definitions of 'psychopathy', with an emphasis on antisocial behaviour, lack of remorse, unreliability and selfishness (Cleckley, 1941), although Henderson (1939) also included those who were predominantly passive or inadequate.

Individuals whose PD is associated with repeated antisocial behaviour come into the province of both law and medicine, providing society with an unresolved dilemma about the concept of personal responsibility for one's actions. However, from a biological perspective, it appears that genetic factors are one type of variable that can predispose individuals to commit aggressive and other antisocial acts.

Definitions

Despite the complexities of the concepts of personality, PDs are established diagnoses in medical practice and are found in the two main recent classifications of mental disorders, the *International Classification of Diseases* (ICD-9 and -10, World Health Organization, 1978, 1992) and the *Diagnostic and Statistical Manual of Mental Disorders* (DSM-III, DSM-III-R, DSM-IV, American Psychiatric Association, 1980, 1987, 1994). But as the characteristics of PD usually differ only in degree or frequency from the features that are present in the majority of the population, the boundaries between normal personality traits and those of a PD are generally arbitrary.

Schneider (1923) stated that PDs are those 'abnormal personalities who suffer through their abnormalities or through whose abnormalities society suffers', while Rado's definition (1953) focussed on the organization of higher mental activity, i.e. 'Disturbances of psychodynamic integration that significantly affect the organism's adaptive life performance, its attainment of utility and pleasure'. More recently, Rutter (1987) considered that PDs are 'a persistent, pervasive abnormality in social relationships and social functioning generally'.

The World Health Organization's definition of PD for ICD-9 (1978) stressed that signs usually appear early in life, and PD was said to consist of

deeply ingrained maladaptive patterns of behaviour generally recognizable by the time of adolescence or earlier and continuing throughout most of adult life, although often becoming less obvious in middle or old age. The personality is abnormal either in the balance of its components, their quality and expression, or in its total aspect. Because of this deviation or psychopathy the patient suffers or others have to suffer and there is an adverse effect upon the individual or on society.

The other main classifactory system, the DSM (i.e. DSM-III, DSM-III-R and DSM-IV) defines personality traits as 'enduring patterns of perceiving, relating to, and thinking about the environment and oneself, and are exhibited in a wide range of important social and personal contexts', and continues: 'it is only when personality traits are inflexible and maladaptive and cause either significant functional impairment or subjective distress that they constitute personality disorders. The manifestations of personality disorders are often recognizable by adolescence or earlier and continue throughout most of adult life, though they often become less obvious in middle or old age' (American Psychiatric Association, 1987). In the DSM-IV, the general diagnositic criteria for a PD consist of: 'an enduring pattern of inner experience and behaviour that deviates from the expectations of the individual's culture' (which is manifested in two or more of the following: cognition, affectivity, interpersonal functioning and impulse control); 'the enduring pattern is inflexible and pervasive across a broad range of personal and social situations'; 'the enduring pattern leads to clinically significant distress or impairment in social, occupational, or other important areas of functioning'; 'the pattern is stable and of long duration and its onset can be traced back at least to adolescence or early adulthood'; 'the enduring pattern is not better accounted for as a manifestation or consequence of another mental disorder'; and 'the enduring pattern is not due to the direct physiological effects of a substance (e.g. a drug of abuse, a medication) or a general medical condition (e.g. head trauma)'.

The 10th revision of the ICD (ICD-10, World Health Organization, 1992) defined a specific PD as

a severe disturbance in the characterological constitution and behavioural tendencies of the individual, usually involving several areas of the personality, and nearly always associated with considerable personal and social disruption. Personality disorder tends to appear in late childhood or adolescence and continues to be manifest into adulthood. These types of conditions comprise deeply ingrained and enduring behaviour patterns, manifesting themselves as inflexible responses to a broad range of personal and social situations. Personality disorders ... are developmental conditions, which appear in childhood or adolescence and continue into adulthood.

In addition, the ICD-10 includes the diagnosis of 'enduring personality changes' that are acquired, usually during adult life, 'following another medical disorder or severely adverse environmental stress'.

The disease concept and PDs

The concept of disease implies maladaptive biological functioning and can be defined in various ways. One of the most basic criteria is an association of disease with excess mortality, and if this is applied to individuals with some types of PDs, there is convincing evidence that the disease concept is justified. For example, antisocial PD was associated with increased risk of unnatural death in a 7 year follow-up of 500 psychiatric outpatients of a psychiatric service; this was related to substance abuse, accidents and suicide (Martin, 1986). But the traditional medical approach of applying no more than a few categorical labels (i.e. 'diagnoses') to an individual patient is not well suited to the identification of PDs, as many patients qualify for several co-occurring PD diagnoses. Therefore, it may be appropriate to modify the traditional format of medical diagnostic systems for the consideration of PDs.

Scadding (1988, 1990) has pointed out that 'diagnosis is the process by which a patient's symptoms and signs are assessed and investigated, with a view to the categorisation of his/her case with others of a similar sort which have been studied in the past, in order that the patient may benefit from the application of established knowledge to the problem'. He has also noted that the concept of 'a disease' is 'logically heterogeneous', as it may refer to a group of signs and symptoms (a syndrome), to the effects of a specific disorder of bodily structure or function, or to the effects of a specified causal agent. The aims of psychiatric research include the investigation of the associations of behavioural syndromes with disorders of bodily structure or function, causal factors, prognosis and efficacy of treatments. A diagnostic label for a disease is always provisional (Mindham, Scadding & Cawley, 1992), as it forms an hypothesis that is 'a conjecture about the relationship between two or more concepts' (Freeman & Tyrer, 1989). Research often leads to revisions of disease concepts, and classification is an essential part of this process.

There is no clear dividing line between normal and abnormal personalities, but it is possible to make reliable arbitrary distinctions, perhaps based on a cut-off score of dimensions that have been measured. However, in practice, the clinician or health-care worker is not concerned with the threshold for a PD diagnosis, but with the questions 'is this person's PD significantly maladaptive?' (i.e. does the individual suffer or do other people suffer?) and, if the answer is 'yes', 'what interventions, if any, are appropriate?'

There have been many criticisms of the disease concept in relation to the use of PD diagnoses; for instance that a PD diagnosis is unreliable and that it is often used as a derogatory label on the basis of inadequate assessment, i.e. 'little more than a moral judgement masquerading as a clinical diagnosis' (Blackburn, 1988). Also, it has been claimed that the process of assigning a PD diagnosis can be used as an excuse to deny patients appropriate help (Lewis & Appleby, 1988) as, in contrast to other mental disorders, a PD diagnosis is not usually considered to take away significant personal responsibility from the patient for his/her actions. As individuals with PD are often disliked because of their behaviour, the use of the PD diagnostic category may have an implicit meaning, namely that the person is not deserving of care and treatment. But while such criticisms of the use of PD categories may sometimes be justified, they should be directed to clinicians and health care workers, rather than to the relevant concepts and classificatory systems.

Assessment

In routine practice, the clinician assesses PD by an interview in which various aspects of the patient's past life and conscious awareness are explored. Various topics are routinely covered but questions are not usually presented in a standard format. If possible, an informant is also seen. It is particularly important to elicit information about the major problems related to PD, which include antisocial behaviour, dependence on others, problems in sustaining relationships and attitudes to other people.

Various methods can be used for a more detailed assessment, in particular for research studies. These may involve self-report questionnaires (for patient and an informant), questionnaires for the clinician (which may involve rating scales), and structured interview schedules.

Whatever the method of PD assessment, other co-occurring abnormal aspects of the patient's mental state may produce distortions of the findings, and these are known as 'trait-state artefacts'. For example, it has been shown that patients who are depressed or anxious often do not provide accurate reports of their previous functioning. However, some assessment methods have been shown to be relatively reliable for some PD features despite variations in anxiety and depression between separate assessments (Loranger *et al.*, 1991; Brown *et al.*, 1992). A further problem is a tendency for patients to acknowledge fewer maladaptive PD traits at a subsequent assessment.

Principles of classification

Classification in medicine has been claimed to be a 'necessary preliminary to almost any useful communication' (Kendell, 1983); however, any classificatory system involves underlying assumptions, which, if incorrect, may hold back the development of knowledge. The various systems have been mainly concerned with disorders that people have but can also be applied to the people (patients) themselves. Any classification involves the definition of membership of a population (e.g. a population of mental disorders) and then, usually, separating its members into two or more groups, which can be called 'types', 'classes' or 'categories'. The main uses of any classification of disorders are to record phenomena, to understand causes and to predict outcome, and it is convenient if one patient is associated with just one class of disorder, particularly in respect of the predictive function. Although a classificatory process always consists of categories, a categorical system (e.g. classifying individuals as below or above a specified height) can be supplemented by complementary dimensional information (e.g. the measured height). A dimension involves the identification of one characteristic (e.g. height in centimetres) among a group of related variables (e.g. a range of heights to the nearest centimetre).

PDs are associated with a wide range of behavioural patterns, and an appropriate classification should aim to include all relevant behaviour, i.e. to provide adequate coverage. Even if PDs consisted of just one class, this would form part of a wider classification of mental disorders and there is evidence that even such a broad diagnostic category of PD has 'satisfactory reliability and reasonable predictive validity', while the 'reliability and temporal stability of most trait-defined subtypes has been shown to be quite poor', except for antisocial PD (Rutter, 1987). Also, for some categories of PD reported in the literature, the internal consistency of the syndromes (i.e. the average covariance among a set of scores) has been low and their validity has been unproven.

The process of defining and classifying personality and PD has been criticized for not paying sufficient attention to mental activity and interpersonal relationships, due to a focus on overt behaviour, and for ignoring the unique aspects of an individual, which are so important in our concept of a human person (Ferguson & Tyrer, 1988). However, a focus on the unique aspects of an individual's PD would not produce knowledge that would be useful to others.

A classification of PDs presents considerable difficulties because of the range, complexity and intercorrelations of relevant behaviours, their interaction with environmental variables and with other mental disorders, and the lack of natural boundaries between the attributes of most people and most of the PD criteria. In addition, boundaries are unclear between various PD subtypes, and between PDs and some other mental disorders. Also, there is some overlap between PDs, as some criteria occur in more than one PD syndrome.

Criteria for PDs are not all constructed on the same basis; some are examples of a trait, i.e. a group of related behaviours, while other criteria consist of relatively specific examples of behaviour. As no list of behaviours for a trait could be exhaustive, there are often difficulties in selecting specific examples of behaviour as diagnostic criteria, as these may be subject to relatively specific effects of variables such as sex or social class.

Methods of classification

Categories

In an ideal classificatory system, each category should contain members that are identical (i.e. all criteria must be met by all members) and should be mutually exclusive (i.e. a member must be in one class only). Also, all the categories should be jointly exhaustive (i.e. there should be one category that is suitable for every member of the population being studied). Disease categories are best suited to populations of disorders in which there are sharp boundaries between the disorders. When PD criteria relate to behaviour that can be found in most individuals (e.g. aggression), an arbitrary dividing line between normality and disorder can only be avoided if there is a point of rarity in the severity or frequency of the behaviour. Thus, if human beings were all either very docile (except in extreme circumstances) or so aggressive that breaches of the law occurred regularly, then a categorical approach could easily be applied because intermediates would be rare. Unfortunately, points of rarity are not found for most PD criteria or most PDs, except, perhaps, for a minority of paranoid, schizotypal, borderline and antisocial PD criteria (Frances, 1982; Livesley & Jackson, 1992).

A 'monothetic' category of disease involves all its members meeting all the criteria, while just a minimum number of positive criteria are needed for membership of a 'polythetic' category. Thus, for the latter, there is a variable level of resemblance to the 'ideal' or 'prototype' member of the class, which meets all the criteria. But a polythetic system is misleading, as a single PD diagnosis is applied to each example of a group of disorders that shows considerable heterogeneity; for example, there are 93 ways in which the DSM-III-R's polythetic criteria for borderline PD can be met.

In a polythetic system it is difficult to determine an appropriate threshold in relation to the number of criteria to be met for diagnosis, and the decision is usually arbitrary. But a variant of a polythetic classificatory system can involve abolition of the threshold concept for an all-or-none diagnosis, and its replacement by a score for each category of disorder, based on the number of criteria met. Also, certain criteria can be designated as essential for class membership or given special weighting.

Dimensions

Data from a population of diseases can be recorded not only by a system of categories but by dimensional scores or ratings, each of which may involve a continuous distribution of the amount of a variable. However, it must be noted that categories and dimensions can be complementary, and that dimensional scores are easily converted into categories; for example, if severity of aggression has been rated on a 10 point scale (10 = very severe), an arbitrary threshold of a score of 6 or more can be used to define a category of aggressive disorder.

PDs have been traditionally described in categorical terms in the psychiatric literature, although the dimensional nature of most PD features has led to an increasing awareness that a more dimensional approach to measurement and classification will be required. But even within recent categorical systems, such as the DSM-III-R, the total score of positive PD criteria for each PD diagnosis can provide a dimensional assessment that may correlate with the degree of social impairment for many patients, although some may show relatively severe disorder restricted to a small number of PD criteria. Threshold values for the number of positive criteria required to produce a categorical diagnosis have been generally arbitrary, but it may be possible to link a cut-off point with clinically-significant variables such as a specified degree of social impairment.

Influential classifications of PDs

The third edition of the American Psychiatric Association's DSM classification, DSM-III (American Psychiatric Association, 1980), was the first internationally-used system that specified criteria for PD diagnoses, although it was often unclear how they should be met. The DSM-III was revised in 1987 (DSM-III-R) and 1994 (DSM-IV), and the first two versions have been the anchor-points for much of the psychiatric literature concerned with PD. The World Health Organization's 9th revision of their *International Classification of Diseases* (World Health Organization, 1978) provided only brief clinical descriptions for its diagnostic categories of PDs, but the 10th revision, the ICD-10 (World Health Organization, 1992), is similar to the DSM-III-R and DSM-IV in providing a set of criteria to be evaluated for each specified PD. The ICD-10 uses a polythetic system in which at least three of the criteria need to be met for each PD diagnosis. Also, diagnostic criteria for research have been published, closely based on the ICD-10 (World Health Organization, 1993).

A diagnostic criterion may require the clinician to make a judgement on a wide range of behaviours (e.g. 'expects, without sufficient basis, to be exploited or harmed by others') or involve relatively specific examples of behaviour (e.g. 'questions, without justification, fidelity of spouse or sexual partner') (American Psychiatric Association, 1987). Also, polythetic criteria may vary in relation to the degree of association with the diagnosis of the disorder, and to their role in distinguishing the syndrome from other disorders.

There are advantages in minimizing the role of clinical judgement for the application of a PD criterion, as this should increase reliability (i.e. repeatability) of assessment, although this may lead to relevant criteria being discarded if they rely heavily on clinical evaluation. This could produce an undesirable reduction in the validity of the syndrome, if the full range of clinically-important phenomena are not being assessed.

Despite the importance of categorical classifications of PDs, their limitations have been recognized, and it is likely that such systems will be increasingly supplemented by dimensional information, both in research and clinical practice. Nevertheless, PD categories have stood the test of time, as they provide simple, convenient, and useful summaries of predominant maladaptive behaviours. Although all-or-none diagnostic PD categories involve arbitrary thresholds and lose information, many decisions in clinical practice are also binary, i.e. to treat/not to treat, or to admit/not to admit, so that the use of all-or-none diagnoses can provide a functional model for these management decisions. On the debit side, the use of various diagnostic categories for PDs can lead to concepts of PDs that are restricted to the various prototypes (i.e. 'ideal' examples of a category); this is misleading as most patients with PD show a mixture of positive criteria from more than one PD syndrome.

Categories of PD in the main international classifications

The DSM-III and its revised version have been the main influences in PD research since 1980 and, like every classification, has underlying assumptions. The DSM-III-R and DSM-IV, with their format of polythetic PD categories, assume that some members of each class are better examples than others, and that the categories reflect natural classes, i.e. 'real-world correlational structure of frequently encountered problematic personality

Table 1.1 *Categories of personality disorder common to the DSM-III-R,*
DSM-IV and ICD-10 classifications

DSM-III-R and DSM-IV category	Corresponding ICD-10 category
Paranoid	Paranoid
Schizoid	Schizoid
Antisocial	Dissocial
Borderline	Emotionally unstable
	Impulsive type
	Borderline type
Histrionic	Histrionic
Obsessive-compulsive	Anankastic
Avoidant	Anxious (avoidant)
Dependent	Dependent
Personality disorder not otherwise specified	Mixed and other

features'. (Also, the PD categories are not assumed to be mutually exclusive, as there is overlap between some of their characteristics.) Further assumptions in DSM-III-R and DSM-IV are that each set of criteria for a specified PD displays a degree of internal consistency, i.e. 'features of the same syndrome should correlate more highly with each other than with features representing a different syndrome' (Morey, 1988), and that the various PD syndromes can be grouped together in three superordinate classes. These are designated as: cluster A, odd or eccentric; cluster B, dramatic, emotional or erratic; and cluster C, anxious or fearful, with the further assumption that each PD syndrome shows greater internal consistency relative to other members of its superordinate group, compared with the other PDs.

DSM-III-R gives 11 criteria sets for PD diagnoses, together with a residual category of 'Personality disorder not otherwise specified' (which corresponds to the 'Mixed and other' category in the ICD-10 classification). There are also two additional 'Proposed diagnostic categories needing further study' – i.e. self-defeating and sadistic PDs. Table 1.1 shows eight of the 11 specified DSM-III-R PD syndromes that closely correspond to syndromes in the 10th revision of the ICD, i.e. paranoid, schizoid, antisocial, borderline, histrionic, obsessive-compulsive, avoidant and dependent PDs. The eight DSM-III-R PD categories shown in Table 1.1 are also found in DSM-IV (American Psychiatric Association, 1994). Several other PD syndromes have been described and are listed in Table 1.2.

Schizotypal, narcissistic, passive-aggressive, self-defeating and sadistic

Table 1.2 *Various categories of personality disorder*
(PD) additional to those shown in Table 1.1

Category of PD	Source
Schizotypal	*DSM-III-R
Narcissistic	*DSM-III-R
Passive-aggressive	DSM-III-R
Self-defeating	DSM-III-R
Sadistic	DSM-III-R
Organic	ICD-10
Enduring personality changes	ICD-10
Accentuation of personality traits	ICD-10
Depressive personality	Various

Note: * and DSM-IV.

PD syndromes are derived from DSM-III-R but do not have equivalent categories in ICD-10. However, the ICD-10 recognizes three further categories: 'organic personality disorder' due to brain disease, damage and dysfunction; 'enduring personality changes', not attributable to brain damage and disease (i.e. after catastrophic or excessive prolonged stress or following a severe psychiatric illness); and 'accentuation of personality traits'. Leonhard (1968) was the first to use the term 'accentuated' to denote personality characteristics that are only maladaptive in an unusually demanding or stressful environment, and this category can be conceptualized as intermediate between normal personality and PD. It should be noted that the ICD-10 categories of 'cyclothymia' and 'schizotypal disorder' are not classified as PDs, but appear elsewhere in sections related to mood disorder and schizophrenia.

Opinions have varied about the validity of a 'depressive personality' category. This was included in ICD-9 but not in the 10th revision, while it is not a DSM-III-R category. However the DSM-III-R's category of 'dysthymia' (a type of depression) is described as chronic and sometimes beginning in childhood, and early-onset dysthymia has been considered by some to be synonymous with 'depressive personality' or 'charactological depression' (Widiger & Shea, 1991). In DSM-IV, 'depressive personality disorder' is included as a criteria set 'for futher study'.

The ICD-10 recommends that its PD categories should be used to reflect the patient's most frequent or conspicuous behavioural manifestations of PD.

Table 1.3 *Possible modifications to a polythetic classification of personality disorders (PDs) as found in the DSM-III-R, DSM-IV and ICD-10 classifications*

1. Changes in the use of existing criteria
    e.g. Specify certain criteria as essential for diagnosis
         Give extra weight to certain criteria
         Change minimum number of positive criteria required for diagnosis
2. Changes in individual criteria or the categories of personality disorders
    e.g. Change individual criteria
         Change overlap between criteria in different PD syndromes
         Change or add exclusion criteria (i.e. criteria which do not allow the
             diagnosis of PD)
         Change the number of PD categories
3. Additional strategies for the classification of personality disorders
    e.g. Add criteria which differentiate PD from other disorders
         Operate an hierarchy in recording co-occurring PDs
         Use compound diagnostic categories (i.e. sub-groups defined by
             additional criteria)
         Add dimensional information
         Add complementary information (e.g. global functioning)

Disadvantages of polythetic PD categories

As the DSM-III-R, DSM-IV and ICD-10 have provided a series of polythetic categories for PD diagnoses, the consequences of such a system must be considered.

A group of individuals who receive such a PD diagnosis are heterogeneous in respect of the relevant disorder, as there are many different combinations of the minimum number of positive criteria required, together with variations in the number of positive criteria above the diagnostic threshold. Also, the minimum number of criteria for diagnosis is arbitrary, and whatever diagnostic threshold is chosen, an all-or-none diagnosis loses information. (However, if all criteria were required to be positive before diagnosis, this would not reflect the heterogeneity that is actually found.) In addition, information is lost by an all-or-none rating for each individual criterion, while different criteria for each PD in DSM-III-R, DSM-IV and ICD-10 are considered to be equally valid, despite apparent variations in clinical importance. Also, the threshold for rating each individual criterion as positive is usually arbitrary.

Many patients fulfil criteria for two or more PD diagnoses, while some criteria contribute to more than one PD. Unfortunately, this is not suited to routine clinical practice, as it is cumbersome to give several PD diagnoses to one patient, and a list of several co-occurring PDs disguises relatively severe maladaptive behaviour in just one category.

Potential modifications to PD categories

As any classification is an hypothesis that invites testing and revision, some possible changes in the most influential polythetic classifications are summarized in Table 1.3.

Firstly, there are several potential changes in the use of existing criteria in DSM-IV and ICD-10. Some 'core' criteria could be specified as essential for the diagnosis and/or given extra weight by increasing the score assigned to their positive rating. Also, the minimum number of positive criteria required for diagnosis could be changed. However, the identification of core criteria is difficult, and core criteria may not exist for some syndromes.

Secondly, changes could be made to the individual criteria and the number of PD categories. The total number of criteria for each PD, together with the minimum number required for diagnosis, are major variables affecting the degree of heterogeneity of a group of diagnosed PDs, while a consideration of the nature of PD criteria must recognize that they consist of a mixture of relatively broad traits and relatively specific examples of behaviour. Some specific behaviours will be better examples of a trait than others, and a choice of several behaviours to indicate a positive criterion will usually give increased reliability compared with the use of just one behavioural example. The assessment of a trait (in contrast to a relatively specific behaviour) requires a greater degree of judgement, and, in a set of criteria, the balance between those that rely heavily on clinical judgement and those that are related to specific behaviour can be reviewed. If the balance is changed in favour of specific behaviours, the reliability is likely to be increased but perhaps at the expense of the validity, if aspects of the disorder that rely heavily on clinical judgement are omitted. Overlap may occur between the various sets of PD criteria; for example, in the DSM-III-R, one criterion is identical in schizoid, schizotypal and avoidant PDs. But, while it would be possible to reduce such overlap by omitting the relevant criterion, this may not be appropriate, if the overlap reflects the reality of these disorders. Thus, excessive pruning of criteria may artefactually restrict the recognition of the syndromes. Exclusion criteria are provided for some PDs in DSM-III-R, and the use of this strategy could be extended. For example, antisocial PD could be excluded as a diagnosis in the presence of manic-depressive disorder, as antisocial behaviour can often be a feature of mania, and if mania is present there is a chance of an incorrect diagnosis of antisocial PD being made. But, although this will reduce co-occurrence of PD diagnosis with other mental disorders, the increased homogeneity of those who receive the diagnosis may not reflect the reality, as different mental disorders can co-occur. However, this approach may be valid for research samples. Other changes in classification might involve the number of PD categories, for instance, various syndromes that have been classed as PDs, such as schizotypal PD and cyclothymic personality, have been increasingly considered to be more closely related to other mental disorders. The relationship between avoidant PD and phobic disorders is another area of uncertainty. It may also be appropriate to combine some of the existing PD categories.

Thirdly, additional strategies for the classification of PDs could be introduced. Criteria could be added with the aim of differentiating a PD syndrome from other mental disorders, and an hierarchy could be introduced for the recording of co-occurring PDs; for example, only one PD could be recorded, perhaps the one that is judged to have the greatest effect on social functioning. The device of the compound diagnostic category could be used to specify, within a group defined by each PD diagnosis, a sub-category associated with another variable, for example, an history of childhood physical or sexual abuse (Mindham *et al.*, 1992). Also, dimensional information could be used to supplement the PD diagnoses, perhaps based on the degree of specific behaviour, the range of related behaviours, the frequency of specific behaviour, and the range of situations in which the behaviour is displayed. For instance, the Personality Assessment Schedule is a system of clinical assessment that is based on dimensional ratings of 24 traits judged to be relevant to PDs (Tyrer & Alexander, 1988), and its ratings can also be converted to categories that correspond to those of the ICD and DSM. This and other systems that have attempted to utilize dimensional information may influence further revisions of the two major international classificatory systems. However, the question of which changes are 'correct' is misleading, as one classificactory system will suit one purpose but not necessarily another. Finally, complementary information such as the severity of the adverse effect of behaviours on social and occupational functioning could be added.

Boundaries between personality disorders and other mental disorders

In addition to problems in defining the boundaries between different PDs, there can be overlap between PDs and other mental disorders when the syndromes share common features.

The nature of the relationships between PDs and other mental disorders is complex and variable; for example, certain PD characteristics, such as antisocial behaviour, may be responsible for adverse life events that are then causal factors for a depressed mood. Also, patterns of conscious mental activity, such as persistent wariness, indecision, suspiciousness or pessimism, may lead to mood disorder involving symptoms of anxiety and depression. These are examples of PD apparently causing mood disorder but the reverse can also occur, as specified in the ICD-10, which notes that 'enduring personality changes' can follow various adverse events, including 'serious psychiatric disorder' such as manic-depressive disorder. Also, although PD and another mental disorder may co-occur independently, the PD may influence the expression or the severity of the other disorder; for example, a patient with an antisocial PD is likely to become increasingly antisocial if he/she develops a schizophrenic illness. Another possible association is when the PD and another co-occurring mental disorder may reflect various features of the same disorder; for instance, it is likely that similar genetic vulnerability can be related to both schizophrenia and schizotypal PD.

Boundaries between PDs and other mental disorders may be unclear because of overlapping diagnostic criteria for the two syndromes under consideration, or because more than one diagnoses has been arbitrarily imposed upon dimensions (e.g. frequency or severity) associated with the relevant behaviours. These issues have been given considerable attention in relation to the interface between PD and depressive or anxiety syndromes. Digman (1990) has pointed out that some features of depression and anxiety have also been generally accepted as features of PDs, for instance, 'neuroticism', involving 'trait depression and trait anxiety'. Some episodic 'states' with features of depression and/or anxiety have produced diagnostic categories that provide meaningful distinctions between some examples of depression or anxiety and PDs (for example, episodic depression in the context of bipolar manic-depressive disorder), but distinct boundaries between PDs and some other examples of depression and anxiety are lacking (Chaplin, John & Goldberg, 1988). Depressive syndromes consist of heterogeneous groups of signs and symptoms that reflect a range of causal factors of varying specificity. For some individuals, genetically-determined vulnerability to abnormal brain function appears to be important and is an example of an 'endogenous' or internal causal factor, although such vulnerabilities may themselves be heterogeneous. There is evidence that environmental life events may precipitate a depressive syndrome in those who have an endogenous vulnerability, although in some patients,

endogenous mood changes can appear 'out of the blue'. Other hypothesized types of causal factors for depressive syndromes include identifiable
biological factors (e.g. brain disease, drug administration, infections,
nutritional factors, and hormonal influences), psychologically meaningful
reactions to (and interactions with) life events, and personality or PD.
There is some evidence that certain features of PDs may make an individual
particularly prone to the development of some depressive symptoms. For
example, borderline PD is associated with emotional instability, a tendency
to develop transient depressed moods, irritability or anxiety, inability to
sustain relationships, and an unstable lifestyle. In addition to mood
disorder being an integral part of this PD, individuals with these characteristics usually experience more stressful life events, which may have additional causal effects for depressed mood or anxiety (Seivewright, 1987).
Also, it has been proposed that certain personality characteristics should be
recognized as a category of 'depressive personality disorder' (Phillips *et al.*,
1990), involving excessively negative and pessimistic beliefs about oneself
and other people, with relatively persistent depressed mood (Hirschfeld &
Shea, 1992).

The hypotheses that give a major causal role for PD in the development
of some depressive syndromes have led to several diagnostic labels for the
corresponding depressive sub-types, i.e. 'characteriological depression'
(Akiskal, Rosenthal & Haykal, 1980), 'affective spectrum disorder'
(Widiger & Shea, 1991; McElroy *et al.*, 1992) and the 'general neurotic
syndrome' (Tyrer *et al.*, 1992).

Before leaving the interface of PD and depressive disorders, mention
must be made of 'cyclothymic' PD which, according to the ICD-9, involves
a pattern of changes of mood involving periods of persistent depression or
persistent elation. But in the subsequent 10th revision of the ICD, cyclothymia was described as 'a persistent instability of mood involving numerous
periods of mild depression and mild elation'. It was considered to be a mood
disorder rather than a PD, and it is likely that this syndrome is genetically
related to the more typical forms of manic-depressive disorder.

While anxiety is often a part of a depressive syndrome, various anxiety
disorders can be diagnosed independently, and there can be difficulty in
defining a boundary between certain features of PDs and certain anxiety-
related syndromes such as social phobia. As described in DSM-III-R, the
latter involves 'a persistent fear of one or more situations in which the
person is exposed to possible scrutiny by others ...' while, in the same
classification, the features of avoidant PD include being unwilling to get
involved with people unless certain of being liked and being reticent in

social situations because of a fear of saying something inappropriate or foolish. It seems likely that these two syndromes are not clinically distinct but reflect overlapping variants along a spectrum of related phenomena (Brooks, Baltazar & Munjack, 1989).

Another group of mental disorders that can be difficult to distinguish from PDs (in particular those PDs with antisocial behaviour) consists of 'impulse-control disorders' (McElroy *et al.*, 1992). These include intermittent explosive disorders (instability of mood with outbursts of anger or violence), kleptomania (a persistent impulse to steal, often without economic motive), pathological gambling, and pyromania (an irresistible impulse to start fires). Also, trichotillomania (an abnormal desire to pull out one's hair) can appear to be similar to some features of obsessive-compulsive PD.

Another boundary problem involves the frequent associations between antisocial PD (variously defined) and substance abuse disorders (Docherty, Fiester & Shea, 1986). The DSM-III-R criteria for antisocial PD include failure to conform to social norms with respect to lawful behaviour and an inability to sustain consistent work behaviour, but these can also occur in syndromes involving substance abuse such as DSM-III-R's 'psychoactive substance dependence'. It appears that either there is considerable overlap between the features of these disorders or that one syndrome is being given more than one diagnosis (Frances, Widiger & Fyer, 1990).

The next area of diagnostic uncertainty involves schizoid, schizotypal and paranoid PDs, schizophrenia and Asperger's syndrome. Schizoid PD involves a relative indifference to personal relationships with social isolation, while schizotypal PD includes features that can appear to be mild forms of some of the features of schizophrenia, for example, odd beliefs, eccentric behaviour, unusual perceptual experiences and odd speech. Evidence has been accumulating that schizotypal PD should be considered as a variant of schizophrenia (Kendler, Eaves & Strauss, 1981) and is classified as such in the 10th revision of the ICD. Asperger's syndrome is characterized by abnormal social interactions and a restricted repertoire of interests and activities in older children but without significant general delay in language or cognitive development. Rutter (1987) noted a possible association between schizoid PD and Asperger's syndrome (and childhood autism), and there is some indication of a familial association between paranoid PD and schizophrenia (Kendler & Gruenberg, 1984).

Finally, the distinction between obsessive-compulsive PD and obsessive-compulsive neurosis can also be arbitrary, for instance, when the former involves excessive attention to detail and organization that can differ only in degree from a compulsive ritual involving clearly abnormal patterns of behaviour.

Further revisions of influential classification of mental disorders may improve the scientific utility of the various diagnoses. If possible, similar syndromes with different names should be merged or the overlap between criteria for two or more diagnoses should be reduced. But this may not always be appropriate if two defined syndromes are both useful despite considerable overlap.

Co-occurrence of personality disorders with other mental disorders

The process of PD diagnosis involves matching signs and symptoms to definitions in a specified classification, and co-occurrence of a PD diagnosis with other PDs, and with other mental disorders, is common. Co-occurrence does not necessarily imply any causal relationships, although there can be complex interactions between PDs, other mental disorders and the social environment.

Common examples of co-occurrence are responsible for some of the problems of defining boundaries between PDs and other mental disorders that have been described, in particular between PDs and some depressive syndromes, anxiety states and substance abuse disorders. As PD can complicate the management of individuals with any other mental disorder, such co-occurrence is of major importance in clinical practice. One of the most common psychiatric diagnoses is a depressive syndrome, and in outcome studies of the treatment of depressive disorders, patients with PDs responded less well to various forms of treatment (Shea *et al.*, 1990; Tyrer *et al.*, 1990). However, as has been described, the problems of defining a boundary between PD and some forms of depression or anxiety can be difficult; Tyrer *et al.* (1992) have argued that, for some depressive syndromes with PD, the PD characteristics of excessive timidity, poor self-esteem, avoidance of anxiety-provoking situations and dependence on others, are invariably associated with depression and anxiety, and that such a patient should be considered to have just one syndrome.

PD has also been reported in association with many other mental disorders, for example (using DSM-III-R terminology) eating disorders, somatization disorders, schizophrenia, manic disorders, sexual disorders, hypochondriasis, paranoid states, dissociative disorders and obsessive-compulsive disorder.

Although there are a number of categories in the main classifications of

PDs, Rutter (1987) has pointed out that the majority of patients with clinically significant PD show a variable mixture of antisocial, borderline, histrionic and narcissistic PDs. Patients with severe PD are often considered to be 'difficult patients' and frequently present with other co-occurring mental disorders, in particular depressive syndromes, episodes of self-harm, anxiety states, substance abuse and eating disorders (Higgitt & Fonagy, 1992).

Epidemiology overview

The DSM-III-R definition of PD is somewhat vague, as it encourages the clinician to decide when aspects of personality 'cause either significant functional impairment or subjective distress'. Therefore the diagnostic threshold is difficult to determine both in practice and in research studies. However, it is generally agreed that PDs are of considerable clinical importance: 'the personality disorders constitute one of the most important sources of long-term impairment in both treated and untreated populations. Nearly one in every 10 adults in the general population and over one-half of those in (psychiatrically) treated populations, may be expected to suffer from one of the personality disorders' (Merikangas & Weissman, 1986).

Prevalence of PD in different settings, estimated by various methods, has been reviewed by Casey (1988). Using a structured interview, PD was found in 13% of an adult urban population (Casey & Tyrer, 1986), while prevalence rates of up to 34% have been reported for populations of patients in primary medical care settings. Bateman (1993) claimed a prevalence rate of about 10% in the general population and 20–30% in patients attending general practitioners. PDs have been commonly found in association with anxiety states, depressive disorders, substance abuse, self-harm episodes and criminal conduct. It was reported that, in England and Wales, 7.6% of psychiatric admissions had a PD diagnosis (Department of Health and Social Security, 1985), which is likely to be an underestimate of the actual prevalence. Other studies have found high rates (up to 50%) in psychiatric inpatient populations, as well as in outpatient samples (20–40%).

Weissman (1993), in a recent review, claimed a lifetime rate for a DSM-III-R PD of 10–13%, and of 2–3% for antisocial PD. For the latter, three different community studies have produced similar rates, and this diagnosis is much more common in males and in younger adults. A decreasing prevalence rate with increasing age has also been found for some other PDs, such as borderline PD, and there appears to be a relatively high prevalence of PDs in urban samples.

Causation

The range of causal variables

Two main classes of causal factors in relation to PDs have been identified, i.e. genetic and socio-cultural (Walton, 1973). But in addition to genetic endowment, other biological influences may be important, such as diet, perinatal trauma and cerebral viral infections. Evidence has been accumulating to indicate the marked influence of genetic factors on both personality and PD, and the effects of such influences may involve the expression of some genetic effects at different stages of life, and several kinds of gene–environment interactions (Kendler & Eaves, 1986). The latter include the effects of some consistent patterns of behaviour on the shaping of social environments.

Various models have been proposed for the effects of environment on personality and PD development, which have led to hypotheses that adverse situations at certain stages in development may have specific effects on the development of the adult personality; for example psychoanalytic theories have postulated three main developmental phases that can be adversely affected by events occurring at certain critical times (Freud, 1962). However, there is no clear evidence that links specific events and situations in childhood to the development of specific adult PD traits. Whitehorn (1952) has provided another model involving four developmental phases leading to maturity, i.e. infantile, when the person expects limitless consideration; childish, when the person is capable of limited commitment and the main need is for security; early adolescent, when the main concern is personal significance; and late adolescent, characterized by loyalty to a cause and to groups of people. Subsequently the mature person is less stereotyped and more flexible in his/her social roles. This appears to reflect the experience of many individuals and, despite the lack of evidence, it seems likely that the timing of various environmental events is of importance for the development of aspects of PD for many individuals.

While the traditional concept of PD is of a developmental disorder, (i.e. with features showing some continuity with childhood behaviour), the latest (10th) revision of the International Classification of Diseases, ICD-10

(World Health Organization, 1992), points out that abnormalities of personality can be acquired later in life 'following severe or prolonged stress, extreme environmental deprivation, serious psychiatric disorder, or brain disease or injury'. But the occurrence of late onset or intermittent PD has not been adequately addressed in the main classifications of mental disorders, despite the fact that the current ideas regarding the interaction of biological and environmental causal factors would predict that patterns of maladaptive behaviour in some individuals would be restricted to periods when the person is in an adverse environment. In clinical practice it is common for individuals to show certain features of PD, such as changeable mood and episodes of self-harm, on an intermittent basis associated with a series of life-crises related to persistent problems with social relationships. The concept of intermittent PD is similar to that of the vulnerable personality (Gelder *et al.*, 1983).

The genotype

The genetic characteristics of an individual reflect his/her genetic inheritance, together with any mutations, and the genetic substrate that influences the development of patterns of maladaptive behaviour is likely to involve many genes whose effects can be additive. Therefore, a search of markers of such genes would be likely to involve several biological and neuropsychological variables.

Non-genetic physical factors

The constitution, which is the biological structure of the individual, may be influenced by a variety of non-genetic physical variables such as brain infections, traumatic cerebral damage, malnutrition, the effects of low birth weight and the effects of alcohol on the foetus *in utero* (Beattie *et al.*, 1983).

Socio-cultural environment

Environmental variables affecting PD, which are mediated by higher mental activity, include those related to parents (or care givers), living group, immediate social milieu and wider cultural influences. It has been noted that, at the age of around 3 months, the human infant begins to discriminate between care givers and to form attachments with a limited number of individuals. This process seems to reflect behavioural patterns seen in higher primates that are necessary for satisfactory social development.

Constitution–environment interactions

Although the biological constitution of an individual may also reflect variables other than genetic factors, particular attention has been paid to genotype–environment interactions, for example, when individuals with different genetic characteristics respond differently to specific environments (Bergeman *et al.*, 1988). It appears that there can be a marked effect of a specified social environment on a minority of subjects who have certain genetic characteristics.

Methods of investigation

Animal studies

Selective breeding for certain behavioural patterns in animals may be relevant to the understanding of human behavioural genetics. For example, strains of rats have been developed that differ in their 'emotional' response to being placed in a brightly lit area, as measured by the frequency of defaecation (Wimer & Wimer, 1985), and 'nervous' pointer dogs appear frightened in the presence of humans, showing immobility (Reese, 1979).

Assessment of biological markers of PD

Genetically or non-genetically determined constitutional factors may be associated with biological 'markers' of personality or PD characteristics. The identification of a biological marker usually involves direct measurement of a biological variable, but can also be considered to include psychological tests of cognitive functions and other higher mental activity. The marker may be directly observable (such as abnormalities in smooth pursuit eye movement in association with schizotypal PD), or be induced by a drug (i.e. a psychopharmacological 'probe'). The latter can include a response of a PD characteristic, such as impulsivity, to a therapeutic trial of medication.

Siever & Davis (1991) have suggested that research into biological markers of PD characteristics should be based on a model of the following four dimensions of maladaptation: problems with cognitive/perceptual organization (shown by some patients with schizoid, schizotypal and paranoid PDs); impulsivity/aggression (shown by some patients with borderline and antisocial PDs, and claimed to be related to an hypothesized reduction in serotonergic neurotransmitter activity); affective instability (shown by some patients with borderline PD and suggested to be related to hypothesized abnormalities of cholinergic and catecholaminergic neuro-transmission); and anxiety/inhibition. It was noted that functioning on these dimensions can also be associated with some non-PD psychiatric disorders (for example, abnormal smooth pursuit eye movements have been associated with schizophrenia), and that such models must recognize that interactions between dimensions are likely to be important. Particular attention has been paid to the biological correlates of schizotypal and borderline PDs.

The comparison of PD assessments in genetically related individuals

The relative importance of genetic and environmental causal variables has been investigated by evaluating PD in identical and non-identical twins reared apart or together, in adoptees, and in several members of the same family. Although many aspects of PD have been considered, the emphasis has been on subjects with prominent antisocial behaviour.

Twin studies provide the best methods for evaluating the effects of genetic and environmental influences, in particular the method of comparing monozygous (MZ) and dizygous (DZ) twins who have been separated from each other and their parents at birth, and raised apart. However, there can be several methodological difficulties in twin studies, including a bias in sample selection and inadequate determination of zygosity. Also, separated twins may have been subject to similar non-genetic perinatal physical influences due, for instance, to poor living conditions, while twins reared together may be exposed to relatively similar treatment compared with twins reared apart, with greater expectations of behavioural similarity.

Results of twin studies on personality characteristics of 'normal' (i.e. non-clinical) subjects have shown the potential of such methodology for the study of clinical populations. Also, as it is generally accepted that most PD characteristics are on a continuum of severity with 'normal' personality traits, the main findings from non-clinical samples are likely to be of relevance to the study of PDs.

Several large twin studies have tried to evaluate the proportions of the variance of 'normal' personality assessments that are related to genetic influences, to shared family environment and to non-familial environmental effects. Bouchard *et al.* (1990) studied 100 twins reared apart and concluded that MZ twins raised apart were as similar as MZ twins raised together. A similar finding, namely, that there is a negligible contribution of a common family environment to the similarity of most measured traits between twin pairs, was reported by Tellegen *et al.* (1988), although there was some effect of common family environment on 'positive emotionality' and 'social closeness'. This study involved 217 MZ and 114 DZ reared-together adult twin pairs, and 44 MZ and 27 DZ reared-apart adult twin pairs. It was concluded that about 50% of measured differences were caused by genetic influences, while the remaining 50% of environmentally-determined variance included measurement error and the influence of transient 'states', such as depression or anxiety. It was also claimed that this study provided evidence of both additive and non-additive genetic effects.

In general, studies of normal personality in related individuals have shown that genetic factors are responsible for between 35% and 60% of the variance for several traits measured by questionnaire; for example, the range of estimates for the genetic contribution to the variance of measurements of extraversion is between 54% and 74% (Livesley *et al.*, 1993).

A further twin study, in a volunteer non-clinical sample, examined genetic and environmental influences on PD (Livesley *et al.*, 1993). Subjects were 90 MZ and 85 DZ twin pairs who completed a 290-item questionnaire. The following dimensions of PD were assessed: affective lability, anxiousness, callousness, cognitive distortion, compulsivity, conduct problems, identity problems, insecure attachment, intimacy problems, narcissism, oppositionality, rejection, restricted expression, self-harm, social avoidance, stimulus seeking, submissiveness, and suspiciousness. Estimates were made for the proportion of the variance of each scale that was accounted for by genetic factors, common (shared) environment and non-shared environment. Additive and non-additive genetic factors were estimated separately, based on comparisons of the correlations between the scores of MZ and DZ twins. The estimates of genetic influence on the variance for 12 of the 18 dimensions were 40% or above. The highest values were 64% for narcissism and 59% for identity problems (i.e. ahedonia, chronic feelings of emptiness, labile self-concept and pessimism), while the lowest values for genetic heritability were for conduct problems (0%) and submissiveness (25%). As in previous studies, the influences of common environment were generally low or non-existent, with the exception of the contributions to conduct problems (53%) and submissiveness (28%). However, marked effects of non-shared environment were generally found. It was concluded that most PD traits involve the extremes of normal variation, and that most aspects of PD are causally related to substantial genetic and non-shared environmental components. But it was pointed out that the relative importance of various causal factors may be different in samples from clinical settings with a diagnosis of PD. Nevertheless, the demonstration that PD traits vary in respect of the relative proportions of

genetic and environmental effects has implications for treatment programmes; for instance, a strong genetic predisposition to a maladaptive
trait may limit the potential for psychological treatments.

Methods to evaluate interactions between causal variables

Evidence of genetic–environmental interactions for personality traits in a
non-patient sample has been provided by Bergeman *et al.* (1988). In their
study of 99 pairs of MZ twins reared apart, perceptions of early rearing
environment appeared to have interacted with genetic factors to influence
personality as assessed during later adult life.

Identification of associations between possible causal variables and PD
features in groups of subjects

Many studies have investigated the correlations (or categorical associations) between hypothesized causal variables (such as abuse in childhood)
and measurement of PD characteristics. However, an association does not,
of course, necessarily reflect a causal relationship.

'Cluster A' PDs (paranoid, schizoid and schizotypal PDs) – evidence of
causation

Evidence from studies of genetically related individuals

A study of schizotypal PD in subjects with a MZ twin showed a concordance rate of 33% (with an absence of borderline PD in co-twins),
compared with 4% in DZ pairs (Torgerson, 1984). Also, an increased
prevalence of schizotypal PD and other 'cluster A' PD psychopathology
has been found in first degree relatives of patients with schizophrenia
(Kendler *et al.*, 1981*a*; Baron *et al.*, 1985; Parnas *et al.*, 1993). Only one
study has failed to demonstrate such a relationship between schizotypal PD
and schizophrenia (Coryell & Zimmerman, 1989). Familial aggregation for
schizotypal PD has also been demonstrated (Livesley *et al.*, 1993). A recent
report of a joint US and Danish project involved 207 offspring of
schizophrenic mothers and 104 controls followed-up for between 15–42
years (Kendler *et al.*, 1993*a, b*) and found that, as well as increased
prevalence in the at-risk offspring of schizophrenia and other psychoses,
there was an excess of schizotypal PD (18.8% versus 5%) and paranoid PD
(2.6% versus 0%).

Evidence from studies of biological markers

Various biological associations with schizotypal and other 'cluster A' PD features have been described. In relation to cognition, attention and information processing (which is believed to reflect dopaminergic neuro-transmission), schizotypal PD features have been associated with impaired performance of tests of eye movements, of 'continuous performance' tasks, and of 'backward masking', and with abnormalities involving 'event-related EEG potentials' (Weston & Siever, 1993). An example of an eye movement disorder is shown by the presence of small 'jumps' when a smoothly-moving target is followed. A 'continuous performance' task may involve monitoring a changing series of letters and making a response when a particular sequence of two letters occurs. 'Backward masking' involves the presentation of two visual stimuli in quick succession; the first, or 'target', stimulus can be more easily identified as the time between the stimuli is increased, and the minimum time associated with recognition of the target stimulus is increased in association with schizophrenia and schizotypal PD. This reflects the speed of information processing. 'Event-related EEG potentials', which are also related to information processing, are EEG recordings of brain activity after, for example, an auditory stimulus. Impaired eye-tracking accuracy has also been found to be associated with schizophrenia (Siever *et al.*, 1990*a*).

Other associations of schizotypal and related PD characteristics have been with reduced platelet monoamine oxidase (MAO), raised homovanillic acid in CSF and plasma, and a characteristic response to an amphetamine 'challenge', in which subjects with co-occurring schizotypal and borderline PDs became transiently worse with amphetamine administration (shown by abnormal cognitions and reduced feelings of well-being), while patients with only a borderline PD diagnosis improved (Schulz *et al.*, 1988). Also, changes in ventricle-to-brain ratio on computerized tomography (CT) scans have been related to schizotypal children of patients with schizophrenia (Schulsinger *et al.*, 1984), and treatment with dopamine receptor antagonist drugs, which are effective in schizophrenia, appear to reduce some of the abnormal cognitions in schizotypal PD.

Freund *et al.* (1992) have reported that, among women with normal IQ who are carriers of the fragile X chromosome abnormality, the degree of fragility (the percentage of cells exhibiting the fragile-X chromosome abnormality) is associated with a range of social and psychological disability, including schizotypal PD features.

Summary

Studies of biological correlates of schizotypal PD have indicated geneti-cally-determined abnormalities in dopaminergic neurotransmission and information processing. Schizotypal PD and schizophrenia appear to be related disorders, and this is consistent with the finding that some patients with schizotypal PD may be helped by low doses of 'neuroleptic' medication.

'Cluster B' PDs (antisocial, borderline, histrionic and narcissistic PDs) – evidence of causation

Evidence from studies of genetically related individuals

Twin studies of antisocial behaviour have been reviewed by Blackburn (1993) and McGuffin & Thapar (1992). Many reports have shown clear differences between a greater concordance for criminal behaviour between MZ twin pairs than between DZ twin pairs for adults, although this difference has not been found in relation to juvenile delinquency. McGuffin & Gottesman (1984) summarized data from seven studies of adult crimina-lity and found mean MZ:DZ concordance of 51%:22%, although it was noted that interpretation must take into account the different methodolo-gies used.

Scandinavian studies have taken advantage of national registers to obtain unselected twin samples; Christiansen (1974, 1977, and re-analysed by Cloninger *et al.*, 1978) studied 3586 twin pairs and reported MZ:DZ concordance for criminality in males of 35%:13% and in females of 21%:8%, while Dalgaard & Kringlen (1976) found a smaller (and non-significant) difference between MZ:DZ concordance rates of 26%:15%, in 31 MZ pairs and 54 DZ pairs.

Therefore, twin studies have shown a definite genetic contribution to adult criminality, but this could not be demonstrated in relation to juvenile crime. This suggests that criminality is, in general, the result of additive combinations of genetic and (substantial) environmental factors. Also, female criminals appear to have, on average, a higher genetic predisposition than male criminals (Cloninger *et al.*, 1978).

Adoption studies in relation to criminality have had various designs, such as identification of criminal parents and comparing their children with those of non-criminal controls, or comparing criminal and non-criminal adoptees in respect of criminality in biological and adoptive parents. The former approach was used by Crowe (1972) in a study of the children of 52 imprisoned female offenders and 52 controls: eight out of the 'at risk' children had arrest records compared with two of the controls. Also, a history of traffic offences in the 'at risk' and control populations was 19:8, and the presence of antisocial PD 6:0. Cadoret (1978) reported similar findings.

Hutchings & Mednick (1975) compared criminal and non-criminal (control) adoptees in their study of 143 subjects and 143 controls. Of the males, 36.2% had become criminal when both biological and adoptive fathers were criminal, 21.4% when the biological father was criminal, 11.5% when the adoptive father was criminal and 10.5% when neither father was criminal. Blackburn (1993) has reviewed how the presence or absence of alcoholism, and pre-adoption factors such as perinatal complications due to poor living conditions, may influence the interpretation of such results.

A further study of 14 427 adoptees included 981 males and 212 females with a criminal record (Mednick, Gabrielli & Hutchings, 1984). When at least one of each pair of biological parents was criminal, 20.0% of sons became criminal compared with 14.7% when an adoptive parent was criminal and 13.5% when no parent was criminal. Therefore, there was a significant effect of a criminal biological parent but not of a criminal adoptive parent, although this effect was related to property offences rather than violent crime.

Cadoret *et al.* (1990), in their study of 286 adult male adoptees, have claimed that their findings suggest that a genetic–environment interaction can be important in the development of antisocial PD. Both alcohol problems and criminality/delinquency in biological parents were associated with increased incidence of antisocial PD in adoptees. Also, the 44 adoptees with antisocial PD were more likely to have alcohol problems. Alcohol problems in a biological parent predicted the same disorder in the adoptee, as did criminality/delinquency, while adverse environmental factors in the adoptive home, namely an alcohol problem, antisocial behaviour or low socioeconomic status, were also shown to increase the risk of antisocial PD in the adoptees, but only when the adoptee had a biological parent with criminality/delinquency.

It appears that while genetic factors are relevant for both antisocial PD and alcoholism, these are separate to some degree (Baron *et al.*, 1985; Dahl, 1993), and Berelowitz & Tarnopolsky (1993) concluded that family studies confirm 'the separateness of borderline and schizotypal personalities, and of borderline personality and major depressive illness'. But there is evidence of a genetic relationship between antisocial PD in men and somatization disorder in women (McGuffin & Thapar, 1992).

Evidence from studies of biological markers

The biological (including neuropsychological) correlates of antisocial PD and criminality have been reviewed by Kilzieh & Cloninger (1993) and Blackburn (1993). There have been claims of frontal and left hemispherical neuropsychological dysfunction in offender groups, including visual–perceptual deficits and impairment of language-related skills (Miller, 1988; Mungas, 1988), and differences from control groups have been reported in relation to EEG findings (including evoked potentials and event-related potentials, i.e. scalp EEG responses to stimuli or events); testosterone levels; autonomic function (including skin conductance levels, skin conductance responses and heart rate) (Raine, Venables & Williams, 1990); blood platelet MAO (monoamine oxidase) activity (Klinteberg *et al.*, 1987; Lykouras, Markianos & Moussas, 1989; Alm *et al.*, 1994); CSF (cerebrospinal fluid) catecholamine metabolites (Virkkunen *et al.*, 1987; Gardner, Lucas & Cowdry, 1990); pre-menstrual tension; minor physical abnormalities (Kandel *et al.*, 1989) and abnormal glucose metabolism. A consistent finding has been that offender populations show electrodermal hyporesponsiveness when anticipating or experiencing aversive stimulation (Blackburn, 1993).

The reported associations between antisocial behaviour, structural brain damage, epilepsy and a proposed 'dyscontrol syndrome' have been inconsistent. A dyscontrol syndrome has been considered to involve explosive outbursts of emotion (usually anger, with minimal triggering events), but with a history of satisfactory social behaviour between episodes. It has been suggested that such a syndrome may sometimes be associated with focal abnormalities of brain structure or function in the temporal lobes or other parts of the limbic system. In relation to epilepsy, the question can sometimes arise as to whether a crime can be committed without awareness, and rare examples of such automatism have been reported. The evidence of an association between temporal lobe epilepsy and non-seizure-related violence is unclear (Blackburn, 1993).

Studies on chromosome abnormalities, such as Kleinefelter's syndrome, suggest that such disorders can sometimes make a non-specific contribution to criminality (as can childhood hyperactivity), and may be mediated by low intelligence, but the explanations for reports of various associations of criminality with physical appearance and relatively muscular body build are unclear (Kumar *et al.*, 1989). In respect of facial appearance, the reaction of others to unattractiveness may sometimes lead to a self-fulfilling prophecy.

There have been many studies of the biological associations of borderline PD (Steiner, Links & Korzekwa, 1988; Lahmeyer *et al.*, 1989; Berelowitz & Tarnopolsky, 1993), although it must be remembered that many subjects with this diagnosis have features of other PDs, particularly the other members of 'cluster B'. Studies have involved the dexamethasone suppression test, the thyrotropic releasing hormone test, sleep studies, electro-encephalography (EEG), platelet MAO (Schalling *et al.*, 1987), platelet adrenergic receptor binding (Southwick *et al.*, 1990; Shekim, Bylund & Frankel, 1990), catecholamine metabolite studies (Linnoila & Virkkunen, 1992), and 'challenge studies', such as the prolactin response to fenfluramine (Halperin *et al.*, 1994), the mood response to methylphenidate (Lucas *et al.*, 1987) or to oral *m*-chlorophenylpiperazine (Hollander *et al.*, 1994), the growth hormone (GH) response to clonidine, and the effects of arecholine on REM (rapid eye movement) sleep latency (Weston & Siever, 1993). Also, antipsychotic drugs, some antidepressant drugs and mood-stabilizing agents such as lithium carbonate and carbamazepine have been found to be of benefit to some patients with affective instability in the setting of PD.

It has been claimed that impulsivity is the most consistent abnormality in 'cluster B' PDs, and may be associated with abnormalities of serotonergic neurotransmitter function, shown by low serotonergic metabolites in the CSF and reduced prolactin response to fenfluramine (Coccaro *et al.*, 1989), together with abnormalities of noradrenergic neurotransmission, shown by an increased growth hormone response to clonidine. Affective instability may also involve abnormalities in acetylcholine neurotransmission (Weston & Siever, 1993). Linnoila & Virkkunen (1992), in their study of an offender group, have suggested that a 'low serotonin syndrome', associated with low 5-hydroxyindoleacetic acid (5HIAA) in the CSF, is related to impulsive, externally-directed aggressive behaviour in some violent offenders, which often occurs under the influence of alcohol, while such CSF changes have also been reported in relation to violent suicide attempts in patients with PD and unipolar depression (Gardner *et al.*, 1990). In the former study, the offender group also showed associations with mild hypoglycaemia, a history of early-onset alcohol and substance abuse, and disturbance in diurnal activity rhythm.

Neuropsychological testing of patients with borderline PD has produced claims of significant impairment, compared with controls, on memory tests of uncued recall of complex recently-learned material (O'Leary *et al.*, 1991).

Sleep EEG studies have been claimed to distinguish patients with borderline PD and a co-occurring depressive disorder from those with borderline PD and other types of co-occurring psychiatric disorder (Lahmeyer *et al.*, 1989).

Evidence from associations within groups of subjects with PD

A number of studies have examined associations and correlations between possible causal variables and PD, in particular environmental variables in relation to borderline and antisocial PDs. Risk of criminality has been shown to be associated with a childhood history of prolonged institutional care, placement out of the family, multiple placements and low socioeconomic status (McGuffin & Thapar, 1992), while both antisocial and borderline PD features have been associated with a history of childhood sexual abuse, physical and emotional abuse, multiple forms of severe and repeated abuse, separation from or death of parents, neglect (i.e. lack of supervision, lack of care and parental unavailability), harsh or rejecting parenting, losses in childhood, maternal overinvolvement combined with inconsistent responses, and witnessing domestic violence or other antisocial behaviour (Bezirganian, Cohen & Brook, 1993; Crowell *et al.*, 1993). Also, a history of sexual abuse has been linked with relatively lethal incidents of self-harm (Van der Kolk, Perry & Herman, 1991; Wagner & Linehan, 1994). Inconsistent parenting can involve a failure to notice and respond positively to desirable behaviour, together with an inability or unwillingness to address and confront antisocial behaviour. In a study of 776 adolescents, it was found that parental inconsistency was associated with subsequent development of borderline PD but only if it was combined with maternal overinvolvement (Bezirganian *et al.*, 1993).

Research has also indicated that consistent and appropriate discipline can be a protective variable, as can a high intelligence (Kandel *et al.*, 1988).

Summary

Studies of related individuals have clearly indicated that genetic factors can predispose an individual to criminal activity. Studies of biological variables have reported that groups of subjects with antisocial PD tend to show hyporesponsiveness when anticipating or experiencing aversive stimulation, while 'challenge' studies, such as the prolactin response to fenfluramine, have shown abnormalities related to borderline PD. Both borderline and antisocial PD have been associated with a history of various aspects of adversity in childhood, in particular repeated abuse involving sexual, physical and emotional aspects. Consistent and appropriate disciplinary practices in the upbringing of children should be encouraged, and may protect against the later development of some aspects of PD in vulnerable individuals. Impulsivity may be helped by serotonergic enhancing drugs, such as fluoxetine, while affective instability may benefit from drugs affecting cholinergic and catecholaminergic neurotransmitter function, such as neuroleptics, lithium and monoamine oxidase inhibitors.

'Cluster C' PDs (avoidant, dependent, obsessive-compulsive PDs and, in DSM-III-R but not DSM-IV, passive-aggressive PD) – evidence of causation

Evidence from studies of related individuals

Evidence of causation is relatively sparse for 'cluster C' PDs, but it has been claimed that avoidant and dependent PDs cluster in families (McGuffin & Thapar, 1992). Genetic evidence for obsessive-compulsive PD is conflicting, but a genetically-determined vulnerability may be linked with Tourette's syndrome (Dahl, 1993).

Evidence from studies of biological markers

Data on biological variables related to the 'anxious' 'cluster C' PDs is limited. However, a few studies have investigated the effects of growth hormone response to clonidine, of lactate infusion, and of inhalation of 7% CO_2 (Weston & Siever, 1993). Also, Joyce, Mulder & Cloninger (1994*a*, *b*) found that temperament, especially dependence and extravagance, was associated with hypercortisolaemia in a group of depressed patients.

Conclusion

A considerable volume of research has identified a range of genetic and environmental causal factors, and their interactions, which must be considered in the development of all PDs. Further studies of biological markers of PD characteristics may lead to improvements in the targeting of both pharmacological and psychological interventions.

Treatability

Unfortunately, 'personality disorder' has often been used as a negative and perjorative term to imply that the individual does not deserve help and that the presenting problems are not the province of medical practice. Also, it has been commonly believed that there are no effective interventions; this can provide an excuse to avoid those patients whose behaviour is unpleasant and difficult to manage. Some patients with PD become poorly tolerated by health care staff as they frequently demand help but reject what is offered. This may be accompanied by complaints, anger, threats and violence.

However, patients with PD can benefit from a variety of interventions, even though the long-term persistence of these disorders usually prevents the clinician from receiving the gratifying feedback of a short-term dramatic cure. However, as the presenting problems often result from an interaction between the PD and the environment, it is often possible to arrange or encourage environmental changes that can lead to a rapid resolution of a crisis. In the longer-term, it is possible for ingrained aspects of PD to become modified, although, in general, any significant changes are gradual, while pronounced traits will never completely disappear or be replaced. Nevertheless, even relatively modest changes (for example, learning to avoid some situations that evoke an outburst of temper) can have significantly beneficial effects.

For many individuals with severe PD, the most helpful strategy is to provide a long-term contact with one or more professionals in the health care and allied services, with back-up measures (e.g. intensive counselling, a short admission to psychiatric hospital, social work intervention, or day care attendance) in times of crisis. Although such a supportive strategy appears deceptively simple, it is often very difficult for the health-care worker to maintain the motivation to continue regular (even if infrequent) contact with a person who is difficult to manage and may be unlikeable. The nature of these contacts, when the conversation may often be very superficial and the clinician may not be using any specific techniques of intervention, may not appear to justify years of professional training. It is tempting not to give another appointment and, of course, this may be quite appropriate, as not everybody with PD needs to be seen over long periods or indefinitely. But for those individuals who are constantly presenting to the psychiatric and other medical services, longer-term support and crisis intervention can be justified, not only because the individual may be helped but also because this may minimize demands on medical services. The specific tasks of the clinician are firstly, to decide on an appropriate format and duration of contact with the psychiatric (or other) services; secondly, to tolerate a lack of response or cooperation; and, thirdly, to override his/her desire to discharge the individual if the contacts evoke anger and frustration in the clinician, when this is not in the patient's interest.

In addition to this supportive approach, there is evidence that more specific interventions can sometimes be of benefit. These include various forms of short-term, intermittent and long-term psychotherapy, the provision of various forms of social and community support, cognitive therapy, different types of group psychotherapy, behaviour therapy and drug treatments, in particular low dose neuroleptics (usually combined with psychological management) for borderline PD.

2

Specified personality disorders: clinical features

J.H. DOWSON

Validity of personality disorder syndromes

For a syndrome to have validity it must be demonstrated that its features are associated with other variables; descriptive validity involves an association with definitions of PD, while concurrent and predictive validity relate PD assessments to measurements of other variables and outcome, respectively.

A PD diagnosis based on a categorical classification of PD is 'inherently imperfect because we can only provide an approximate match to an hypothetical construct' (Widiger & Frances, 1985a), and the main polythetic diagnostic systems give rise to PD syndromes that have a variable degree of resemblance to the 'ideal' or 'prototype' disorders. Also, there can be overlap between diagnoses if similar or identical features occur in more than one syndrome, and co-occurrence of several PDs may be present in the same individual. Furthermore, when two or more PD syndromes co-occur, it cannot be assumed that they are independent, as interactions will occur.

The DSM-III-R and DSM-IV claim that PD syndromes can be grouped into 'clusters', which implies that if one PD member of the cluster is present, features of the associated PDs are more likely to co-occur than features of PDs in other clusters. The first cluster includes paranoid, schizoid and schizotypal PDs, and people with these syndromes often appear odd or eccentric. Antisocial, borderline, histrionic and narcissistic PDs form a second cluster, leading to dramatic, emotional or erratic behaviour, while the third cluster consists of avoidant, dependent, obsessive-compulsive and passive-aggressive PDs (the latter is omitted in DSM-IV). Individuals with the latter disorders often appear anxious or fearful.

This chapter will summarize the clinical features of categories of PD based on various sources, but it must be remembered that all classifications are provisional, and the major classifications of mental disorders are subject to regular revisions. Although the many problems of classification and assessment of PD might lead a pessimist to conclude that PD diagnoses are unlikely to be useful, many have persisted in clinical practice.

A particular definition of a PD syndrome can be evaluated in several ways, for example, by using the criteria to divide a group of patients into cases (with the disorder) and non-cases; also, each individual diagnostic criterion can be evaluated in relation to frequency of positive ratings in the cases (sensitivity), rarity of positive ratings in non-cases (specificity) and association of positive ratings with a diagnosis (positive predictive power). Other ways in which the properties of a PD can be investigated include a comparison of the defined syndrome with the descriptions in the literature (i.e. descriptive validity), and examination of concurrent validity, reliability (i.e. inter-rater agreement and temporal stability of diagnosis), the degree of overlap with other PD syndromes and the frequency of co-occurrence with other disorders. It is also important to consider if the application of the diagnosis is subject to prejudice (such as racial or sexual) or if its use (such as for sadistic or antisocial PD) could lead to unfortunate legal consequences. Finally, the value of a PD diagnosis is partly reflected by its level of acceptance among those who are professionally concerned with personality disordered individuals.

Many of the syndromes to be described are useful to clinicians as a convenient summary of the main PD features for individual patients. Although most individuals with PD fulfil criteria for more than one PD, many such individuals show predominant features (i.e. those judged to cause the most problems) that relate to just one PD diagnosis. In psychiatric practice, the features of borderline PD are important as a frequent origin of many crises and of 'difficult to manage' patients, while in primary medical care, other PDs, such as histrionic and obsessive-compulsive PDs, are relatively more important as causes of common complaints such as anxiety and some depressive symptoms. In forensic practice, antisocial PD is of particular relevance.

Paranoid personality disorder

Main features

These include excessive sensitivity to rebuff, insecurity, suspiciousness and mistrust of others.

Clinical origins

Kretchmer (1918) described a 'sensitive' personality, which involves excessive suspiciousness and exaggerated reactions to setbacks, and these features have been incorporated into all the versions of the DSM classification. But despite general agreement among clinicians that such a syndrome does exist, it is relatively uncommon in clinical practice and has attracted little research. However, there is evidence from family and adoption studies that, together with schizoid and schizotypal PD, paranoid PD has a genetic link with schizophrenia (Kendler *et al.*, 1984). For example, increased risks of schizophrenia, paranoid PD and schizotypal PD were found in relatives of a sample selected on the basis of the presence of schizotypal PD (Siever *et al.*, 1990*b*).

Main definitions

The DSM-III-R considers that the essential feature of paranoid PD is a 'pervasive and unwarranted tendency . . . to interpret the actions of people as deliberately demeaning or threatening' and four of the following are required for the diagnosis:

(1) expects, without sufficient basis, to be exploited or harmed by others, (2) questions, without justification, the loyalty or trustworthiness of friends or associates, (3) reads hidden demeaning or threatening meanings into benign remarks or events, (4) bears grudges or is unforgiving of insults or slights, (5) is reluctant to confide in others because of unwarranted fear that the information will be used against him or her, (6) is easily slighted and quick to react with anger or to counterattack, (7) questions, without justification, fidelity of spouse or sexual partner.

The DSM-IV contains minor modifications; for example, the first criterion becomes: 'suspects, without sufficient basis, that others are exploiting, harming, or deceiving him or her'.

The ICD-10 criteria show considerable overlap with the above, but also include the following: a combative and tenacious sense of personal rights out of keeping with the actual situation; a tendency to experience excessive self-importance, manifest in a persistent self-referential attitude; and preoccupation with unsubstantiated 'conspiratorial' explanations of events both immediate to the patient and in the world at large.

Clinical features

Paranoid PD is characterized by a marked distrust of others and sensitivity to rebuff. These features appear to relate to an underlying insecurity and are accompanied by a watchful alertness.

Such individuals are suspicious, tense, emotionally cold and rigid in their thinking. There is often a fear of losing independence, a resentment of those in authority and a fear of intimate relationships. They see themselves as victims of mistreatment and abuse, although this is associated with a disdain for weakness or disability in others. There is an excessive sense of personal rights and self-importance. Jealousy may be marked and directed towards those with power and influence as well as to colleagues and sexual partners. It may be felt that others have been responsible for preventing the achievement of the person's potential.

These attitudes lead to a variety of interactive behaviours. Such persons seem touchy, argumentative and hostile with a tendency to counterattack at minimal provocation; they are guarded and secretive, being reluctant to disclose personal information and having an excessive concern about confidentiality; they may appear devious, stubborn and unwilling to compromise; they lack humour, capacity for enjoyment and tender feelings; and they have difficulty in expressing doubts and insecurities. Anger may be provoked by a positive regard as this is seen as only conditional, while a grudge is accompanied by vindictiveness. Not surprisingly, these individuals tend to generate unease, fear and hostility in others. They are often not fully aware of the effects of their behaviour. Faced with a new situation, the person may search for confirmation of his/her expectations and become convinced of hidden motives on the basis of inadequate evidence, without being able to appreciate the total context of the situation. Criticism is very difficult to accept and there is a low tolerance threshold with a tendency to try and avoid any blame. Because of the combination of insecurity and self-importance, groups of people are avoided, unless the person is in a dominant position. Under times of stress they may experience transient 'psychosis-like' phenomena, such as ideas of reference, which may involve a feeling that others are taking special notice of him/her.

Presentation to medical services

Individuals with paranoid PD seldom seek help for the features of their syndrome; however this disorder may be the origin of secondary symptoms such as anxiety, some depressive symptoms, or substance abuse. These may be in the context of occupational problems such as conflicts with those in authority, or relationship difficulties within the family. As these individuals tend to be secretive and guarded, evidence of paranoid PD features may only emerge gradually within a series of interviews or treatment sessions.

It appears that paranoid PD can, more specifically, lead to the development of other psychiatric syndromes, although these are 'final-common-pathways' that may also reflect other disorders such as schizophrenia.

Some individuals with paranoid PD, the so-called 'paranoid litigants', become heavily involved with legal activities, tribunals or complaints procedures. It is useful to be able to predict the likelihood of such behaviour, so that particular care can be taken to provide detailed explanations to the patient and to keep adequate written records. Others with paranoid PD may develop a delusional preoccupation with a part of the body, usually a facial feature, which is known as 'dysmorphophobia'. For example, a chance remark about the size of a patient's nose at the age of 14 led to a discrete delusional preoccupation that his nose was severely deformed and attracted ridicule. Such people may present to surgeons with requests for cosmetic operations, but these are not indicated unless there is a clear and widely accepted need for corrective surgery. Finally, the syndrome of 'morbid jealousy', which involves a delusional preoccupation with a partner's supposed infidelity, may also arise in the context of paranoid PD, although this can also occur in association with schizophrenia or alcohol abuse.

Associated features
Reference has been made to the evidence that suggests that individuals with paranoid PD can share some genetic factors with those showing schizotypal PD, schizoid PD or schizophrenia. The DSM-III-R has claimed that paranoid PD is more frequently diagnosed in men.

Current status
Despite the relative lack of empirical research, the category of paranoid PD has a long clinical tradition. The phenomena associated with this diagnosis can undoubtedly be of clinical significance in patient groups. The genetic relationships between paranoid PD, the other PDs in DSM-III-R's cluster A (schizotypal and schizoid PDs) and various types of schizophrenia, require further investigation.

Schizoid (and schizotypal) personality disorder

Main features
The main features of schizoid and schizotypal PDs will be considered together; these include social withdrawal, lack of emotional rapport, sensitivity, a preoccupation with an internal world of cognitive processes

involving fantasy, and odd thoughts, appearance and behaviour. There is evidence that a group of individuals with such features is associated with a genetic predisposition that is related to genetic causes of schizophrenia.

Clinical origins

Although Bleuler (1908) drew attention to that part of any personality that involves the direction of the person's attention to the inner mental life and away from the external world, the concept of schizoid PD originated from observations that social withdrawal and eccentricity appeared to have an increased prevalence among relatives of patients with schizophrenia and among the patients' premorbid personalities (Widiger *et al.*, 1988; Vaglum & Vaglum, 1989). The vivid internal mental world that can accompany social withdrawal was recognized by Kretchmer (1925), who described persons who loved books, were impractical and lazy, yet could act with passionate energy in certain areas. Despite social withdrawal, deep friend-ships could sometimes be developed with a select few.

The revisions of the third edition of the DSM classification in 1980 were of critical importance to the more recent concepts of the schizophrenia-related PDs, and, prior to 1980, the DSM subdivided a schizoid PD category into schizoid, avoidant and schizotypal PDs; schizoid PD denoted social withdrawal in the context of an apparent indifference to social relationships, together with a reduced range of emotional experience and expression, while, in contrast, individuals with avoidant PD were thought to have the desire to relate socially with more capacity for social relation-ships. In avoidant PD there was also a pervasive social discomfort due to fear of humiliation and disapproval. The third of the pre-1980 subcategor-ies, schizotypal PD, was reserved for those features that appeared, on the evidence of the Danish adoption studies of schizophrenia, to be the most specific indicators of genetic linkage with schizophrenia, namely odd or eccentric thoughts and behaviour (Kendler *et al.*, 1984; Modestin, Foglia & Toffler, 1989). However, detailed evaluation of the range of PD features in relatives of patients with schizophrenia has also identified an increased prevalance of emotional detachment, unsociability and suspiciousness (Kendler, 1985), which indicates that features in the DSM-III's definition of schizoid PD were also related to schizophrenia. Another controversial and confusing aspect in the classifications of these PDs has been the claim that 'schizophrenia-like' features can also be found in borderline PD.

Other syndromes, which are described as 'developmental' as they become apparent in childhood, appear to be linked to schizoid (and schizotypal) PD in adults; these are schizoid PD of childhood (Wolff, 1991), autism, and Asperger's syndrome (Tantam, 1988). (The latter incorporates schizoid PD of childhood in the ICD-10.)

Schizoid PD of childhood occurs more in boys than girls in a ratio of 4:1. While autism is usually evident before the age of 3, schizoid PD of childhood occurs later and, in general, patients are less disabled than those with either autism or Asperger's syndrome, although the boundaries between these disorders are not clear. Schizoid PD of childhood involves solitariness, impaired empathy, emotional detachment, rigidity of mental set with single-minded pursuit of special interests, increased sensitivity, odd styles of communication (including overcommunicativeness), odd gaze and gestures, and unusual fantasies. This is usually in the setting of average or superior intelligence but there may be specific developmental delays, especially of language-related skills. Such children present problems to teachers and parents; they do not conform socially and react to constraints with outbursts of weeping, rage or aggression. Follow-up studies have shown that features of this disorder persist to at least early adult life and it appears that biological causal factors, such as genetic influences, are implicated. The risk of the subsequent development of schizophrenia may be increased but is still relatively low at an estimated 1 in 10, but in a follow-up study (Wolff, 1991), in which the mean age of patients was 27, 75% fulfilled DSM-III criteria for schizotypal PD and there were significantly increased prevalences of both schizoid and schizotypal PDs compared with a control group. Also, the patient group had more impairment related to social integration, heterosexual relationships and sensitivity, together with unusual modes of communication, involving odd thoughts, overtalkativeness, unguarded communications, abnormal eye contact, abnormal smiling, single-minded pursuits of special interests and poor work adjustment. There was a greater incidence of attendance at psychiatric services and two patients had developed schizophrenia. Wolff (1991) has hypothesized that schizoid PD of childhood may be related to autism, Asperger's syndrome and schizophrenia, in an association that may involve the sharing of a genetically based predisposition that requires additional genetic and other factors for the development of the latter three disorders.

Autism is also more common in boys and is usually apparent before the age of 3. Most affected individuals have significant learning difficulties and there is poor communication with a pattern of restricted repetitive behaviour. It has been reported that parents of such children show increased schizoid PD features (Wolff, 1991) and that follow-up indicates a probable increased incidence of schizoid PD and schizophrenia (Szatmari, Barto-lucci & Bremner, 1989).

Asperger's syndrome is also apparent in early childhood and more common in boys but there is usually no widespread delay or retardation in language or cognitive development; features include poor empathy, poverty of non-verbal expression, pedantic repetitive and circumstantial speech that may lack appropriate intonation, an inflexible routine some-times involving intense interests, clumsy gait and posture, and difficult peer relationships (Mawson, Grounds & Tantam, 1985). The ICD-10 notes a tendency for these abnormalities to persist into adolescence and adult life.

Main definitions

DSM-III-R considers that the essential features of schizoid PD are a pervasive pattern of indifference to social relationships and a restricted range of emotional experience and expression. At least four of the following criteria are required:

(1) neither desires nor enjoys close relationships, including being part of a family (authors' note: the lack of desire for relationships has been questioned), (2) almost always chooses solitary activities, (3) rarely, if ever, claims to experience strong emotions, such as anger or joy, (4) indicates little or no desire to have sexual experiences with another person (age being taken into account), (5) is indifferent to the praise and criticism of others, (6) has no close friends or confidants (or only one) other than first-degree relatives, (7) displays constricted affect, e.g. is aloof, cold, rarely reciprocates gestures or facial expressions, such as smiles or nods.

The DSM-IV criteria combined criteria 3 and 7 to form the criterion: 'shows emotional coldness, detachment, or flattened affectivity', and has given an additional criterion: 'takes pleasure in few, if any, activities'.

DSM-III-R classifies schizotypal PD as a separate disorder although criterion 6 for schizoid PD is included in the schizotypal PD syndrome. Also, criterion 8 for schizotypal PD: 'inappropriate or constricted affect, e.g. silly, aloof, rarely reciprocates gestures or facial expressions, such as smiles or nods', is very similar to criterion 7 for schizoid PD.

The essential features for schizotypal PD are considered to be peculiari-ties of ideation, appearance and behaviour, as well as deficits in interperso-nal relations. The DSM-III-R criteria are:

(1) ideas of reference (excluding delusions of reference), (2) excessive social anxiety, e.g. extreme discomfort in social situations involving unfamiliar people, (3) odd beliefs or magical thinking, influencing behaviour and inconsistent with subcultural

norms, e.g. superstitiousness, belief in clairvoyance, telepathy, or 'sixth sense', 'others can feel my feelings' (in children and adolescents, bizarre fantasies or preoccupations), (4) unusual perceptual experiences, e.g. illusions, sensing the presence of a force or person not actually present (e.g. 'I felt as if my dead mother were in the room with me'), (5) odd or eccentric behaviour or appearance, e.g. unkempt, unusual mannerisms, talks to self, (6) (same as criterion 6 for schizoid PD – see above), (7) odd speech (without loosening of associations or incoherence) e.g. speech that is impoverished, digressive, vague, or inappropriately abstract, (8) inappropriate or constricted effect, e.g. silly, aloof, rarely reciprocates gestures or facial expressions, such as smiles or nods (similar to schizoid PD criterion 7 – see above), and (9) suspiciousness or paranoid ideation.

It should be noted that criteria 3 and 4 involve cognitive-perceptual distortions which, although not included in the DSM-III-R criteria for borderline PD, have been claimed to be found in this disorder. The DSM-IV criteria are similar but more explanation is given for criterion 2, i.e. 'excessive social anxiety that does not diminish with familiarity and tends to be associated with paranoid fears rather than negative judgements about self'.

The ICD-10 also separates schizoid PD and schizotypal disorder, although the latter is classified with schizophrenia and not as a PD. The criteria for ICD-10 schizoid PD show considerable overlap with those of DSM-III-R, but also include 'excessive preoccupation with fantasy and introspection' (an attribute that has often featured in clinical descriptions), and 'marked insensitivity to prevailing social norms and conventions'.

The ICD-10 criteria for schizotypal disorder show some overlap with DSM-III-R's schizotypal PD, but the former also specifies 'depersonalization, derealization, occasional transient quasi-psychotic episodes with intense illusions, auditory or other hallucinations and delusion-like ideas, usually occurring without external provocation, and obsessive ruminations without inner resistance, often with dysmorphophobic, sexual or aggressive contents'.

Clinical features

The features of schizoid (and schizotypal) PD result in various degrees of social withdrawal and eccentricity, but individuals in whom these characteristics are predominant are relatively rare in psychiatric practice, although Tantam (1988) has described 60 patients from the severe end of the spectrum. In this group, men outnumbered women 6 to 1, 25% had criminal convictions, while half had a history of antisocial behaviour. Nearly half had another psychiatric diagnosis and only a few lived independently. In contrast, individuals with less severe schizoid (and schizotypal) PD features are usually capable of steady work and the traits can sometimes be adaptive, for instance, in academic and other intellectual pursuits that can be compatible with social detachment and a focus on isolated mental activity. For the purpose of this chapter, schizoid and schizotypal PDs have been considered together, despite their separation in DSM-III-R, DSM-IV and ICD-10, as features from both syndromes appear to be genetically related to schizophrenia; it has also been suggested that if sufficient schizotypal features are present, schizoid features are invariably present (Livesley & Schroeder, 1990).

Individuals can appear self-sufficient, detached, aloof, and self-absorbed, seeming preoccupied with their thoughts. They are usually socially withdrawn with little emotional responsiveness, tenderness, warmth and humour. In extreme cases there can be a callous disregard for the suffering of others. There is relatively poor empathy, with little apparent concern for the opinions of others. Interests tend to be solitary, but at times there can be an emotional investment in specific and narrow activities or pursuits that may involve a passionate preoccupation, although this may fluctuate or disappear.

It has long been recognized that a detached unemotional exterior can hide a rich and complex pattern of mental activity and the following features of schizoid (and schizotypal) PD have been described: extreme sensitivity, suspicious vigilance, curiosity about others, rigidity of thinking, omnipotent and vengeful fantasies, depersonalization and derealization (i.e. as if self, body or world are unreal) and idiosyncratic moral or political views with a tendency towards mystical and spiritual interests. There are different views in the literature as to whether individuals with pronounced schizoid (and schizotypal) features do not wish for close relationships or are emotionally needy; but evaluation depends on the definitions and concepts used, and it is likely that these attributes may vary. For example, an individual with reduced capacity and desire for close relationships may still feel the 'need' for positive feelings and concern for others in the context of a rather immature dependency.

As previously described, schizoid (and schizotypal) PD originated with an attempt to describe and identify features that seemed to be more prevalent in the premorbid personalities of individuals who developed schizophrenia and in their close biological relatives. Three main categories of such features have been described: transient psychotic episodes, involving delusions and/or hallucinations; odd appearance and behaviour, which can affect dress, hairstyle and mannerisms; and cognitive-perceptual distortions. The latter include odd speech that is mildly disjointed, superstitious ideas, an interest in clairvoyance and telepathy, odd or illogical reasoning, ideas of reference, chronic suspiciousness and unusual religious beliefs. Although these features are not specific to the schizoid (and schizotypal) PD syndrome, as they can be found in the borderline PD syndrome, they appear to be less prevalent and enduring in the latter (Sternbach *et al.*, 1992).

While social withdrawal is the main overt feature of schizoid (and schizotypal) PD, a small number of enduring relationships may be formed that may involve significant emotional reactivity; also, as has been described, passionate interest in certain organizations or pursuits can occur. Males tend not to be involved in enduring heterosexual relationships, although females may passively accept courtship and the subsequent relationship. An affected individual often appears quiet, suspicious, lethargic, uninteresting and unassertive. There may be poor social skills, little eye contact and a lack of self-disclosure. Speech may be vague, for instance, involving a lack of clarity in the person's goals.

In severely affected individuals, especially if antisocial PD features are also present, bizarre crimes may be committed. In men, the lack of sexual relationships may be accompanied by deviant sexual fantasies, an interest in voyerism and pornography, excessive masturbation and, at times, associated criminal behaviour.

Presentation to medical services

Schizoid (and schizotypal) PDs alone, or as the predominant clinical features, are rare in psychiatric practice, and when such patients do present, they usually have other PDs and/or other psychiatric disorders such as substance abuse, a depressive syndrome or anxiety. This means that the schizoid (and schizotypal) features of those individuals who are identified in family studies of schizophrenia may be different in many respects from those who present to general medical or psychiatric services. Schizoid (and schizotypal) features are often present in individuals who have committed odd or bizarre crimes in the absence of a mental disorder other than PD. Bornstein *et al.* (1988) reported ten patients with DSM-III schizotypal PD and found higher prevalences of drug abuse and major affective disorders than in a comparison group with other disorders; the patients with schizotypal PD also had a history of more self-harm and hospitalization.

Associated features

Associations between schizoid (and schizotypal) PD and schizophrenia have already been noted. There appears to be an increased prevalence of these PD features in the premorbid personalities of those who subsequently develop schizophrenia, and despite the heterogeneity of the schizophrenia category and the use of various definitions of schizophrenia and schizoid (and schizotypal) PD, such an association has often been reported. Cutting's review of retrospective studies (1985) found an overall prevalence of premorbid schizoid (or schizotypal) PD in 26% of patients with schizophrenia, while Foerster *et al.* (1991) also found good evidence of this association, especially in males. Another reported association is between schizoid (and schizotypal) PD (and also paranoid PD) and schizophrenia in genetically-related individuals. This has been found in studies involving adopted and non-adopted subjects, which have indicated that genetic but not familial-environmental variables are responsible for the relationship of schizoid (and schizotypal) PD to schizophrenia (Kendler, 1988). In a large study of relatives of patients with schizophrenia, and of controls, DSM-III-R schizotypal PD had a significantly increased prevalence in relatives of patients with schizophrenia, and there were more modest increased prevalences for paranoid, schizoid and avoidant PDs (Kendler *et al.*, 1993*a,b*). The prevalence rate of schizotypal PD was greater in parents than in siblings of schizophrenic patients. In another family study, certain features of schizotypal PD, such as odd speech, inappropriate mood and odd behaviour, together with excessive social anxiety, were more common in relatives of patients with schizophrenia than in relatives of those with major depression (Torgerson *et al.*, 1993). Although Squires-Wheeler *et al.* (1989) reported that the rates of schizotypal traits in children of parents with affective disorders were as high as those found in the children of subjects with schizophrenia, Pica *et al.* (1990) found a difference between premorbid PDs in relation to bipolar affective disorders compared with schizophrenia. But other studies have suggested that schizotypal PD is increased in relatives of patients with psychoses other than schizophrenia (Silverman *et al.*, 1993; Thaker *et al.*, 1993).

The associations between schizoid (and schizotypal) PD and various syndromes in childhood (i.e. schizoid PD of childhood, autism and Asperger's syndrome), have also been described. Also, follow-up of patients with these childhood disorders into adult life has led to the claim that some individuals may develop increasingly narcissistic PD features, which is of interest as some clinical descriptions of schizoid individuals have also included grandiosity.

The 'schizophrenia-like' features of schizoid (and schizotypal) PD have, as has been noted, caused some controversy in the major classifications of psychiatric disorders, as it has been unclear whether some of these should be considered as relatively specific as markers of a genetic vulnerability that is shared with schizophrenia. Also, such features have caused problems in defining borderline PD, as claims that brief 'psychotic' episodes are important characteristics of borderline PD were not reflected in the criteria in DSM-III and DSM-III-R (George & Soloff, 1986). But there is evidence that so-called 'cognitive-perceptual distortions' as well as brief episodes involving delusions and/or hallucinations, often occur in the setting of a diagnosis of borderline PD, and that individuals can qualify for DSM-III-R diagnoses of both schizotypal PD and borderline PD (McGlashan, 1987). However, cognitive-perceptual distortions appear to be more enduring in schizoid (and schizotypal) PD than in borderline PD (Sternbach *et al.*, 1992). In a follow-up study of individuals with a mixture of schizoid (and schizotypal) and borderline PD features, it was found that odd or illogical thinking, suspiciousness and social isolation (but not the other features of borderline PD), predicted the development of schizophrenia (Fenton & McGlashan, 1989).

Current status

Although ICD-10, DSM-III-R and DSM-IV separate schizoid PD from schizotypal PD (or schizotypal disorder, in ICD-10), the original pre-1980 broad concept of schizoid PD incorporated both categories and there is evidence that features from both syndromes are associated with schizophrenia. It has been recently suggested that schizoid PD and schizotypal PD 'may be slightly different variants ... or different points along a schizophrenia spectrum' (Widiger *et al.*, 1988).

The controversy and confusion about the separation of certain 'schizophrenia-like' features of schizoid and schizotypal PDs into categories such as 'transient psychosis' (i.e. involving delusions and hallucinations) and 'cognitive-perceptual distortions' continues. Such features have also been considered to be part of the syndrome of borderline PD, but may be less enduring in this disorder. The status of those individuals with both schizoid (or schizotypal) PD and borderline PD is unclear. It has been suggested that, for schizoid (and schizotypal) PD, the criteria should be modified to require that cognitive-perceptual distortions must not be limited to discrete periods of affective symptomatology, such as depression, anxiety and anger. Another suggested modification to the schizoid and schizotypal PD DSM-III-R criterion 'has no close friends or confidants . . .', is to add 'due primarily to lack of desire, pervasive discomfort with others or eccentricities', which takes into account the claims that lack of desire for relationships is generally found (Siever, Bernstein & Silverman, 1991).

The overlap between schizoid (and schizotypal) PD and the DSM-III-R category of avoidant PD is another area of uncertainty. It has been stated that there is no clear boundary between the syndromes as, contrary to some descriptions, schizoid (and schizotypal) PD can also be associated with anxiety and discomfort in social situations (Overholser, 1989).

Antisocial personality disorder

Main features

Enduring patterns of antisocial behaviour have been classified in a medical context by various sets of criteria, identified by terms such as 'psychopathy' (or psychopath or psychopathic PD), 'sociopathy' (or sociopath or sociopathic PD) and 'antisocial' PD. But there has been controversy about the degree to which specified antisocial behaviours should be part of any set of defining criteria, as it has been claimed that the most characteristic features are traits such as lack of empathy and remorse, unreliability, failure to make loving relationships, failure to learn from adverse experience and impulsive actions (Cleckley, 1976). Craft (1965b) considered that the two main features are a lack of feeling for others and a liability to act on impulse.

Despite the heterogeneous nature of the PDs of the individuals identified by criteria sets based mainly on specified antisocial behaviours, follow-up studies of children with 'conduct disorder' into adult life have established the validity of the concept of enduring patterns of antisocial behaviour, even though most children who are identified as having conduct disorders do not go on to exhibit clinically or socially significant maladaptive adult behaviour (Guze, 1976; Robins, 1978).

Clinical origins

Pinel (1809) has been credited with the earliest influential suggestion that repeated, aimless antisocial behaviour may be a mental disorder. This led to the term 'manie sans délire' (mania without delusions) and was the precursor of Prichard's 'congenital deficiency of the moral sense' or 'moral insanity' (1835), which provided an hypothesis that a diseased 'moral faculty' could account for antisocial behaviour. But Koch (1891) believed that there could be biological causes, describing abnormal behaviour that was not insanity as 'constitutional psychopathic inferiority'. Walker & McCabe (1973) have noted that the term 'psychopathic' first appeared in the mid-19th century German literature to mean 'psychologically damaged', and encompassed all forms of psychopathology.

In this century, Cleckley has provided an influential clinical description in his book *The Mask of Sanity* (5th edition, 1976) in which the following 16 features of psychopathy were identified:

superficial charm and good intelligence; absence of delusions and other signs of irrational thinking; absence of nervousness or psychoneurotic manifestations; unreliability; untruthfulness and insincerity; lack of remorse or shame; inadequately motivated antisocial behaviour; poor judgement and failure to learn by experience; pathological eccentricity and incapacity for love; general poverty in major affective relations; specific loss of insight; unresponsiveness in general interpersonal relations; fantastic and uninviting behaviour with drink and sometimes without; threats of suicide, rarely carried out; sex life impersonal, trivial, and poorly integrated; and failure to follow any life plan.

In spite of these features, even if pronounced, the person may present with a convincing 'mask of sanity', i.e. with apparent normality. In Cleckley's view, the psychopath (or sociopath) has an impaired learning ability with relative unresponsiveness to social reinforcement, so that these individuals do not react with appropriate affect (mood) to situations that would normally produce an emotional response. Although there is awareness of social values, these do not influence motivation, resulting in irresponsibility, unreliability, poor judgement and a relative inability to profit from experience.

Various subtypes of antisocial PD have been described; Karpman (1948) separated 'primary' psychopaths, who were similar to those identified by Cleckley's criteria, from 'secondary' psychopaths, who were characterized by the presence of other disorders, particularly anxiety. It was claimed that a generally low level of anxiety is a characteristic of the primary psychopath and is associated with a relative lack of effect of social constraints and punishments for selfish and impulsive acts, as these do not produce significant anxiety or guilt. The category of secondary psychopathy has also attracted other labels such as 'neurotic' or 'symptomatic' (Hare, 1970), and it has been suggested that, for such individuals, the motivations, personality, response to treatment and outcome is often very different compared to those with primary or 'true' psychopathy (Blackburn, 1988).

The classification of patterns of antisocial behaviour must also take into account the prevalence of such behaviour in the population under study or in certain subcultural groups. West (1983) has pointed out that in a non-clinical sample of males from a low socioeconomic background in London, over a third had criminal convictions by the age of 24. But the incidents of conviction declined after the age of 18, and it appeared that delinquency in young men may usually be self-limiting. Also, there are delinquent subcultures in which antisocial behaviour (mainly defined in terms of criminal behaviour) is condoned and rewarded. If antisocial behaviour is perceived as 'normal' within the subculture, 'antisocial' individuals may still have satisfactory relationships and show appropriate guilt and remorse in their social context. Such persons have been called 'subcultural delinquents' (Hare, 1970).

These ideas have led to definitions of two overlapping categories of disorder, the first related to a lack of feelings for others with impulsivity, and the second to specified antisocial behaviour. Sets of defining criteria for PD syndromes associated with antisocial behaviour have incorporated varying proportions of items from these two categories. Therefore, for any criteria set for antisocial PD, in particular when mainly based on specified antisocial behaviour, an heterogeneous group of individuals is identified in respect of their personality. As there is a variety of PD psychopathology that is associated with chronic antisocial behaviour, Blackburn (1988) has concluded that a concept of antisocial or psychopathic PD that is even partly based on socially deviant behaviour is unsatisfactory and 'little more than a moral judgement masquerading as a clinical diagnosis'. However, this appears to overstate the case, as there is evidence that impulsive, aggressive and relatively unemotional personality characteristics characterize a subgroup of individuals who present with repeated antisocial acts. But such individuals will form part of a larger, heterogeneous group defined by an history of antisocial behaviour, and this group will contain individuals with a variety of personality structures. There will also be variability in relation to anxiety, the influence of a delinquent subculture, other co-occurring mental disorders and other co-occurring PDs involving borderline, histrionic and narcissistic features.

Despite the problem in the diagnosis of PD on the basis of antisocial behaviour, in England and Wales the Mental Health Act 1959 defined 'psychopathic disorder' as 'a disorder or disability of mind . . . which results in abnormally aggressive or seriously irresponsible conduct on the part of the patient, and requires or is susceptible to medical treatment'. However, this issue was addressed in the UK by the Butler Committee (Home Office, Department of Health and Social Security, 1975), which stated: 'the class of persons to whom the term "psychopathic disorder" relates is not a single category identifiable by any medical, biological or psychological criteria'.

The first edition of the DSM in 1952 contained the term 'sociopathic personality disturbance' but this was a broad category that also included sexual deviations and addictions. 'Antisocial personality' as defined by DSM-II in 1968 was, however, based on Cleckley's concept:

this term is reserved for individuals who are basically unsocialized and whose behaviour pattern brings them repeatedly into conflict with society. They are incapable of significant loyalty to individuals, groups or social values. They are grossly selfish, callous, irresponsible, impulsive and unable to feel guilt or to learn from experience and punishment. Frustration tolerance is low. They tend to blame others or offer plausible rationalizations for their behaviour. A mere history of repeated legal or social offences is not sufficient to justify this diagnosis.

The next revision of the DSM, DSM-III (1980), used a similar term, i.e. 'antisocial personality disorder', but this was derived from a broader concept as the emphasis was on specified criminal behaviour which captured a wide range of PD and other disorders. In the DSM-III-R (1987) the balance between specified antisocial behaviour and PD traits was partially redressed in favour of the latter, but did not include many of the features derived from clinical descriptions, such as selfishness, egocentricity, callousness, manipulativeness and lack of empathy. As a result, DSM-III-R antisocial PD appeared to be both too broad and too narrow; a wide range of criminals and antisocial persons were included without the characteristic PD traits, while some of those with these traits were excluded if they had not shown examples of the specified antisocial behaviours (Hare, Hart & Harpur, 1991).

An alternative to the DSM criteria has been 'The Psychopathy Checklist' (PCL) (Hare, 1980) and the revised version, the PCL-R (Hare, 1991), which were related to Cleckley's descriptions. This concept of psychopathy is associated with early onset, long-term maladaptive functioning, and social dysfunction or disability. Unstable personal relationships and poor occupational record is accompanied by an increased risk of criminal activity. Features are usually noticeable by middle to late childhood and generally persist into adult life, although there may be some improvement in social adaptation after the fourth decade (Hare, McPherson & Forth, 1988).

The PCL-R was developed for use in male forensic populations, and factor analysis of its 20 items has identified two factors, each involving associations between subgroups of items. The first, which corresponds to Cleckley's concept, is associated with egocentricity, lack of remorse and callousness, as well as with features of narcissistic and histrionic PDs, while there is a negative association with empathy and anxiety. In contrast, the second factor is positivity correlated with the DSM-III-R category of antisocial PD, as both are associated with criminal behaviour. The second factor is also positively correlated with socioeconomic problems and self-report measures of antisocial behaviour in the context of an impulsive, antisocial and unstable lifestyle (Hare *et al.*, 1991). Therefore, the PCL-R includes items related to both the DSM-III-R antisocial PD syndrome and the PD traits such as those described by Cleckley. Most of the PCL-R items require the clinician to make a judgement about the degree of a trait with the help of a manual, which gives a description and some examples of associated behaviour. Psychopathy as defined by PCL or PCL-R has been associated with several aspects of criminality; such individuals are charged with a greater number and variety of criminal offences compared with other offender groups, and show a higher incidence of violent and aggressive crimes, physical violence, verbal abuse, threats and intimidation (Hare & McPherson, 1984). Murders and serious assaults committed by PCL-R psychopaths were less likely to occur in the setting of a domestic dispute or emotional arousal and their victims were more likely to be men and to be relatively unknown to them. It has been estimated that PCL-R psychopathy is a narrower concept than DSM-III-R's antisocial PD, and that a majority of PCL-R items are present in about 25–30% of prison populations, compared with a prevalence for antisocial PD of about 60–70% (Hare *et al.*, 1991).

Main definitions

The DSM-III-R criteria for antisocial PD require evidence of conduct disorder with an onset before the age of 15, as indicated by a history of three or more of the following: 'truancy, running away, fights, using weapons, forcing sexual activities on others, physical cruelty to animals, physical cruelty to people, destruction of others' property, fire-setting, lying, stealing without confrontation of a victim, and stealing with confrontation of a victim'. In DSM-IV there are three additional behaviours: 'often bullies, threatens, or intimidates others; has broken into someone else's house, building or car; and often stays out at night despite parental prohibitions, beginning before age 13 years'. Also, a pattern of irresponsible and antisocial behaviour since the age of 15 is needed, as indicated by at least four of the following ten criteria:

unable to sustain consistent work behaviour; failure to conform to social norms with respect to lawful behaviour; is irritable and aggressive; repeatedly fails to honour financial obligations; fails to plan ahead, or is impulsive; has no regard for the truth; is reckless regarding his or her own or others' personal safety; if a parent or guardian, lacks ability to function as a responsible parent; has never sustained a monogamous relationship for more than one year; and lacks remorse (feels justified in having hurt, mistreated or stolen from another).

Various examples of some of these criteria are specified, the current age must be at least 18, and the occurrence of antisocial behaviour must not be exclusively during the course of schizophrenia or manic episodes. In the DSM-IV, the number of adult criteria are reduced to seven; one of these, 'consistent irresponsibility, as indicated by repeated failure to sustain consistent work behaviour or honour financial obligations', incorporates DSM-III-R's criteria 1 and 4, while the DSM-III-R criteria which specify behaviour as a parent or guardian and relate to a monogamous relationship for more than one year, are omitted.

In the ICD-10 the equivalent category is 'Dissocial PD', which is much closer to the PCL-R criteria and to Cleckley's concept than is the DSM-III-R's antisocial PD. As with all the specified PDs in the ICD-10, a diagnosis of dissocial PD requires:

a minimum age of 16; markedly disharmonious attitudes and behaviour usually involving several areas of functioning; that the abnormal behaviour pattern is pervasive and clearly maladaptive to a broad range of personal and social situations; that the above manifestations always appear during childhood or adolescence and continue into adulthood; that the disorder leads to considerable personal distress but this may only become apparent late in its course; and that the disorder is usually, but not invariably, associated with significant problems in occupational and social performance.

At least three of the following specific criteria are required for a diagnosis of dissocial PD:

callous unconcern for the feelings of others; gross and persistent attitude of irresponsibility and disregard for social norms, rules and obligations; incapacity to maintain enduring relationships, though having no difficulty in establishing them; very low tolerance to frustration and a low threshold for discharge of aggression, including violence; incapacity to experience guilt and to profit from experience, particularly punishment; and a marked proneness to blame others, or to offer plausible rationalizations, for the behaviour that has brought the patient into conflict with society.

Persistent irritability is an associated feature, while conduct disorder during childhood and adolescence may further support the diagnosis although it is not invariably present.

The Revised Psychopathy Checklist (PCL-R) (Hare, 1991) consists of the following 20 items: glibness/superficial charm; grandiose sense of self-worth; need for stimulation/proneness to boredom; pathological lying; cunning/manipulative; lack of remorse or guilt; shallow affect; callous/lack of empathy (i.e. a lack of a normal range and depth of emotions); parasitic lifestyle; poor behavioural controls (i.e. violent behaviour or threats and verbal abuse in response to frustration, failure, discipline or criticism); promiscuous sexual behaviour; early (i.e. childhood) behaviour problems; lack of realistic, long-term goals; impulsivity (i.e. behaviour that is carried out suddenly, without preparation or consideration); irresponsibility; failure to accept responsibility for own actions; many short-term marital relationships; juvenile delinquency; revocation of conditional release; and criminal versatility (i.e. involving many different types of offence). Hare *et al.* (1991) have developed a ten-item criteria set for psychopathic PD based on the PCL-R, each being rated on a 3-point scale; the 10 items are: 'glib and superficial; inflated and arrogant self-appraisal; lacks remorse; lacks empathy; deceitful and manipulative; early behaviour problems; adult antisocial behaviour; impulsive; poor behavioural controls; and irresponsible'.

Clinical features

Hare *et al.* (1991) have distinguished between interpersonal, affective and behavioural features of psychopathy. Individuals with antisocial PD often seem grandiose, self-centred, manipulative, dominant and unfeeling, and find long-lasting relationships difficult. They may show labile emotions, which lack consistency or depth, and a lack of empathy, anxiety, guilt and remorse. Their behaviour is characterized by impulsivity and sensation-seeking which is often antisocial and may involve criminality, substance abuse and social irresponsibility.

The common features of antisocial PD in adolescence have been described by West (1983); aggressiveness may be shown by defiance of parents and authorities, destructiveness, quarrels and fights with peers, cruelty and bullying, disgruntled and resentful attitudes, fierce temper and intolerance of frustration. Failure to acquire social skills is shown by carelessness and slovenliness, poor educational attainment in comparison with measured intelligence, clumsiness and uncooperativeness in team efforts, restlessness and inattentiveness in school, and frequent absences from class. There is a lack of patience and sustained mental effort so that they seem lazy and poorly motivated. Social rules are broken, involving theft, vandalism, driving away vehicles, reckless risk-taking, truancy, drug and alcohol use, early and irresponsible sexual behaviour or misconduct, running away from home, and staying out at night. There are difficulties in relationships shown by chronic conflicts with parents, distrust of others, a restriction of peer relationships to those with similar characteristics and an unwillingness to take part in organized leisure activities. Discipline evokes hostility and there is stubbornness, unresponsiveness to punishment, and lack of guilt or remorse. The first signs of conduct disorder in females who develop antisocial PD usually appear at puberty, while in males these are generally obvious in earlier childhood (American Psychiatric Association, 1987).

In a small minority of individuals with features of antisocial PD or PCL-R psychopathy, aspects of mental functioning and behaviour may be severely dangerous or bizarre, for instance, involving serious and/or unprovoked aggression, fire-setting or murderous fantasies. In those individuals whose serious aggression or fire-setting is associated with PD, men are much more common than women, and, within this group, men show more aggression while women have a history of more arson and property damage.

For individuals with PD involving antisocial behaviour in secure hospitals, associations have been reported with a history of incest, being in institutional care as a child, childhood conduct disorder, social deprivation, criminality and other PDs. Borderline, paranoid and narcissistic PD traits have been noted, while some severely dangerous or bizarre individuals with PD do not have antisocial PD or PCL-R psychopathy but rather borderline, schizoid and/or schizotypal PD features.

One of the characteristic features of antisocial PD is an inability to sustain close relationships due to self-centredness, lack of empathy and callousness. In severe cases, the latter may involve the regular infliction of pain and degradation. The lack of commitment to sexual partners is often associated with a pattern of violence and separation.

Presentation to medical services

Although one of the characteristics of an individual with severe antisocial PD can be lack of anxiety, many antisocial individuals present with complaints of tension and depression. The motive for medical consultation often comes from pressure from others such as the courts, an employer or the person's sexual partner who may threaten to leave unless 'treatment' is sought. Many presentations to medical services involve the complications of substance abuse (including drunken violence), self-harm episodes and demands for medication. When contact is made there may be threats, verbal abuse or actual violence. It has been estimated that antisocial PD as defined by DSM-III-R occurs in 3% of American men but less than 1% of women.

Differential diagnosis can sometimes be difficult; for example, mania can be associated with antisocial behaviour and this form of mood disorder can present in relatively mild and chronic forms. However, the absence of conduct disorder in childhood and an episodic nature of the antisocial behaviour can be distinguishing features. Also, when adult antisocial behaviour is mainly restricted to events associated with substance use disorder (such as theft to obtain drugs or assaults when intoxicated), a diagnosis of antisocial PD is often not justified.

Associated features

Males are at much greater risk than females, and other associations with the diagnosis include young age (under 45), lower socioeconomic status, urban residence and homelessness (North, Smith & Spitznagel, 1993). Race does not appear to be related to risk (Jordan *et al.*, 1989).

Robins (1978) has shown that while antisocial PD is clearly associated with a history of childhood conduct disorder, most children with conduct disorder do not go on to develop antisocial PD. If a subject gave a history of several types of conduct disorder, this was a predictor of antisocial PD, while social class was a poor predictor of serious adult criminality. Loeber (1990) found that the pattern of childhood conduct disorder can predict later delinquency, and that a high risk was associated with relative frequency and variety, occurrence in multiple settings and relatively early onset. Other risk factors in children for later aggressive offences were hyperactivity, impulsive behaviour, attention problems, poor social skills, poor peer relationships, academic problems and male sex. Subsequent non-aggressive crime was associated with a history of non-aggressive conduct disorders and female sex. Also, the DSM-III-R has claimed that antisocial PD, as defined in this classification, is associated with low socioeconomic class, abuse as a child, removal from the home and growing up without parental figures of both sexes.

Family studies of antisocial PD involving biological children and adoptees have shown that 'both genetic and environmental factors contribute to the risk of this group of disorders' (American Psychiatric Association, 1987). It has been reported that antisocial PD as defined by DSM-III-R is about 5 times more common among first-degree biological relatives of males with the syndrome than among the general population, while the risk to the first-degree biological relatives of females with the disorder is nearly 10 times greater. Within a family that includes a member with antisocial PD, there is an increase of antisocial PD, substance use disorder and somatization disorder (involving multiple complaints of physical symptoms without obvious cause) in both males and females, compared with the general population (American Psychiatric Association, 1987). In addition, individuals with antisocial PD have a reduced life expectancy due to increased rates of self-harm episodes, substance use disorders, violence and risk-taking behaviour.

The relationship between substance use disorders and antisocial PD is complex; Brooner *et al.* (1992), in a study of 237 intravenous drug abusers, found that the 44% with DSM-III-R antisocial PD were generally more deviant and impaired than the rest. Twenty-four per cent fulfilled only the adult criteria for antisocial PD and it was suggested that this reflected a late-onset and less severe form of antisocial PD. Seven per cent fulfilled criteria only for the childhood criteria for antisocial PD, while the remaining 25% did not fulfil sufficient criteria for the diagnosis of either childhood or adult antisocial disorder.

Current status

Definitions of antisocial PD that are based mainly on specified antisocial behaviour have been validated by long-term follow-up of children with conduct disorder, although this concept, as exemplified by DSM-III-R's category of antisocial PD, has been criticized for emphasizing identifiable antisocial acts at the expense of personality traits (Hare *et al.*, 1991). Also, there is increasing support for the recognition of a subgroup of individuals with repeated antisocial behaviour that is mainly restricted to the context of drug and alcohol abuse (Ferguson & Tyrer, 1991).

Borderline personality disorder

Main features

Borderline PD involves widespread instability in behaviour, shown by intense and stormy relationships, impulsivity with destructive or otherwise antisocial actions, self-harm and suicidal behaviour, self-mutilation or substance abuse, labile mood (in particular with anger and depression), and an inconsistent self-image.

When such features are pronounced, a patient is often considered as 'difficult to manage' and generally displays various other psychiatric syndromes, such as affective disorder, substance abuse and somatization disorder.

Clinical origins

Stern (1938) used the term 'borderline' to refer to patients who were usually receiving regular psychotherapy and appeared severely disturbed and difficult to manage, although not persistently out of touch with reality due to delusions and hallucinations. However, the severity of the disorder 'bordered on' the generally-recognized serious mental disorders, such as schizophrenia and manic-depressive disorder, and some authors believed that the behaviour of such patients was related to the 'psychoses', i.e. the most severe forms of mental illness, in particular to schizophrenia (Knight, 1953). This hypothesis was supported by reports that many patients developed transient 'psychotic-like' symptoms (i.e. involving a departure from reality) when sufficiently stressed.

Kernberg's (1967) description of the 'borderline personality organization' involved a different perspective; the focus was not on a syndrome of behaviour but on characteristics of mental functioning, such as a poor capacity to tolerate anxiety, to control impulses and to develop socially-productive ways of behaving, together with a tendency to have irrational thinking patterns and to use certain psychological defence mechanisms. The latter refer to ways of thinking that have the effect of making a person less aware of feelings and attitudes; for instance, other people may be categorized into 'all-good' or 'all-bad', so that any relationship is either idealized or devalued, perhaps associated with a denial of contradictory ideas or memories. Such 'splitting' may be partly recognized by the individual and this can contribute to a feeling of insecurity in which he or she continually feels neglected, hating those on whom he or she is dependent. It has been claimed that another common defence associated with borderline PD is 'projection', in which one's own unacceptable feelings and attitudes are perceived as belonging to someone else. The concept of borderline personality organization also involved 'identity disturbance' with a lack of consistency about interests, values and desired relationships, and it was believed to frequently co-occur with various other psychiatric disorders such as anxiety, obsessive-compulsive disorder, hypochondriasis, sexual disorders, substance abuse and impulsive, antisocial or self-harm behaviour.

The DSM-III (1980) incorporated two of the previous uses of the term 'borderline'; features that were considered to be associated with schizophrenia contributed to the category of 'schizotypal PD', while 'borderline PD' reflected Kernberg's linkage of 'borderline' with personality and was also based on the work of Gunderson and colleagues (Gunderson & Singer, 1975). Gunderson's concept of borderline PD included low achievement, impulsivity, manipulative suicide attempts, intense mood changes, transient loss of reality, high socialization, and disturbed close relationships, which were evaluated by the Diagnostic Interview for Borderline Patients (Gunderson, Kolb & Austin, 1981). This consisted of a semistructured interview with 29 items, covering instability in social functioning, poor impulse control, disturbances of depression and anger, interpersonal difficulties, and transient 'psychotic-like' disturbances, such as derealization, depersonalization, depressive delusions and paranoid delusions. The core features of the DSM-III concept of 'borderline PD' were impulsive, unstable and intense relationships with inappropriate and intense anger, but the criteria did not include the 'psychotic-like' features that had been considered as important in the earlier clinical descriptions and in the criteria of Gunderson and colleagues. The revisions that led to the DSM-III-R reduced the co-occurrence of the diagnosis of borderline and schizotypal PDs, as, with the DSM-III-R, depersonalization and derealization, (which can occur in borderline PD, as well as in other disorders and in non-clinical populations), were no longer examples of unusual experiences for the diagnosis of schizotypal PD, as had been the case in DSM-III. Also, 'odd behavior' was added as a criterion for this latter diagnosis. But it is of note that both DSM-III and DSM-III-R criteria for borderline PD did not include 'psychotic-like' features.

Main definitions

DSM-III-R claimed that the main feature of borderline PD is a pattern of instability involving relationships, mood and self-image. For the diagnosis to be made, at least five of the following are required:

(1) A pattern of unstable and intense interpersonal relationships characterized by alternating between extremes of overidealization and devaluation. (2) Impulsiveness in at least two areas that are potentially self-damaging, e.g. spending, sex, substance abuse, shoplifting, reckless driving, binge eating. (3) Affective instability:

marked shifts from baseline mood to depression, irritability, or anxiety, usually lasting a few hours and only rarely more than a few days. (4) Inappropriate, intense anger or lack of control of anger, e.g. frequent displays of temper, constant anger, recurrent physical fights. (5) Recurrent suicidal threats, gestures, or behaviour, or self-mutilating behaviour. (6) Marked and persistent identity disturbance manifested by uncertainty about at least two of the following: self-image, sexual orientation, long-term goals or career choice, type of friends desired, preferred values. (7) Chronic feelings of emptiness or boredom. (8) Frantic efforts to avoid real or imagined abandonment.

The DSM-IV contains an additional criterion: 'transient, stress-related paranoid ideation or severe dissociative symptoms'.

ICD-10 has an equivalent category of 'emotionally unstable personality disorder' and describes two variants, impulsive and borderline types, which both show impulsiveness and lack of self-control. The impulsive type is characterized by outbursts involving anger or violence, while the borderline type is a wider concept involving many of the features of the equivalent DSM-III-R borderline PD. It should be noted that both these classifications did not specify the 'psychotic-like' features which were noted in early clinical descriptions associated with the 'borderline' term, although these are referred to in the DSM-IV criteria. However, the Diagnostic Interview for Borderline Patients includes 'psychotic' phenomena such as derealization, depersonalization, brief psychotic depressive episodes, and brief paranoid experiences.

Clinical features

Patients whose predominant problems are related to the features of borderline PD are common in psychiatric practice, and present considerable difficulties in management due to volatile moods, impulsivity, substance abuse and self-harm. It has been claimed that the associations between these various features produce three clusters, i.e. self-damaging acts with impulsivity; anger, labile mood and stormy relationships; and identity disturbance, emptiness and intolerance of being alone (Hurt *et al.*, 1988). However, the last cluster is the least specific to the borderline PD syndrome. Other psychiatric disorders often co-occur, such as affective disorders, substance abuse, eating disorders and short-lived 'psychotic-like' features including non-delusional, paranoid experiences (such as ideas of reference and marked suspiciousness), dissociative experiences, superstitiousness, magical thinking and a 'sixth sense' (Gunderson & Zanarini, 1987).

The instability of self-image (i.e. identity disturbance) consists of uncertainty related to concepts of self in various circumstances, involving a lack of clarity of goals, beliefs, interests and values. Also, uncertainty in sexual orientation is claimed in DSM-III-R, although it is unclear if this has any specific association with borderline PD. But if sexual difficulties co-occur with any PD, they are likely to contribute to an exaggeration of problem behaviour. Such features of 'identity disturbance' are often found in the context of a fear of being alone, and the patient may also complain of often feeling empty, bored, uninterested, lonely, hopeless, and despairing. Personal relationships are characterized by feelings that alternate between extremes of overidealization or devaluation. Devaluation involves a tendency to discredit or undermine the 'important others'; there is often a wish for an exclusive relationship, together with anger when this ideal is not realized. Such anger may be triggered by limit setting, confrontations or separations that are actual or anticipated. There may be a sustained fear of being abandoned, which can contribute to episodes of extreme panic when alone. As a consequence of a tendency to devalue relationships, unless in a phase of idealization, it is difficult for the individual to build up a store of positive memories or fantasies about important people in his/her life in the past or present. Instead, feelings and concepts about others tend to be negative and associated with anger. This can be contrasted with a type of 'aloneness' which may be experienced by a person without obvious PD, when there is a longing to regain a lost relationship or experience, accompanied by positive feelings in relation to the memories (Adler, 1981). Mood is subject to rapid and frequent shifts, which may involve depression with thoughts of self-harm and suicide, irritability, anxiety, and chronic, intense anger. Chronic anger is accompanied by bitterness, sarcasm and unreasonable demands (Gardner *et al.*, 1991). The mood component of the range of features of depressive disorders consists of a variety of experiences, and it has been claimed that depression in borderline PD can have a characteristic quality with thoughts of sustained emptiness and destructiveness, associated with a 'conflicted' dependency, involving mixed feelings of hostility and dependency on an important person or situation. In contrast, when an unconflicted dependency (i.e. without the hostility) is affected by loss (or anticipated loss), the resulting features of depression have a different quality and a better outcome (Gunderson & Zanarini, 1987).

Various studies have investigated the prevalence and nature of 'psychotic-like' phenomena in samples of individuals selected on the basis of borderline PD or of various other psychiatric disorders, and in non-clinical populations. But the term 'psychotic-like' is confusing; taken at face value it indicates phenomena which resemble certain features, namely delusions

Table 2.1 *Features of the mental state and/or history involving 'departures from consensual reality' associated with borderline personality disorder (PD)*

Feature	Degrees of specificity of the associations of mental state features with borderline PD compared with other PDs	% of subjects with borderline PD who had a history of the phenomena shown (Zanarini et al., 1990)
Cognitive-perceptual distortions:	+ + (except in relation to schizotypal PD)*	
(i) Odd or illogical reasoning (e.g. marked suspiciousness, illogical thinking, belief in telepathy and sixth sense)		68% (Controls 24%)**
(ii) Unusual perceptions (e.g. recurrent illusions, depersonalization, derealization, body-image distortions)		62% (Controls 20%)
(iii) Non-delusional paranoia (e.g. undue suspiciousness, ideas of reference, other paranoid states)		100% (Controls 66%)
Transient psychotic experiences, i.e. delusions and/or hallucinations for periods usually less than 2 days (or if for longer, may be atypical compared with other 'psychotic' disorders)	+ + + +	40% (Controls 2%)
Prolonged delusions and hallucinations (Note: usually secondary to co-occurring mental disorders other than PDs)	+	14% (Controls 4%)

Notes:
* Schizotypal PD has a higher prevalence of associated cognitive-perceptual distortions compared with borderline PD (Sternbach *et al.*, 1992).
** The control group consisted of patients with other PDs and contained 14.5% with a paranoid, schizoid or schizotypal PD.

and hallucinations, of the so-called 'psychoses', such as schizophrenia, manic-depressive disorder or dementia. However, a delusion, as usually defined, can also occur in other disorders, for example, obsessive-compulsive disorder. It can be argued that a better term than 'psychotic-like' phenomena is 'departures from consensual reality', when reality is defined as a consensus opinion of a group of individuals (such as clinicians) who are drawn from the non-patient population. Table 2.1 outlines the main 'departures from consensual reality' that have been considered to be part of the syndrome of borderline PD. These are divided into three categories; the first, 'cognitive-perceptual distortions', includes odd or illogical reasoning, unusual perceptions and non-delusional paranoia such as undue suspiciousness. These features have been described as occurring more frequently with borderline and schizotypal PDs (especially the latter) compared with other PDs. The second category consists of 'transient psychotic experiences', and usually involves hallucinations and delusions for relatively short periods of less than two days. If they last longer in borderline PD, these phenomena would be likely to affect only a discrete part of the patient's functioning or differ from the major psychotic disorders by having a banal or fantastic content. Zanarini *et al.* (1990) found that, in their sample with borderline PD, a history of transient hallucinations was more common than of transient delusions, i.e. 26% and 20% respectively, and in another sample with borderline PD, Sternbach *et al.* (1992) reported that the ratio of transient auditory to visual to olfactory hallucinations was 90:30:9. Although histories of transient 'psychotic' experiences are relatively specific to borderline PD (i.e. they are rarely found with other PDs or in non-clinical populations), Zanarini *et al.* (1990) found that these phenomena had been present in the previous two years in only 40% of the sample with borderline PD. The third category of 'departures from consensual reality' includes delusions and/or hallucinations which are prolonged. Although these can occur in association with borderline PD, they are rare, and are usually associated with a co-occurring mental disorder.

Because individuals with borderline PD find being alone difficult to tolerate, they tend to seek out company and support. Gunderson & Zanarini (1987) have described the developmental cycle that often affects such relationships; a clinging dependent style develops in the context of sustained dysphoria, and when the relationship is disrupted, perhaps by limit-setting, confrontation or separation, this leads to threats of self-harm, somatic complaints and misleading communications. The dependency, which may be transiently idealized, is then replaced by an angry devaluation. Perceived or actual loss of support then leads to panic, with attempts to ward off feelings of aloneness by impulsive actions involving substance abuse, promiscuity and recklessness.

Some common behaviours associated with borderline PD have already been described. These include suicidal threats and impulsive self-damaging behaviour such as drug overdoses, wrist cutting and episodic substance abuse, together with promiscuity, sexual deviance, aggression and leaving home. Also, self-mutilation may occur, commonly taking the form of multiple small cuts on the forearms; individuals usually recognize that this is not an attempt at suicide, but rather a response to feelings of extreme tension and anger, which may be relieved by the episode. Often the threats or episodes of self-harm appear to be designed to elicit a supportive and saving response from 'significant others', but such episodes must not be dismissed on this account. Whatever the underlying motivation, repeated self-harm puts the patient at a significantly increased risk of completed suicide.

Coid (1993*b*) described 72 females detained in English maximum-security hospitals under the Mental Health Act 1983 under the legal category of 'psychopathic disorder' who fulfilled criteria for borderline PD, and suggested that such women had a distinct affective syndrome. The women showed mood-related self-harm behaviour with a feeling of compulsion, which seemed to relieve the original mood symptoms.

Presentation to medical services

Patients with borderline PD often demand urgent help in a crisis and are difficult to manage because of their instability of mood, threats of self-harm, self-harm episodes including self-mutilation without obvious suicidal intent, and intense anger. Also, they often present with a variety of somatic complaints for which no obvious cause or effective treatment can be found, or with other psychiatric disorders including depression, anxiety and substance abuse. Violence may be a feature of the presentation, especially if associated with antisocial PD features and substance abuse.

Associated features

Borderline PD has often been reported to co-occur with schizotypal, histrionic, antisocial and narcissistic PD features, as well as with substance abuse and affective disorders (Higgitt & Fonagy, 1992; Oldham *et al.*, 1992). Also, families of patients with borderline PD had greater prevalences of depressive, substance abuse and antisocial disorders (Goldman *et al.*, 1993).

Co-occurrence with these other PDs is due, in part, to some overlap in the criteria for definition, as antisocial PD involves unstable relationships, histrionic PD is associated with rapidly shifting emotions, and schizotypal PD includes cognitive-perceptual distortions. But, in addition, co-occurrence of the other features of these PDs is common in clinical populations (Gunderson, Zanarini & Kisel, 1991*b*).

In this chapter, schizoid and schizotypal PD have been considered together, but even if they are separated, there is evidence from follow-up studies that borderline PD is distinct from schizoid and/or schizotypal PD. Borderline PD is not genetically related to schizophrenia (McGlashan, 1983), although borderline, schizoid and schizotypal PDs may show certain features that can also occur in schizophrenia, such as suspiciousness, ideas of reference, odd beliefs, illogical thinking, and unusual perceptual experience. Cognitive-perceptual distortions appear to be more common and more enduring in schizoid (and schizotypal) PD, compared with borderline PD (Sternbach *et al.*, 1992).

Co-occurrence of borderline PD with histrionic and antisocial PD features has often been reported (Gunderson & Zanarini, 1987), and there is evidence that this adversely affects outcome. Narcissistic PD features have also been found to be common in individuals with borderline PD.

While there is an undoubted association between some features of depressive disorders and borderline PD, the nature of such relationships remains to be clarified (Tarnopolsky & Berelowitz, 1987).

Current status

Although the borderline PD syndrome was not introduced into one of the main classifications of mental disorder until 1980, the subsequent decade saw more publications related to this disorder than to any other PD. The features of borderline PD are of considerable importance in clinical populations, and appear to be the basis of some of the most severe and enduring problems in routine clinical practice.

Follow-up studies suggest that the syndrome shows a degree of temporal stability, although improvement generally occurs by the fourth decade. Genetic studies suggest that borderline PD is not related to schizophrenia, while the relationships with various types of affective disorder require further study (Gunderson & Elliot, 1985). Future revision of the main classifications will need to take into account the frequent and relatively specific occurrence of transient, and possibly stress-related, delusions and hallucinations, as well as the less specific cognitive-perceptual distortions, in patients with borderline PD. Modifications to present criteria could involve a recognition that mood changes usually appear reactive to relationship and environmental changes (Gunderson *et al.*, 1991*b*).

Histrionic (or hysterical) personality disorder

Main features

Individuals with DSM-III-R's histrionic PD often show attention-seeking behaviour, self-centredness, rapidly shifting and exaggerated emotional reactions, sexual provocativeness and an excessively impressionistic style of speech. But this diagnosis is a concept that has been criticized as possibly representing a prejudiced male view of women – 'a caricature of femininity' (Ferguson & Tyrer, 1988).

Clinical origins

Easser & Lesser (1965) have described how Sigmund Freud recognized a relationship between what in the DSM-III-R would be termed 'somatization disorder' or 'conversion disorder' (i.e. involving physical complaints that apparently are not due to a recognizable disease) and the 'erotic personality, whose major goal in life is the desire to love or above all to be loved'. There is a resemblance between this description and DSM-III-R's criteria for histrionic PD, which include: 'is inappropriately sexually seductive in appearance and behaviour'. Also, the DSM-III-R claims that 'brief reactive psychosis' (which may involve hallucinations and/or delusions in the context of a dissociative disorder), 'conversion disorder' and 'somatization disorder' are possible complications. Thus, the idea of a link between a specified personality disorder and a vulnerability to so-called 'hysterical disorders' (i.e. somatization disorder, conversion disorder and dissociative disorders) has endured.

Histrionic PD represents a concept that has had an evolving clinical tradition over many decades, based mainly on clinical descriptions, although there are some supporting data (Pfohl, 1991). However, the terms histrionic or hysterical PD have often been applied without precision; Lazare (1971) noted that 'hysterical is commonly used in a perjorative sense to describe a patient who is self-engrossed, incapable of loving deeply, lacking depth, emotionally shallow, fraudulent in affect, immature, emotionally inconsistent, and a great liar ... The presence of just one of these traits together with a tired resident, may result in the diagnosis of "just hysterical"'.

Kernberg (1967) outlined features that were considered to distinguish histrionic or hysterical PD from other disorders; these were: emotional lability; overinvolvement; dependent and exhibitionistic needs; pseudohypersexuality; sexual inhibition; competitiveness; and masochism. In a review of pre-1966 literature, Lazare, Klerman & Armor (1966) identified the suggested features of dependence, egocentricity, emotionality, exhibitionism, fear of sexuality, sexual provocativeness and suggestibility, while a factor analytic investigation of hysterical personality (Lazare *et al.*, 1966; Lazare, Klerman & Armor, 1970), based on a self-report rating scale (the Lazare–Klerman Trait Scale), obtained a factor that resembled clinical descriptions of hysterical PD. This involved aggression, emotionality, exhibitionism, egocentricity and sexual provocativeness. It should be noted that such a factor is a construct that is not a single directly measurable variable, but is derived from the association between the measurement of other, directly observable variables.

The DSM-I of 1952 did not include an histrionic PD category, although some of the above features contributed to the broader concept of 'emotionally unstable personality'. However, the DSM-II, in 1968, included 'hysterical personality' (and the alternative term 'histrionic PD'), which was claimed to be 'characterized by excitability, emotional instability, overreactivity, and self-dramatization. This self-dramatization is always attention-seeking and often seductive, whether or not the patient is aware of its purpose. These personalities are also immature, self-centred, often vain, and usually dependent on others. This disorder must be differentiated from Hysterical neurosis'. But the DSM-III revision of the histrionic PD category, in 1980, did not include seductiveness, and the overlap with the criteria for borderline PD led to further changes in DSM-III-R (1987) in which some of the overlapping criteria such as 'prone to manipulative suicide attempts' were omitted. Also, two new criteria were added i.e. 'is inappropriately sexually seductive in appearance or behaviour', and 'has a style of speech that is excessively impressionistic and lacking in detail'. (The resulting DSM-III-R criteria are similar to the syndrome obtained by Lazare and colleagues by factor analysis.)

The various definitions of hysterical or histrionic PD have been associated with a greater prevalence of these diagnoses in women, and there has been concern that this may sometimes reflect a prejudiced tendency for the clinician to make the diagnosis more often in women, perhaps as a result of not giving this diagnosis to similar features in men. Some studies have indicated that the application of the histrionic PD diagnosis may indeed be subject to such bias, although additional reasons may contribute to a greater prevalence in women, and it has been suggested that there may be sex-related differences in the features of histrionic PD (Pfohl, 1991). It is of interest that a twin study indicated a genetic contribution for histrionic PD in women but not in men (Torgerson & Psychol, 1980). But the possibility that histrionic PD is a diagnostic category that is liable to be misused by some clinicians as a perjorative label, reflecting negative attitudes and the denial of appropriate treatment, needs to be kept under review.

Main definitions

For the DSM-III-R's histrionic PD, four or more of the following eight criteria are required:

constantly seeks or demands reassurance, approval, or praise; is inappropriately sexually seductive in appearance or behaviour; is overly concerned with physical attractiveness; expresses emotion with inappropriate exaggeration, e.g. embraces casual acquaintances with excessive ardour, uncontrollable sobbing on minor sentimental occasions, has temper tantrums; is uncomfortable in situations in which he or she is not the centre of attention; displays rapidly shifting and shallow expressions of emotions; is self-centred, actions being directed toward obtaining immediate satisfaction – has no tolerance of the frustrations of delayed gratification; and has a style of speech that is excessively impressionistic and lacking in detail, e.g. when asked to describe mother, can be no more specific than, 'She was a beautiful person'.

The DSM-IV criteria omit DSM-III-R criteria 'constantly seeks or demands reassurance, approval or praise' and 'is self-centred . . .', which are replaced by two new criteria, i.e. 'is suggestible, i.e. easily influenced by others or circumstances', and 'considers relationships to be more intimate than they actually are'.

The ICD-10 also has a category of histrionic PD. This has six criteria, five of which have similar counterparts in DSM-III-R, i.e. self-dramatization, theatricality, exaggerated expression of emotions; shallow or labile affectivity; continued seeking for excitement, and activities in which the patient is the centre of attention; inappropriate seductiveness in appearance or behaviour; and over-concern with physical attractiveness. The remaining ICD-10 criterion, i.e. 'suggestibility, easily influenced by others or by circumstances', is also included in the DSM-IV criteria. Associated features are described as egocentricity, self-indulgence, continuous longing for appreciation, feelings that are easily hurt, and persistent manipulative behaviour to achieve own needs.

Clinical features

Many features have already been noted. The characteristics of attention-seeking behaviour incorporate exhibitionism (i.e. drawing attention by dress, speech or behaviour) and exaggerated expressions of emotion, at times resembling a theatrical performance. Such individuals may be good company, welcome guests, good at public speaking and accomplished in amateur dramatics. Some cases are reminiscent of Jaspers' description (1946) of a personality that seems to have lost its core and consists entirely of a series of shifting masks.

Other features include a craving for novelty and excitement, short-lived enthusiasms, a tendency to become bored, a lack of consideration for others, excessive vanity and concerns with physical appearance, self-centred behaviour involving excessive demands of others with angry scenes or demonstrative self-injury, and a readiness to display exaggerated emotion easily, perhaps involving angry tantrums or dramatic despair with rapid recovery. The latter behaviour is often manipulative, in that it is designed to influence the feelings or behaviour of others. This may present with overdoses or other forms of self-harm, which seem mainly motivated by anger and a wish to punish partners or family members. Such individuals may be seen in a very angry and distressed state, perhaps leading to hospital admission, but this rapidly improves. Sometimes it is difficult to reconcile the calm, composed individual in the hospital with the clinical notes of the emotionally-fraught admission the previous day.

Inappropriate seductive behaviour, involving flirting and sexual advances, may be part of a pattern in which the person with histrionic PD finds it difficult to relate to the preferred sex in a non-sexual way (Livesley & Schroeder, 1991). Such individuals tend to try and control the other person in a relationship or to enter a dependent relationship, so that interactions tend to have a child–parent or parent–child quality. A mature, adult relationship involves considerable flexibility of roles with give-and-take, which is difficult for those with histrionic PD to achieve. Such individuals may be relatively successful in looking after or relating to old people, children or adults with handicaps as, in all these instances, the relationship is relatively structured, with a parent–child element. There is a tendency to indulge in romantic fantasy, and the quality of sexual relationships varies from promiscuity through normality to unresponsiveness. Sometimes the recipient of seductive behaviour is a doctor or another health care worker who is in a professional relationship with the patient. If these advances are reciprocated the patient is likely to tell her (or his) spouse or partner, which can then lead to a formal complaint. It seems that the motivation behind this behaviour is often the gratification from the attention that this situation provides.

An excessively impressionistic style of speech is not invariable but, when present, can be strikingly obvious during interview, when it is very difficult to obtain details about any topic. A further description is provided by Pfohl (1991), i.e. a 'cognitive style dominated by formation of poorly delineated global impressions without consideration of details that support or contra- dict their opinion, e.g. believes a particular professor is a fantastic teacher but cannot provide details about how the professor's technique differs from others and is unable to identify areas that could use improvement'. Such people may have creative talents but are unlikely to be good at thinking that involves logical analysis.

The first DSM-III-R criterion for histrionic PD, 'constantly seeks or demands reassurance, approval or praise', is often found when this diagnosis is made but is also common in patients with other PDs. Pfohl (1991) has recommended that this should be omitted in future revisions of the DSM-III-R criteria (as, indeed, has occurred in the DSM-IV criteria) or that a more detailed evaluation of the relevant behaviour is undertaken to distinguish the behaviour in histrionic PD from similar behaviour in other PDs.

The clinician will often notice that these patients take extra time and energy, as they require reassurance and approval on matters that may go well beyond the expertise of the clinician. The patient shows minimal interest in being taught how to independently evaluate his/her performance and expresses the need to have someone stronger provide a stamp of approval for his/her decisions. This contrasts with the related criterion for narcissistic PD where the need for attention and admiration suggests that the individual views him/herself as equal or superior to the person providing the attention.

Pfohl (1991) also recommends that a second change be made to the DSM-III-R criteria for histrionic PD, in relation to the criterion: 'is self- centred, actions being directed toward obtaining immediate satisfaction; has no tolerance for the frustration of delayed gratification'. Pfohl noted that four studies have found that a positive rating for this criterion was common in relation to other PDs and that it really consists of two separate items. A suggested alternative was: 'is intolerant of, or frustrated by, situations involving delayed gratification', which would refer to just one of the two traits. However, both parts of the criterion have been omitted from the DSM-IV criteria. In addition, Pfohl (1991) also introduced a proposed new criterion based on clinical experience, i.e. 'tends to view relationships as possessing a greater level of intimacy than is actually the case, e.g. refers to someone he/she recently met as a "dear, dear friend", refers to doctors and other professionals by first name and talks about a "special" relation-ship when referring to a doctor known on a casual professional level'. (As has been noted, this suggestion was included in the DSM-IV criteria.) It has been pointed out that while a person with narcissistic PD may also talk about 'special' friendships, the important status of these friends is empha-sized rather than the special nature of the intimacy.

Presentation to medical services

There is evidence that histrionic PD often co-occurs with other PD diagnoses, in particular borderline, antisocial and narcissistic PDs, and with somatization disorder, which involves a history of many physical complaints with no biological changes to account for the symptoms (Pollack, 1981; Kaminsky & Slavney, 1983; Lilienfeld *et al.*, 1986).

Individuals with histrionic PD may also present with symptoms of anxiety and depression, manipulative self-harm in the context of relation-ship difficulties and, as with many individuals with PD, substance abuse. Also, it is probable that there is an increased vulnerablity to conversion disorder and dissociative disorders, which can include certain types of delusions and hallucinatory experiences.

Associated features

The co-occurrence of histrionic PD with borderline, antisocial and narcis-sistic PDs, and with somatization disorder, conversion disorder and dissociative states, has been noted. Histrionic PD appears to be diagnosed more frequently in women and has been claimed to be more common among first-degree relatives of people with the disorder than among the general population (American Psychiatric Association, 1987).

Although some features of histrionic PD overlap with those of borderline PD (i.e. both are associated with unstable mood and dependent or 'clinging' behaviour), histrionic PD is generally associated with more stability in relationships and roles, relative absence of cognitive-perceptual distortions and transient psychotic experiences, better self-esteem linked to sexual desirability, less hostility and a more vague way of thinking (Gunderson & Zanarini, 1987).

Current status

Despite a long clinical tradition in the descriptive literature, the diagnosis of 'histrionic' PD requires further research to determine whether it merits a separate category. However there is no doubt that the above features appear to be relevant to the problems of many patients with PD in psychiatric practice, although it may be that, in general, they co-occur with prominent features of other PDs. Poor test–retest reliability has been reported, in particular with an unstructured clinical interview (Pfohl, 1991), and sex-related differences in the use of the diagnosis require further investigation.

Narcissistic personality disorder

Main features

The main features have been described as 'a pervasive pattern of grandiosity (in fantasy or behaviour), lack of empathy, and hypersensitivity to the evaluation of others' (American Psychiatric Association, 1987).

Clinical origins

Narcissism has been defined as 'an interest in (or focus on) the self' (Bursten, 1989), and while Sigmund Freud's paper 'On narcissism' appeared in 1914 (Freud, 1955), it was not until 1968 that Kohut introduced the term 'narcissistic personality disorder' to describe disturbances in several areas including grandiosity and pronounced angry reactions. The inclusion of narcissistic PD in DSM-III, in 1980, was largely due to reports in the psychoanalytic psychotherapy literature, derived from descriptions of subjects for whom narcissistic behaviour was predominant and discrete, that is, not accompanied by other significant psychopathology (Akhtar & Thomson, 1982). Despite its appearance in DSM-III, there had been little experimental evidence to justify its inclusion, while subsequent research using DSM-III and DSM-III-R criteria has mostly involved patients who, although eligible for the diagnosis of narcissistic PD, are dissimilar from the patients (many in fee-paying psychotherapeutic relationships), whose characteristics led to the original descriptions of the syndrome. The 1987 revisions, which led to DSM-III-R, substantially increased the number of patients who fulfilled diagnostic criteria for narcissistic PD (Gunderson *et al.*, 1991*a*).

The DSM-III-R criteria for narcissistic PD have been assessed by a semi-structured interview, the Diagnostic Interview for Narcissism (DIN) (Ronningstam & Gunderson, 1989, 1990), by structured interviews for the assessment of all DSM-III-R PDs (Stangl *et al.*, 1985; Loranger *et al.*, 1987; Zanarini *et al.*, 1987), and by the revised version of the Personality Diagnostic Questionnaire (PDQ-R), which is a self-report instrument (Hyler *et al.*, 1990). Additional methods of identification relate to other definitions of narcissism (Dowson, 1992*a*).

The DSM-III-R states that the essential feature is 'a pervasive pattern of grandiosity (in fantasy or behaviour), hypersensitivity to the evaluation of others, and lack of empathy', while a previous comparison of three diagnostic systems, including DSM-III, concluded that 'in differential diagnosis, the most outstanding and specific narcissistic characteristics are grandiosity and entitlement' (Ronningstam, 1988). Studies with the DIN and its precursor compared a group of patients, characterized by discrete clinically-identified narcissistic psychopathology, to groups of subjects with other PDs (Ronningstam & Gunderson, 1988, 1990, 1991). These studies indicated that four criteria, i.e. 'reacts to criticism with feelings of rage, shame or humiliation ...'; 'is interpersonally exploitative ...'; 'lack of empathy ...'; and 'is preoccupied with feelings of envy ...', did not discriminate significantly between the groups, while aspects of grandiosity were the most distinctive aspects of the narcissistic group.

A study of 291 patients with various PDs, based on data from a questionnaire completed by clinicians, found that 22% received the DSM-III-R diagnosis of narcissistic PD (Morey, 1988), while a study which used the PDQ-R self-report questionnaire reported a diagnosis of narcissistic PD in 34% of 87 patients applying for inpatient treatment of severe PD (Hyler *et al.*, 1990). Two semistructured interviews were also applied in the latter study and produced narcissistic PD diagnosis in 17% and 22% respectively. Also, there are many claims of co-occurrence of narcissistic PD, as defined by DSM-III or DSM-III-R, with other PDs (Dowson, 1992*a*).

As one of the aspects of narcissism involves difficulties in the subject viewing himself/herself realistically (Gunderson, Ronningstam & Bodkin, 1990), an informant's view might be expected to be important in assessment. However, there is little empirical evidence; a study using DSM-III criteria and semistructured interviews of 66 depressed patients and their informants reported low diagnostic agreement for all PDs (Zimmerman *et al.*, 1988). Informants reported more pathology, but while narcissistic PD was not diagnosed on the basis of any patient's data, this diagnosis was made in only three subjects on the basis of informants' data. But, in a study of DSM-III-R narcissistic PD evaluated by patients' and informants' self-report questionnaire, one criterion, i.e. 'has a sense of entitlement ...', showed 'fair to good' reliability when patients' and informants' ratings were compared (K = 0.62) (Dowson, 1992*a*). It was concluded that the identification of a sense of entitlement by the patient may be a relatively reliable and valid indicator of narcissism, when data are obtained from a patient's self-report questionnaire or from the clinical interview.

Main definitions

Narcissistic PD is not represented in the ICD-10 classification but the DSM-III-R provides nine criteria, five or more of which are needed for diagnosis, i.e.

reacts to criticism with feelings of rage, shame, or humiliation (even if not expressed); is interpersonally exploitative: takes advantage of others to achieve his or her own ends; has a grandiose sense of self-importance, e.g. exaggerates achievements and talents, expects to be noticed as 'special' without appropriate achievement; believes that his or her problems are unique and can be understood only by other special people; is preoccupied with fantasies of unlimited success, power, brilliance, beauty or ideal love; has a sense of entitlement; unreasonable expectation of especially favourable treatment, e.g. assumes that he or she does not have to wait in line when others must do so; requires constant attention and admiration, e.g. keeps fishing for compliments; lack of empathy: inability to recognize and experience how others feel, e.g. annoyance and surprise when a friend who is seriously ill cancels a date; is preoccupied with feelings of envy.

The DSM-IV criteria omit the first of the above criteria (i.e. 'reacts to criticism ...') and include a new criterion, i.e. 'arrogant, haughty behaviors or attitudes'. Also, the fourth DSM-III-R criterion is expanded to: 'believes that he or she is "special" and unique and can only be understood by, or should associate with, other special or high-status people (or institutions)'.

Clinical features

Ronningstam & Gunderson (1990) identified the following characteristics as significantly more common in a sample based on features of narcissistic PD compared with another comparison group: a sense of superiority with arrogant haughty behaviour and a sense of uniqueness; exaggeration of talents, boastful and pretentious behaviour and grandiose fantasies, although often with high achievement; self-centred and self-referential behaviour; and need for attention and admiration.

A sense of superiority, with arrogant and haughty behaviour, involves an unrealistic view that he/she is better than other people. Bad aspects of self are forgotten, and there is a tendency to forgive oneself too easily, with an exaggerated view of a perceived insult when the subject's superiority is not acknowledged. Other people may be viewed with disdain as inferiors, while their successes are downgraded (Livesley & Schroeder, 1991). Feelings of superiority may also involve a sense of entitlement, in which special favours, rights or privileges are expected. In the medical context this may involve an unrealistic expectation of 'total cure' in which all problems will be solved. However, such superiority is usually accompanied by a fragile self-esteem and hypersensitivity to criticism. It is as if a completely unconditional positive regard is expected and anything short of this is unacceptable, giving rise to anger. Horowitz (1989) has described various forms of anger, the most severe of which is an explosive (i.e. sudden and severe) self-righteous even 'towering' or 'blind' rage, perhaps triggered by an insult. This may be characterized by verbal abuse or physical violence. In extreme cases the person feels completely justified in having such feelings, at least during the state of anger, as others are viewed as subhuman without a right to exist. But as some guilt and shame may be present at the time or subsequently, this can lead to a mixture of anger and shame at aspects of self (such as a tendency to irrational anger), together with anxiety that is related to fear of loss of emotional control. Also, a state of chronic embitterment may occur, with ideas that the person has been treated unfairly; this may present as a 'blustery-outgoing' or 'sullen-withdrawing' behaviour pattern. A sense of uniqueness describes a belief that the self is special and that few others have much in common. Such individuals often complain of being misunderstood, as they consider that only someone very special would be able to understand them.

Exaggeration of talents and achievements is often accompanied by boastful and pretentious behaviour, which can be the most obvious sign of narcissistic PD features in social interactions, including the clinical interview. The activities of such individuals are constantly referred to and they may draw attention to themselves in ways that assume their importance. Grandiose fantasies may involve unlimited success, power, beauty, wealth or ideal love, and sometimes there is a history of periods of success that may be seen as a justification of their superiority. Ronningstam & Gunderson

(1990) pointed out that such individuals are more likely to be seen in private practice rather than hospital-based services.

Self-centred and self-referential behaviour involves the person appearing self-preoccupied with a tendency to assign personal meaning to events that are unrelated to them. It has also been observed that although they lack interest in the personal opinions and reactions of others, this may be associated with the previously-mentioned hypersensitivity to criticism. Although the usual pattern is one of self-absorption and preoccupation with ideas of superiority, this equilibrium can be upset by events, such as criticism, which challenge these assumptions. Relationships are character-ized by selfishness and a lack of input in the form of empathy and positive regard for others (Horowitz, 1989). Other people are used to further the person's aims, perhaps involving 'social climbing' or occupational advan-cement, while another person may be exploited when, if the relationship has adverse effects on the other individual, this is accepted or ignored by the narcissistic subject. People are often discarded as friends when the relation-ships are no longer useful. If the person with PD does not have special abilities, another individual with talent may be selected for a dependent relationship that has been termed a 'mirror transference' (Horowitz, 1989); loss of such a person may lead to a severe, hopeless grief. Finally, a need for attention and admiration can be reflected by an excessive concern with grooming and appearance, 'fishing for compliments' or exhibitionist behaviour. Sometimes, physical disfigurement can lead to a severe and prolonged depressive reaction.

Evaluations of the specificity of individual DSM-III-R criteria for narcissistic PD, in relation to patients with narcissistic PD and comparison groups, has indicated that those criteria related to grandiosity perform best, while the following three perform poorly: 'reacts to criticism with feelings of rage, shame or humiliation'; 'lack of empathy'; and 'is preoccupied with feelings of envy' (Gunderson *et al.*, 1991*a*). Angry reactions to criticism are also commonly found in relation to paranoid and borderline PDs, and it was suggested that the related criterion for narcissistic PD might be reworded to: 'reacts to criticism, defeat, or rejection with sustained feelings of disdain, shame or humiliation (even if not expressed)', although this ignores the fact that rage can occur in narcissistic PD. With regard to lack of empathy, Ronningstam & Gunderson (1989) noted that this is difficult to evaluate, particularly in a single interview, and is also commonly associated with antisocial and passive-aggressive PDs. The third problem criterion, which is related to envy, was found to be relatively uncommon and also associated with histrionic and avoidant PDs.

Ronningstam & Gunderson (1990) claimed that narcissistic PD often includes three features that are not fully covered by DSM-III-R criteria, namely 'boastful and pretentious behaviour, arrogant and haughty behaviour, and self-centred and self-referential behaviour'. Other non-DSM features were described in a study by Morey (cited in Gunderson *et al.*, 1991*a*) and consisted of the following: egocentricity, dominance, interpersonal disdain, preoccupation with status, petulant anger and fragile self-concept. Also, the following associated features have been noted: acts arrogantly; self-assured and confident; has sense of high self-worth; viewed as vain and self-indulgent; and views self as gregarious and charming. It has been suggested that a new criterion for narcissistic PD might be 'arrogant, haughty behaviour and/or attitudes', which can often be identified in single interviews and is not usually found with histrionic, antisocial or borderline PDs (Gunderson *et al.*, 1991*a*). This has been included in the DSM-IV criteria.

Presentation to medical services

Narcissistic PD, as defined in DSM-III-R, does not often occur in patients who do not fulfil criteria for other PDs, although in some individuals, particularly in private psychotherapeutic practice, narcissistic features may be predominant.

Individuals with a PD which includes significant narcissism may seek help because of depressive symptoms and anxiety in a social crisis or in relation to events that challenge feelings of superiority. The presentation may involve shame, panic, helplessness, depressed mood, hypochondriasis, self-destructiveness, envy, rage (which occasionally can lead to very serious physical violence), excessive demands, and substance use disorder. He or she may feel humiliated about being depressed, and discomfort is not well tolerated; the exceptional quality of the despair may be stressed. The faults of others may be cited together with the uniqueness of the patient's problems.

Often there are unrealistic expectations of what help can be given; the patient appears to believe that because a special or unique problem has been presented, he or she is then entitled to its complete resolution. Anything less than this goal or the unlimited efforts of others is unacceptable; for example, the patient may feel he or she should be seen on a daily basis and will not accept a delay for a further appointment.

Associated features

Gunderson *et al.* (1991*a*) have reviewed 11 studies based on DSM-III and DSM-III-R definitions of narcissistic PD, which showed that it is rare for patients who meet criteria for this disorder not to meet criteria for other PDs, in particular histrionic, borderline and antisocial PDs, but also passive-aggressive, paranoid and schizotypal PDs. In a study of 60 patients evaluated for DSM-III-R PDs by self-report questionnaire, narcissistic PD scores (i.e. the number of positive narcissistic PD criteria for each subject) were significantly correlated with histrionic, borderline and passive-aggressive PD scores (Dowson, 1992*a*).

Current status

While many of the features of narcissistic PD occur in patients with various PDs, it is likely that most of the patients who are eligible for the DSM-III or DSM-III-R diagnosis are dissimilar from those whose characteristics originally prompted the development of this diagnostic category. It remains to be determined if the syndromes identified by DSM definitions will be shown to be related to causal factors or outcome. But grandiosity, which has been considered to be the most reliable and discriminating aspect of narcissism, and which can be identified by a sense of entitlement, is commonly found in clinical practice, and narcissistic features often appear to contribute to the development of a depressed mood.

Avoidant personality disorder

Main features

The main characteristic is an avoidance of social contact, despite a wish for relationships, in the context of social discomfort, low self-esteem and a fear of failure, rejection, criticism, ridicule or of the experience of strong feelings.

Clinical origins

The term 'avoidant personality' was introduced by Millon (1969), and 'avoidant PD' appeared in the DSM-III in 1980. But there had been several previous descriptions involving the avoidance of other people because of various fears; Kretschmer (1925) described those whose 'life is composed of a chain of tragedies ... (the person) behaves shyly, or timidly, or distrustfully ... seeks as far as possible to avoid and deaden all stimulation from the outside'. Horney (1945) described a 'detached type' in whom 'there is intolerable strain in associating with people and solitude becomes primarily a means of avoiding it ... the underlying principle here is never to become so attached to anybody or anything so that he or it becomes indispensable ... better to have nothing matter much'. Subsequently, Horney (1950) gave a further description:

on little or no provocation he (or she) feels that others look down on him, do not take him seriously, do not care for his company, and, in fact, slight him. His self-contempt ... makes him ... profoundly uncertain about the attitudes of others toward him. Being unable to accept himself as he is, he cannot possibly believe that others, knowing him with all his shortcomings, can accept him in a friendly or appreciative spirit'.

Another theoretical perspective for such behaviour was provided by Burnham, Gladstone & Gibson (1969) who described a 'need-fear dilemma'; i.e.

he (or she) has an inordinate need for external structure and control ... existence depends upon his maintaining contact with objects (which include social relationships). The very excessiveness of his need for objects also makes them inordinately dangerous and fearsome since they can destroy him through abandonment. Hence, he fears and distrusts them. One way to avert or alleviate the pain for his need-fear dilemma is ... object avoidance ....

Although 'avoidant PD' was retained in DSM-III-R, and 'anxious (avoidant) PD' is the equivalent in ICD-10, the clinical usefulness of a separate category for these features is uncertain, as other features of PD are often present and there is overlap between the features of avoidant PD, schizoid PD and social phobia (Millon, 1991). However, it has been claimed that avoidant PD can be distinguished from these other disorders by the presence of several features including a wish for relationships, a wider range of feared social and interpersonal situations and low self-esteem.

Main definitions

The DSM-III-R provides seven criteria for avoidant PD, four or more of which are required for diagnosis, i.e.

is easily hurt by criticism or disapproval; has no close friends or confidants (or only one) other than first-degree relatives; is unwilling to get involved with people unless certain of being liked; avoids social or occupational activities that involve significant interpersonal contact, e.g. refuses a promotion that will increase social demands; is reticent in social situations because of a fear of saying something inappropriate or foolish, or of being unable to answer a question; fears being embarrassed by blushing, crying, or showing signs of anxiety in front of other people; exaggerates the potential difficulties, physical dangers, or risks involved in doing something ordinary but outside his or her usual routine, e.g. may cancel social plans because she anticipates being exhausted by the effort of getting there.

However, the DSM-IV criteria show several changes: two of the criteria, i.e. 'avoids occupational activities that involve significant interpersonal contact, because of fears of criticism, disapproval, or rejection', and 'is unwilling to get involved with people unless certain of being liked' resemble their precursors, but the following new criteria are suggested:

shows restraint within intimate relationships because of the fear of being shamed or ridiculed; is preoccupied with being criticized or rejected in social situations; is inhibited in new interpersonal situations because of feelings of inadequacy; views self as socially inept, personally unappealing, or inferior to others; is unusually reluctant to take personal risks or to engage in any new activities because they may prove embarrassing.

Four of the six ICD-10 criteria for anxious (avoidant) PD are similar to those in DSM-III-R, i.e. 'excessive preoccupation with being criticized or rejected in social situations; unwillingness to become involved with people unless certain of being liked; restrictions in lifestyle because of need to have physical security; and avoidance of social or occupational activities that involve significant interpersonal contact because of fear of criticism, disapproval, or rejection'. The two remaining ICD-10 criteria are: 'persistent and pervasive feelings of tension and apprehension'; and 'belief that one is socially inept, personally unappealing, or inferior to others'.

Clinical features

The timidity and widespread avoidance of an appropriate degree and quality of social contact is associated with a chronic state of anxiety when with others, ideas of poor self-worth, an expectation of humiliation or rejection, and, sometimes, a belief that strong feelings are unacceptable (Beck & Freeman, 1990). But at the same time there is a strong wish for affection and acceptance in relationships.

Several studies of the prevalence of DSM-III and DSM-III-R avoidant PD in various patient groups gave an average of around 10% (Millon, 1991), which confirms clinical impressions that these features are not uncommon in clinical settings. Millon noted that while avoidant PD shares social withdrawal with schizoid (and schizotypal) PD, shares low self-esteem with dependent PD, and shares social anxiety with the non-PD diagnostic category of 'social phobia', the motivations and pattern of symptoms may differ between the various disorders. For example, although social anxiety is found with both avoidant PD and social phobia, the anxiety with avoidant PD is usually related to a wider range of interpersonal situations, while social phobia may coexist with a number of satisfying social relationships. But a person with avoidant PD has few or any close relationships, despite the desire for them, because others are not trusted without excessive reassurance. This has been summarized by Millon (1991): 'avoidant PD is essentially a problem of relating to persons; social phobia is largely a problem of performing in situations', and several studies suggest that groups of patients can be identified in which the two disorders can be distinguished, the person with avoidant PD having more severely impaired social skills and being likely to have more severe anxiety and depression (Turner *et al.*, 1986).

Low self-esteem in the context of dependent PD is usually due to a feeling that he/she is incompetent rather than to a fear of social interaction. Indeed, social contact makes the person with dependent PD feel more secure and not more anxious as it does with avoidant PD. The dependent PD person is anxious at the prospect of interpersonal loss, while someone with avoidant PD can be afraid of becoming too closely involved (Trull, Widiger & Frances, 1987).

The lack of social engagement in both avoidant PD and schizoid (and schizotypal) PD appears to reflect different underlying thoughts and feelings. It has been generally believed that avoidant PD is characterized by interpersonal anxiety, low self-esteem and self-consciousness, but with a desire for relationships, while schizoid (and schizotypal) PD is not related to poor self-esteem and reflects relative indifference to achieving closeness to others.

Various recommendations have been made to improve the DSM-III-R criteria for avoidant PD (Millon, 1991), which have influenced the changes in the DSM-IV criteria. The first DSM-III-R criterion ('is easily hurt by criticism and disapproval') could be amended to 'frequently anticipates and worries about being criticized or disapproved of in social situations'. Such a change would make the revised criterion more specific for avoidant PD, as the original version also reflects a feature of dependent PD. The second criterion ('has no close friends or confidants ...') could be modified to: 'has few friends despite the desire to relate to others'. The fifth and sixth criteria ('is reticent in social situations ...' and 'fears being embarrassed') could be condensed and reformulated as: 'development of intimate relationships is inhibited (despite desire) owing to the fear of being foolish and ridiculed, or being exposed and shamed'. It was also proposed that the seventh criterion ('exaggerates the potential difficulties ...') be deleted, as it was relatively uncommon in relation to the other features of avoidant PD and was often found with obsessive-compulsive disorder, dependent PD and schizotypal PD. Finally, a new criterion was suggested: 'possesses low self-esteem because he or she feels socially inept and/or unappealing'.

Beck & Freeman (1990) have described some hypothetical cognitions in relation to avoidant PD that are based on characteristic statements in clinical practice, i.e.

I am socially inept and undesirable; other people are superior to me and will reject or think critically of me if they get to know me; I can't handle strong feelings; you'll think I'm weak; if I give in to these feelings they will go on forever, if I ignore them, it might get better some day; I'm unattractive, boring, stupid, a loser and pathetic; I don't fit in'.

Presentation to medical services

Depressive features, anxiety and frustration with oneself are common in the context of restricted social relationships and impairment of occupational functioning. Also, in common with most PDs, avoidant PD may be a risk factor for substance abuse.

Associated features

Social phobia and avoidant PD may co-occur, but the nature of any causal relationships are uncertain. DSM-III-R claims that avoidant disorder of childhood or adolescence, and disfiguring physical illness, predispose to the development of avoidant PD.

Current status

Avoidant PD is a relatively new category dating from 1980, consisting of phenomena which are relevant to some patients with PD in clinical populations who can present with depressive features, anxiety or substance abuse. Features of other PDs are often present and it can be difficult to distinguish some features of avoidant PD from other disorders, particularly schizoid PD, dependent PD and social phobia.

Dependent personality disorder

Main features

The main characteristic of dependent PD is a pervasive pattern of dependent and submissive behaviour in the context of an excessive need to be taken care of, and fears of separation.

Clinical origins

A degree of dependency and attachment is part of the normal range of adaptive human characteristics but excessive dependency can cause serious problems. Some theories have linked adult patterns of dependency with past events related to the infant's instinctive initial reliance on the mother, while others have claimed that elements of dependency should be viewed as a learned behaviour in a social context.

Early clinical descriptions were derived from psychoanalytic psychotherapy literature; for instance Abraham (1924) wrote: 'some people are dominated by the belief that there will always be some kind person – a representative of the mother, of course – to care for them and to give them everything they need. This optimistic belief condemns them to inactivity . . . they make no kind of effort, and in some cases they even disdain to undertake a bread-winning occupation'.

In the DSM-I, in 1952, the concepts of dependent and passive-aggressive behaviours were linked, so that passive-dependent personality was defined as a subtype of passive-aggressive personality, and related to helplessness and indecisiveness, with a tendency to cling to others like a dependent child to a supporting parent. No distinct category or description was provided by DSM-II, but the DSM-III in 1980 described three characteristics of the 'passive-dependent' PD, i.e. such a person passively allows others to assume responsibility for major areas of life because of inability to function independently; subordinates his or her own needs to those persons upon whom he or she depends in order to avoid any possibility of having to rely on self; and lacks self-confidence. In 1987, the DSM-III-R modified the term to 'dependent' PD, and expanded the description by providing nine criteria, five or more of which were required for diagnosis. Most were related to passivity and subordination, which had been features in DSM-III, but criteria associated with anxious attachment and sensitivity to criticism were added.

An equivalent category of 'asthenic' PD was provided by the ICD-9 in

1978. This denoted an individual who could be described as weak-willed, widely compliant and falling in with the wishes of others, having little capacity for enjoyment, and avoiding responsibility with a lack of self-reliance. It was noted that such persons may persuade others to help them but may drift down the social scale if unsupported.

Main definitions

The DSM-III-R requires at least five of the following criteria for a diagnosis of dependent PD, in the context of a pervasive pattern of dependent and submissive behaviour:

is unable to make everyday decisions without an excessive amount of advice or reassurance from others; allows others to make most of his or her important decisions, e.g. where to live, what job to take; agrees with people even when he or she believes they are wrong, because of fear of being rejected; has difficulty initiating projects or doing things on his or her own; volunteers to do things that are unpleasant or demeaning in order to get other people to like him or her; feels uncomfortable or helpless when alone or goes to great lengths to avoid being alone; feels devastated or helpless when close relationships end; is frequently preoccupied with fear of being abandoned; and is easily hurt by criticism or disapproval.

However, the last criterion is omitted in the DSM-IV criteria, and the seventh criterion becomes: 'urgently seeks another relationship as a source of care and support when a close relationship ends'.

The ICD-10 also includes a dependent PD category, with similar features, characterized by three or more of the following:

encouraging or allowing others to make most of one's important life decisions; subordination of one's own needs to those of others on whom one is dependent, and undue compliance with their wishes; unwillingness to make even reasonable demands on the people one depends on; feeling uncomfortable or helpless when alone, because of exaggerated fears of inability to care for oneself; preoccupation with fears of being abandoned by a person with whom one has a close relationship, and of being left to care for oneself; and limited capacity to make everyday decisions without an excessive amount of advice and reassurance from others.

Clinical features

The DSM-III-R's concept of dependent PD emphasizes dependent and submissive behaviour. Such persons are passive, docile, self-effacing and tend to put their faithful trust in those they rely on. Excessive advice is sought together with reassurance that their actions are correct. Responsibility is transferred to others, they find it difficult to initiate tasks, and there is a constant fear of being rejected or abandoned, associated with clinging behaviour.

Although the features of dependent PD show some overlap with other syndromes, in particular with borderline, avoidant and histrionic PDs, even overlapping aspects can show distinctive characteristics if carefully evaluated (Hirschfeld, Shea & Weiss, 1991). For example, while fear of abandonment can be found with both dependent and borderline PDs, in the latter it produces anger and manipulative behaviour, in contrast to submissive and clinging behaviour in dependent PD. With dependent PD, feeling uncomfortable or helpless when alone may be related to 'exaggerated fears of being unable to care for himself or herself' (according to the DSM-IV criteria), while in borderline PD, this characteristic is not usually associated with such thoughts. Also, compared with those with borderline PD, those with dependent PD are more tolerant of being alone if they know they have access to support and they do not give a history of such intense and unstable relationships.

Dependent and avoidant PDs share feelings of inadequacy and sensitivity to criticism, but the excessive need for attachment, fear of separation, submission and clinging behaviour in dependent PD is in contrast to the fear of humiliation and rejection, timidity and withdrawal in avoidant PD.

A need for reassurance and approval is a feature of both dependent and histrionic PDs, but, in the former, reassurance is required because the person doubts whether his or her actions are correct, while in histrionic PD it is associated with the need for approval and praise as an end in itself.

Studies of the DSM-III-R criteria for dependent PD have shown that the criteria: 'is easily hurt by criticism or disapproval', and 'feels devastated or helpless when close relationships end', are non-specific, as they often occur with other PDs and are not consistently associated with the other features of dependent PD. (As noted, the former criterion has been omitted from the DSM-IV). Also, endorsement rates for these two criteria were high in patients with no diagnosis of PD. The criterion with the lowest endorsement rate in those who qualified for the dependent PD diagnosis was: 'volunteers to do things that are unpleasant or demeaning in order to get other people to like him or her' (Hirschfeld *et al.*, 1991).

Several investigations have separated the features of dependent PD into two associated subgroups related to emotional reliance on significant others (attachment), and a more general lack of social self-confidence (general dependency). Livesley, Schroeder & Jackson (1990) described five features of attachment, i.e. fear of loss of an attachment figure; need for affection; need for proximity to the attachment figure; feelings of security based on physical presence of the attachment figure; and strong protest at separation from the attachment figure. These authors also provided five features of general dependency, i.e. low self-esteem; need for advice and reassurance; need for constant reassurance and approval; need for care and support; and submissiveness.

Hirschfeld *et al.* (1991) have reviewed the DSM-III-R criteria for dependent PD; the first two criteria were supported, but it was suggested that the third, i.e. 'agrees with people ...' should be rewritten as: 'has difficulty expressing disagreement with others because of fear of their anger or loss of support'. A modification was also suggested for the next criterion, i.e. that 'has difficulty initiating projects ...' be developed by adding 'this is due to a lack of self-confidence in judgement and not to a lack of motivation or energy'. The final criterion, i.e. 'is easily hurt by criticism or disapproval', was recommended for deletion, as it is commonly found in other PDs and other psychiatric disorders, while the remaining criteria were reworded as follows:

has difficulty independently initiating projects or doing things on his or her own. This is due to a lack of self-confidence in judgement and not to a lack of motivation or energy; goes to excessive lengths to obtain nurturance and support from others, to the point of volunteering to do things that are unpleasant; feels uncomfortable or helpless when alone, because of exaggerated fears of inability to care for him/ herself; when close relationships end, indiscriminatingly seeks another relationship to provide nurturance and support; and is frequently preoccupied with fears of being left to take care of himself/herself.

These recommendations have contributed to the changes in DSM-IV.

Presentation to medical services

A depressive syndrome is commonly associated with dependent PD (Reich & Noyes, 1987), and although definitions of dependent PD and depressive disorders can overlap, with both involving lack of initiative, feeling helpless and difficulty making decisions (Zuroff & Mongrain, 1987; Overholser, Kabakoff & Norman, 1989), it appears that there may be a causal relationship between dependent PD and some forms of depressive disorder. Also, an individual with dependent PD may have an increased vulnerability to the development of other disorders, such as panic attacks and phobias, alcoholism and substance abuse. Individuals with dependent PD are particularly vulnerable to worry and anxiety about being unsupported, so that panic attacks may be precipitated by new responsibilities, while phobias are reinforced by avoidance and any increased care from others.

Reich, Noyes & Troughton (1987*b*) found that dependent PD was the most frequent PD diagnosis in patients with panic disorder, particularly in the subgroups with phobic avoidance, when the prevalence was about 40%.

Associations have also been claimed between dependent PD and somatic complaints. Hill (1970), in an early study of 'passive-dependent' individuals, found that all subjects had reported somatic complaints which had often led to a great deal of medical attention. Often medical treatments were considered as their main source of support, when their problems became viewed in bodily rather than in psychological terms. For those with dependent PD, seeking comfort from a variety of sources may also lead to a higher incidence of obesity and tobacco dependence.

In a counselling or psychotherapeutic relationship, the engagement of such individuals is readily achieved, but thereafter there is a tendency to resist the clinician's efforts to encourage more autonomy and to discharge them from treatment. This may lead to what appears to be a permanent commitment, which may not be compatible with the demands of a clinical service.

Associated features

DSM-III-R's dependent PD has been shown to commonly co-occur with other PDs, in particular borderline PD, but also with avoidant, histrionic and schizotypal PDs (Reich, 1990*b*). The proportion of patients with PD who had a diagnosis of dependent PD ranged from 7 to 47% in five studies with a median of 20% (Hirschfeld *et al.*, 1991).

The possibility of prejudicial sex bias in the use of the dependent PD diagnosis has aroused controversy, but this should not prevent the evaluation of any genuine sex differences. While Kass, Spitzer & Williams (1983) found that dependent PD (based on clinicians' DSM-III diagnoses with no standardized assessment), was diagnosed over 2.5 times more often in women, Reich (1987) did not confirm this finding using standardized interview and self-report instruments. This limited evidence suggests that clinicians' attitudes to the association between dependent PD and gender requires further study. However, there may be genuine gender-related differences in the prevalence of submissive behaviour resulting from both genetic and environmental factors.

Finally, the DSM-III-R has claimed that chronic physical illness may predispose to the development of dependent PD in children and adolescents.

Current status

Dependent PD is a common disorder in psychiatric practice. It is associated with depressive and anxiety disorders and usually co-occurs with other PDs, in particular, borderline and avoidant PDs. Excessively dependent behaviour in medical settings can impose inappropriate and unsustainable demands on available resources.

Obsessive-compulsive personality disorder

Main features

The essential feature has been described as 'a preoccupation with perfectionism, mental and interpersonal control, and orderliness at the expense of flexibility, openness, and efficiency' (Pfohl & Blum, 1991).

Clinical origins

In the early part of this century, Sigmund Freud (1959) described certain individuals with so-called anal character as 'orderly, parsimonious and obstinate ... Orderly covers the notion of bodily cleanliness, as well as conscientiousness in carrying out small duties and trustworthiness ... Parsimony may (include) ... avarice; and obstinacy can go over into defiance, to which rage and revengefulness are easily joined'.

Abraham (1921) provided further descriptions, which have been summarized by Pfohl & Blum (1991), i.e. pleasure in indexing, compiling lists, and arranging things symmetrically; superficial fastidiousness masking disarray or lack of cleanliness underneath; pleasure in possessions with an inability to throw away worn out or worthless objects; a tendency to postpone every action and unproductive perseverance; preoccupation with preserving correct social appearances; in close personal relationships refuses to accommodate to others and expects compliance; produces exaggerated criticism of others and insists on controlling interactions with others; and a generally morose or surly attitude. Some of these features, i.e. perfectionism, excessive scrupulousness, rigidity and hoarding, contributed to Kahn's description (1928) of the 'anankastic' person, a term which is retained in ICD-10.

In 1952, the DSM-I included a description of 'compulsive' personality and a similar account was retained in DSM-II, although the category was termed 'obsessive/compulsive personality', involving excessive concern with conformity and adherence to standards of conscience. Such individuals were rigid, overinhibited, overconscientious and unable to relax easily. Subsequently, DSM-III provided a fuller description in the form of five criteria, of which four were necessary for diagnosis, while the DSM-III-R expanded the features to nine criteria, of which five were required. This increase in criteria produced a greater variety in the syndrome, and it has been estimated that DSM-III-R criteria would produce about twice as many diagnoses of obsessive-compulsive PD compared with those of DSM-III, in a given population (Pfohl & Blum, 1991).

Most of the features described by Freud and Abraham are reflected by the DSM-III-R criteria, with the exception of a pattern of anger and hostility. The clustering of the various features was investigated by Lazare *et al.* (1966, 1970) using factor analysis of a self-report rating scale. One factor involved orderliness, strong conscience, perseverance, obstinacy, rigidity, rejection of others, parsimony and emotional constriction. This and other studies using self-report inventories have not provided evidence for marked anger as part of an obsessive-compulsive factor (Pfohl & Blum, 1991).

Main definitions

DSM-III-R requires at least five of the following nine criteria:

perfectionism that interferes with task completion; preoccupation with details, rules, lists, order, organization, or schedules to the extent that the major point of the activity is lost; unreasonable insistence that others submit to exactly his or her way of doing things, or unreasonable reluctance to allow others to do things because of the conviction that they will not do them correctly; excessive devotion to work and productivity to the exclusion of leisure activities and friendships (not accounted for by obvious economic necessity); indecisiveness – decision making is either avoided, postponed, or protracted . . . (do not include if indecisiveness is due to excessive need for advice or reassurance from others); overconscientiousness, scrupulousness and inflexibility about matters of morality, ethics, or values (not accounted for by cultural or religious identification); restricted expression of affection; lack of generosity in giving time, money, or gifts when no personal gain is likely to result; inability to discard worn-out or worthless objects even when they have no sentimental value.

The DSM-IV criteria omit the features related to indecisiveness and restricted expression of affection, and include a new criterion: 'rigidity and stubbornness'.

The equivalent category in ICD-10 is 'anankastic' PD, which requires three of eight criteria, in addition to the general criteria for PD. Five of the criteria closely resemble DSM-III-R features, i.e.

preoccupation with details, rules, lists, order, organization or schedule; perfectionism that interferes with task completion; excessive conscientiousness, scrupulousness, and undue preoccupation with productivity to the exclusion of pleasure and interpersonal relationships; excessive pedantry and adherence to social conventions; and unreasonable insistence by the patient that others submit to exactly his or her way of doing things, or unreasonable reluctance to allow others to do things.

The three remaining are: 'feelings of excessive doubt and caution; rigidity and stubbornness; and intrusion of insistent and unwelcome thoughts or impulses'.

Clinical features

The central feature of perfectionism is often associated with the feeling 'I should', together with deliberate, purposeful activity, reflecting a focussed, stimulus-bound style of thinking (Beck & Freeman, 1990). Beck & Freeman have itemized various hypothetical characteristic thoughts, e.g.

There are right and wrong behaviours, decisions and emotions; I must avoid mistakes to be worthwhile; to make a mistake is to have failed; to make a mistake is to be deserving of criticism; I must be perfectly in control of my environment as well as of myself; loss of control is intolerable; if something is or may be dangerous, one must be terribly upset by it; one is powerful enough to initiate or prevent the occurrence of catastrophes by magical rituals or obsessional ruminations; if the perfect course of action is not clear, it is better to do nothing; without my rules and rituals, I'll collapse in an inert pile.

Such individuals may appear preoccupied with unimportant detail, humourless, rigid, dogmatic, obstinate and indecisive. However, it must be remembered that obsessional traits that are relatively moderate can be an asset in many occupations, and that many 'normal' individuals with such attributes would attract positive descriptions such as dependable, precise, punctual, having high standards, persistent, stable and determined.

Persons with problematic obsessive-compulsive traits lack adaptability to new situations and fail to take opportunities. Their perfectionism may lead to occupational inefficiency because they get side-tracked by trivial detail or postpone actions due to indecision. One patient would spend several hours trying to compose a short letter, although he could manage to complete other parts of his work that involved a structured routine. There may be a lack of humour, of expressions of affection and of enjoyment.

Opinions tend to be based on moral principles and others are often judged harshly. Meanness is associated with a lack of enjoyment in giving or receiving. There is a tendency to worry and to be sensitive to criticism as they expect to be judged as severely as they judge themselves. Although they appear unemotional, this may hide resentment, anger and, perhaps, aggressive fantasies. Indeed, such persons can experience a range of emotions such as love and loyalty to a select group of friends or family, concern, guilt, mourning and sadness (Akhtar, 1987).

The various DSM-III-R criteria for obsessive-compulsive PD have been reviewed by Pfohl & Blum (1991). Two criteria, i.e. 'unreasonable insistence that others submit to exactly his or her way of doing things, or unreasonable reluctance to allow others to do things because of the conviction that they will not do them correctly', and 'indecisiveness: decision making is either avoided, postponed or protracted ...' have often been found in persons without a diagnosis of obsessive-compulsive PD, which indicated that the sensitivity of these criteria was low. Pfohl & Blum recommended that the latter criterion should be excluded in DSM-IV and that the former be modified to identify the specific feature of the trait, i.e. 'reluctant to delegate tasks or to work with others'. Also, possible new criteria were suggested, namely, 'periods of rigid adherence to authority are punctuated by great irritation or overt anger when authority figures are perceived as bending the rules; argues stubbornly with others who have a different political or philosophical viewpoint and considers opposing opinions utterly without merit; critical and judgemental of others, e.g. prone to make biting and sarcastic remarks'. As has been noted, the DSM-IV has been influenced by these suggestions.

Presentation to medical services

The features of obsessive-compulsive PD are common origins for presentation to primary care physicians or to psychiatric services, as associated social and occupational difficulties may cause anxiety, depressive disorders or hypochondriasis.

Associated features

There have been many claims that obsessive-compulsive PD is related to obsessive-compulsive disorder (OCD), which, despite the similarity of the terms, can be distinguished by the presence of obsessions, with or without compulsions. Obsessions and compulsions consist of distressing and time-consuming thoughts and behaviour, which may significantly interfere with the person's normal routine, occupational functioning, usual social activities or relationships with others. Obsessions are recurrent and persistent ideas, thoughts, impulses, or images that are usually experienced, at least initially, as intrusive and senseless; while compulsions are repetitive, purposeful and intentional behaviours that are performed in response to an obsession, or according to certain rules or in a stereotyped fashion (American Psychiatric Association, 1987).

However, such an association is difficult to evaluate as the boundary between the two disorders can be indistinct and arbitrary; not all patients with OCD give a history of experiencing their phenomena as 'intrusive or senseless', and the distinction between, for example, a marked preoccupation with detailed organization and a compulsion involving a series of actions performed in a particular order or in a stereotyped manner, may not be possible. Pollack (1979, 1987) has reviewed earlier (pre DSM-III) studies and considered that 'clearly there is no necessary one-to-one relationship between obsessional personality (i.e. obsessive-compulsive PD) and obsessional neurosis (OCD), despite the occasional findings that more obsessive-compulsive neurotics than would be expected by chance show evidence of a premorbid obsessional personality'. The studies in relation to DSM-III and DSM-III-R have led to a similar conclusion and have been reviewed by Pfohl & Blum (1991), who stated

the majority of patients with obsessive-compulsive disorder (OCD) do not meet criteria for obsessive-compulsive PD. Among patients with OCD who do have a personality disorder, several other personality disorders may be just as common or more common than obsessive-compulsive PD. It is not possible to determine at this time whether patients with OCD are more likely to meet criteria for obsessive-compulsive PD than patients with other Axis I diagnoses.

The other PDs that were commonly found as co-occurring with OCD were dependent, mixed, histrionic and avoidant PDs, and it has been noted that obsessive-compulsive PD is common among patients with depressive and anxiety disorders.

Pfohl & Blum (1991) have also reviewed the co-occurrence of other PDs with obsessive-compulsive PD. Co-occurrence rates involving paranoid, histrionic, borderline, narcissistic and avoidant PDs were 'unexpectedly high'; for example, for three studies related to DSM-III-R criteria, the average percentages for the co-occurrence of the above five PDs with obsessive-compulsive PD were 55%, 24%, 29%, 40% and 57% respectively. The rates for borderline PD are surprising, as aspects of the personality structures of the two disorders, such as impulsiveness and perfectionism, appear to be incompatible. Pfohl & Blum (1991) pointed out that other PDs may be associated with some behaviours which are characteristic of obsessive-compulsive PD, such as lack of generosity, but that these may be related to different motivations. However, it is possible that co-occurrence of obsessive-compulsive PD with some features of other PDs will be shown to contradict current concepts of the relevant cognitive processes in this disorder.

In a non-patient community study, DSM-III's 'compulsive PD' had a prevalence of 1.7% in the sample of the population studied, and it was claimed that this was associated with a vulnerability to the development of anxiety disorders (Nestadt *et al.*, 1991).

In the DSM-III-R it is claimed that obsessive-compulsive PD is more frequently diagnosed in males, and is apparently more common among first-degree relatives of those with this disorder than among the general population.

Current status

Obsessive-compulsive PD consists of features that have long been part of clinical descriptions and are common origins of anxiety, some depressive disorders and impaired occupational functioning in patient groups. The relationship with obsessive-compulsive disorder is uncertain, despite the similarity of the terms, and there appears to be a high degree of co-occurrence with other PDs.

Passive-aggressive personality disorder

Main features

The most characteristic feature is a pattern of passive resistance to external demands, with obstructive behaviour and poor performance both socially and occupationally. Affected individuals avoid being assertive, although they may be irritable, sulky or argumentative. They resent interference and control, and express their resistance by such behaviour as delaying tactics, providing a poor quality of work, forgetfulness, stubbornness, and sabotaging the efforts of others.

Clinical origins

The term 'passive-aggressive' was used in a 1949 US Joint Armed Services Technical Bulletin, to describe soldiers who displayed features such as passiveness, obstructionism or aggressive outbursts (Beck & Freeman, 1990) and the first edition of the DSM, in 1952, contained a 'passive-aggressive' category divided into three subtypes: passive-aggressive, passive-dependent and aggressive. Using these DSM-I categories in a study of 400 outpatients, Whitman, Trosman & Koenig (1954) found 19% with the passive-aggressive subtype. DSM-II, in 1968, gave this term the status of a separate diagnosis and this remained the situation in DSM-III. However, it has also been claimed that passive-aggressive behaviour should be viewed as a transient reaction that can be shown by most people in situations when they feel helpless. Although the early concepts of passive-aggressive PD were narrowly based, i.e. on resistance to external demands, Millon (1981) noted associated characteristics such as irritability, low frustration tolerance, pessimism, and sulking behaviour. Some of these are represented in the augmented criteria found in the DSM-III-R, but the category is not represented in the ICD-10.

Main definitions

In the DSM-III-R, five of the following nine criteria are required for diagnosis of passive-aggressive PD:

procrastinates, i.e. puts off things that need to be done so that deadlines are not met; becomes sulky, irritable, or argumentative when asked to do something he or she does not want to do; seems to work deliberately slowly or to do a bad job on tasks that he or she really does not want to do; protests, without justification, that others make unreasonable demands on him or her; avoids obligations by claiming to have 'forgotten'; believes that he or she is doing a much better job than others think he or she is doing; resents useful suggestions from others concerning how he or she could be more productive; obstructs the efforts of others by failing to do his or her share of the work; and unreasonably criticizes or scorns people in positions of authority.

The category is omitted from the DSM-IV except as a criteria set 'provided for further study', characterized by: 'passively resists fulfilling routine social and occupational tasks; complains of being misunderstood and unappreciated by others; is sullen and argumentative; unreasonably criticizes and scorns authority; expresses envy and resentment toward those apparently more fortunate; voices exaggerated and persistent complaints of personal misfortune; and alternates between hostile defiance and contrition'.

Clinical features

The starting point for such behaviour in passive-aggressive PD is resentment towards the demands of others, in the context of a wish for autonomy, negative attitudes based on the assumptions that others are trying to control them and take advantage of them, and a belief that they are misunderstood or unappreciated. This is accompanied by a failure to engage in direct assertion, conflict or expressions of anger, often due to a fear of disapproval or to concern that this will lead to more interference and control by others. Such people are often sulky, irritable, or argumentative when asked to do something, and protest to others how unreasonable the demands are. They resent useful suggestions and unreasonably criticize and blame those in authority as being arbitrary and unfair (American Psychiatric Association, 1987).

Such people find it difficult to accept that it might be better to state their case and try and modify requests from others, and that their own behaviour has contributed to social and occupational difficulties. They tend to be dependent, lack self-confidence and are pessimistic about the future. There is a tendency towards a negative view of most situations based on the idea that others are trying, unreasonably, to control them. While a person with paranoid PD may suspect hidden motives, with passive-aggressive PD anything that disturbs his or her autonomy is considered to be unfair and unreasonable. Beck & Freeman (1990) have described various characteristic thoughts: 'How dare they tell me what to do; nobody gives me credit for the work I do; people take advantage of me; rules are arbitrary and stifle me; being direct with people could be dangerous; people take advantage of you if you let them; and it doesn't matter what you do – nothing works out anyway'.

If his or her behaviour is challenged, the individual may respond with further obstructive acts, although there may be occasional overt anger. In clinical settings there may be lateness, non-attendance, poor cooperation – perhaps with inadequate answers to questions, and irritability.

Presentation to medical services

Common complications include depressive disorders and alcohol abuse (American Psychiatric Association, 1987), often in the setting of relationship difficulties (Small *et al.*, 1970). Patients may present because of complaints and pressure from employers or spouses. It is likely that a chronically pessimistic outlook makes such individuals liable to develop secondary depressive symptoms. As autonomy is important, such patients may resent having to answer questions and can appear irritated and uncooperative. They may complain that nothing works out and that this is the fault of others.

Associated features

There is some overlap with the features of avoidant, paranoid and dependent PDs. The diagnosis of passive-aggressive PD usually co-occurs with other PDs and may contribute to the causation of certain types of depression and alcohol abuse.

Current status

Passive-aggressive PD is rarely found as a discrete diagnosis for patients in psychiatric practice, but the features often appear to contribute to presentations to medical services.

Self-defeating personality disorder

Main features

The DSM-III-R describes the essential feature as 'a pervasive pattern of self-defeating behavior ... The person may often avoid or undermine pleasurable experiences, be drawn to situations or relationships in which he or she will suffer, and prevent others from helping him or her'. But the diagnosis is not made if self-defeating behaviours occur exclusively in response to, or in anticipation of, being physically, sexually or psychologically abused, or only when the person is depressed. Also, this diagnosis has been suggested 'for those who repeatedly place themselves in abusive, detrimental and injurious situations despite the opportunity to avoid them' (Widiger *et al.*, 1988). Therefore, this disorder involves active participation on the patient's part in producing and maintaining adverse situations.

Clinical origins

In 1983, 'masochistic' PD was proposed as a category for future revisions of the DSM in an attempt to incorporate behaviour that had been noted in the literature of several disciplines, including psychoanalytic psychotherapy. However, this attracted criticism and controversy, related to concern that such a diagnosis could be misused, for example by blaming a woman for remaining in an abusive relationship if no alternative can be readily achieved (Kass *et al.*, 1989). There has also been anxiety that this concept could be used unfairly to discriminate against women when fitness to look after children is at issue. Additional controversy about the relevance of psychoanalytic concepts of female masochism, with the implication that the person may derive unconscious pleasure from suffering, led to the name of the proposed new category to be changed to 'self-defeating' PD in 1985 (Fiester, 1991).

In the DSM-III-R, 'self-defeating PD', was defined by eight criteria, and was one of the 'proposed diagnostic categories needing further study' (it is not included in DSM-IV). But only four of the original ten criteria for masochistic PD had been retained in a similar form. The term 'masochism' had been used by Krafft-Ebing (1901) to describe a psychosexual disorder in which pain and suffering coexisted with sexual gratification, while Freud (1961) extended the concept to include self-imposed suffering, i.e. persistent self-reproach and a pattern of contributing to unnecessary failures and accidents, perhaps in the context of being exploited. Other chronic features that have been claimed to be related to these attributes have included unfounded or exaggerated feelings of suffering or of exploitation; frequent complaints and demands about being mistreated; passive self-abasement; an attitude of poor self-worth; a tendency to provoke rejecting responses; to be rejecting of help; feeling ethically or morally superior; responding to positive events by a negative reaction; rejecting opportunities for pleasure; pessimism; self-punishing, self-destructive behaviour, involving self-inflicted pain or adversity; sabotaging goals; a lack of interest in those who treat him/her well; and sacrificial or martyred behaviour (Kass *et al.*, 1989). Two self-defeating PD criteria (i.e. 'rejects or renders ineffective the attempts of others to help him or her', and 'following positive personal events, e.g. new achievement, responds with depression, guilt, or a behaviour that produces pain, e.g. an accident') can be reflected by specific doctor–patient problems, namely, the patient sabotaging the clinician's efforts and a 'negative therapeutic reaction', in which any progress may be cancelled out by its subsequent negative effect on the patient.

The self-defeating PD criteria provide a variety of behaviours to be evaluated, and Spitzer *et al.* (1989) invited each of 2000 clinicians to rate one of their patients with self-defeating PD behaviour and another with other PD features. Fifty-one per cent of respondents thought there was a need for the proposed self-defeating PD category, and 222 patients who were selected as examples of those who show some self-defeating PD criteria were rated and compared with 222 patients with other PDs. Although the eight self-defeating PD criteria were often found in the control group, all were considerably more common in the self-defeating PD, in particular the first criterion, i.e. 'chooses people and situations that lead to disappointment, failure or mistreatment ...'. In another study of over 1000 patients with PD (each clinician was asked to rate the first patient who came to mind with PD), self-defeating PD was found in 42% of females and 28% of males (Spitzer *et al.*, 1989). But it was the sole diagnosis in just 4% and was usually associated with borderline and dependent PDs. Spitzer *et al.* (1989) also reported on 85 patients 'who had at least one DSM-III-R PD' assessed by a structured interview; the diagnosis of self-defeating PD was made in 21%. Two further studies report on patients evaluated by self-defeating PD criteria: 18% of 76 cocaine abusers who were assessed by a structured interview received a diagnosis of self-defeating PD (Kleinman *et al.*, 1990), while in another study of 110 outpatients rated by clinicians, self-defeating PD was a diagnosis in 14%, and one-third of these patients had no other PD (Nurnberg *et al.*, 1991). Although several other studies have reported self-defeating psychopathology, these were related to earlier criteria for maso-chistic PD (Kass, MacKinnon & Spitzer, 1986; Reich, 1990*a*).

Main definitions

Self-defeating PD is one of the 'proposed diagnostic categories needing further study' in DSM-III-R, but is not found in DSM-IV or in ICD-10. There are two exclusion criteria, namely that the disorder does not occur exclusively in response to, or in anticipation of, being physically, sexually or psychologically abused, and that it does not occur only when the person is depressed. Five of the following eight criteria are required:

chooses people and situations that lead to disappointment, failure, or mistreatment even when better options are clearly available; rejects or renders ineffective the attempts of others to help him or her; following positive personal events (e.g. new achievement), responds with depression, guilt, or a behaviour that produces pain (e.g. an accident); incites angry or rejecting responses from others and then feels hurt, defeated, or humiliated (e.g. makes fun of spouse in public, provoking an angry retort, then feels devastated); rejects opportunities for pleasure, or is reluctant to acknowledge enjoying himself or herself (despite having adequate social skills and the capacity for pleasure); fails to accomplish tasks crucial to his or her personal objectives despite demonstrated ability to do so, e.g. helps fellow students write papers, but is unable to write his or her own; is uninterested in or rejects people who consistently treat him or her well, e.g. is unattracted to caring sexual partners; and engages in excessive self-sacrifice that is unsolicited by the intended recipients of the sacrifice.

Clinical features

DSM-III-R describes how a person with self-defeating PD can repeatedly enter relationships with others (or place him or herself in situations), that are self-defeating and have adverse consequences, even when better options are clearly available. For example, a woman may appear to choose to repeatedly enter relationshps with men who have alcohol dependence, or a man with employment skills may persist with jobs where these are not used. Reasonable offers of assistance from others, including medical services, are rejected, for example by not following-up on an agreed treatment plan. The person's reaction to positive events, including the relief of symptoms, or encouragement, may be a worsening of a depressed mood, perhaps with feelings of guilt. However, such persons usually do not appear to be engaged in deliberate sabotage, as they do not seem to be fully aware of the motivations associated with their actions. An adverse event such as an 'accident', or losing something, may seem to others to follow a clear pattern, but the individual is not necessarily aware of deliberate intent. Often, a person's behaviour, such as making unreasonable demands from medical services, invites anger and rejection, and this produces a feeling of hurt and humiliation. Opportunities for pleasure may be avoided, or enjoyment is denied in situations where this would be expected. He or she may seem to avoid taking available opportunities, so that any achievements are not in keeping with his or her potential, while people who treat the person well may be experienced as uninteresting, so that friends or partners are chosen who are bound to disappoint. There can be a tendency to do things for others that involve excessive self-sacrifice, but this does not make the person feel better and often makes the recipients feel guilty and rejecting.

It has been noted that several criteria for this diagnosis require a high degree of judgement for their application, for example, 'engages in excessive self-sacrifice . . .', 'rejects people who consistently treat him/her well . . .', and '. . . when better options are clearly available' (Fiester, 1991). The evaluation of the latter is particularly problematic in a setting of poverty, substance abuse, crime and violence.

Self-defeating PD should be distinguished from self-defeating behaviour that is found only in the context of physical, sexual or psychological abuse, as such behaviour can sometimes be viewed as a coping strategy for a woman to avoid the further violence that would result if she asserted herself or finished the relationship. Also, the diagnosis of self-defeating PD should not be made if the behaviour is only found in the presence of a depressive disorder, although this distinction can be difficult to make.

It has been suggested that to qualify as a 'diagnosis', a syndrome must be capable of defining a group of patients in whom the features are relatively discrete (or predominant) and that this group should be distinguished from other groups, taking course and outcome into account (Robins & Guze,

1970). Evidence for the justification of self-defeating PD as a diagnostic category on this basis is lacking, as few patients with a discrete self-defeating PD have been described, and positive self-defeating PD criteria have been commonly found in association with other PDs (Spitzer *et al.*, 1989). However, the concept of self-defeating PD as a syndrome could still have a reality, even in a population of patients with co-occurring PDs, if there is a greater correlation (or association) between its component items, compared with the degree of correlation (or association) of its component items with items from other PD syndromes. However, a study using a self-report questionnaire based on DSM-III-R PDs indicated that the criteria for self-defeating PD had a greater correlation with other PD syndromes than with the self-defeating PD syndrome itself (Dowson, 1994).

Presentation to medical services

As with many PD diagnoses, self-defeating PD features are seldom discrete, but they can contribute to the development of some depressive disorders and other common psychiatric symptoms.

Associated features

The limited evidence suggests that the diagnosis of self-defeating PD is made more frequently in women than men in clinical samples (Fiester, 1991), and in view of concerns about the possible potential for the misuse of this category, the reasons for the apparent sex difference in the frequency of its use are of particular importance. If such a difference exists, it may be due to three possible causes or their combinations (Sprock, Blashfield & Smith, 1990). The first involves a 'gender bias' on the part of the clinician, reflecting socially-determined ideas about which types of behaviour are healthy or pathological for males versus females. The second involves gender bias in the way clinicians apply the criteria, while the third reflects real differences in the prevalences of the disorders in males and females, due to different susceptibilities, based on biological, genetic, social or environmental factors. Fiester's review of the limited data (1991) concluded that there was no clear evidence of gender bias in the application of the criteria, although further studies are required.

The nature of an association between self-defeating PD and depressive disorders has also been controversial, and it has been suggested that self-defeating PD should be considered to be related to the spectrum of depressive disorders, rather than to the other PDs. A concept of a 'depressive-masochistic' personality has been a feature of the psychoanalytic literature, and it can be difficult to distinguish self-defeating PD features due to personality traits from those secondary to chronic depressive disorder.

Additional associations of self-defeating PD have also been claimed, namely with other co-occurring PDs (in particular with borderline, avoidant and dependent PDs), increased prevalence in the relatives of subjects with the disorder, and an increased frequency of an history of physical, sexual or psychological abuse in childhood (Fiester, 1991).

Evidence for concurrent or predictive validity for self-defeating PD is sparse, but McCann *et al.* (1991), in a study of bulimic patients that included PD assessment by a structured interview, claimed that those who showed self-induced vomiting scored higher on the narcissistic, self-defeating and borderline scales.

Current status

The features of self-defeating PD have been found in clinical descriptions for several decades, and are present in many patients with PD in psychiatric practice, although they usually co-occur with other PDs. While they should be evaluated in a PD assessment, the provision of a distinct diagnostic category cannot be justified as there is insufficient evidence that it describes features that are relatively discrete or that the criteria are associated with each other more than with the features of other PDs. Despite this, clinicians in psychiatric practice are aware that, for a few patients who are among the most difficult to help, their self-defeating behaviour appears to be the most disabling aspect of their PD psychopathology.

Sadistic personality disorder

Main features

The DSM-III-R describes the essential feature as 'a pervasive pattern of cruel, demeaning, and aggressive behaviour directed toward other people, beginning by early adulthood. The sadistic behaviour is often evident both in social relationships (particularly with family members) and at work (with subordinates), but seldom is displayed in contacts with people in positions of authority or higher status'. Also, 'The diagnosis is not made if the sadistic behaviour has been directed towards only one person (e.g. a spouse) or has been only for the purpose of sexual arousal (as in sexual sadism).'

Clinical origins

Sadism was a term originally used by Krafft-Ebing (1901) to describe the desire to inflict pain upon a person who was the sexual 'object'. But while Freud (1957) also considered that aggressiveness or a desire to subjugate was associated with the biological substrate of sexuality in males, he believed that there were two aspects of sadism, a generalized aggressive and violent attitude towards the sexual object, and a more specific sexual sadism, involving sexual satisfaction that is dependent on the humiliation and mistreatment of the sexual partner. Subsequently, the psychoanalytic literature has tended to consider that sadism is related to masochism (which is the desire to have pain inflicted by the sexual object), and that both are related to biological sexual instincts (Fiester & Gay, 1991). These ideas have been extended beyond sexual relationships; for example Horney (1950) has described the 'vindictive sadist' who shows a repeated tendency to dominate, deprecate, humiliate, blame and cruelly criticize others, but not in the context of sexual gratification.

As a category in a major classification, 'sadistic PD' first appeared in the DSM-III-R in 1987, but only as one of the 'proposed diagnostic categories needing further study', together with self-defeating PD. Both these proposed disorders were controversial; some considered that self-defeating PD reflected culturally-determined ideas of how women should behave, and that sadistic PD had been included to placate such criticisms by 'balancing the ticket', as cruelty, anger and aggression were supposedly associated with a culturally-sanctioned male role. The DSM-III-R concept of sadistic PD specifies that the associated behaviour has not been aimed solely at the purpose of sexual arousal, and Fiester & Gay (1991) have reviewed several studies that suggest that sexual sadomasochists generally limit sadistic and masochistic behaviour to their sexual encounters, and are rarely involved with more generalized sadistic interactions.

One of the main reasons why sadistic PD was included in DSM-III-R was that several forensic psychiatrists believed that there was a need for such a category, particularly in forensic settings, in relation to people who showed a pattern of cruel and aggressive behaviour towards others but whose behaviour was not adequately encompassed by the antisocial PD diagnosis. Such individuals showed pronounced aggressive and domineering behaviour, in the relative absence of a history of childhood conduct disorder and adult criminality.

The addition of this new proposed diagnostic category to DSM-III-R gave rise to concern that it might be used to mitigate or excuse violent crime, in particular repeated violence and sexual abuse to a child, spouse or partner. As Spitzer *et al.* (1991) noted: 'the medicalization of evil deeds becomes an avenue of excuses'. But many other diagnoses have the potential to be exploited to interfere with the aims of a criminal justice system and such a potential should not be an argument for the suppression of a valid diagnostic category. As Spitzer *et al.* (1991) have pointed out, it is possible to have specific laws precluding the use of PD diagnoses as mitigating factors in criminal proceedings, and such laws have been enacted in several states in the USA in respect of the diagnosis of antisocial PD. But although it is understandable, and perhaps inevitable, that a society has very different attitudes to a murderer with a schizophrenic illness involving florid delusions, compared to a murderer with antisocial or sadistic PD, a clear distinction between illness and normality in relation to this example cannot be justified from a biological perspective, as genetic and other biological factors are major causal variables in respect of both schizophrenia and PDs. It can be argued that a logical approach to the detention and supervision of dangerous individuals with PD would not be based mainly on concepts of blame and responsibility, and that the risk of the continuation of antisocial behaviour should be given more consideration despite the difficulties in prediction.

Main definition

DSM-III-R includes sadistic PD as one of the 'proposed diagnostic categories needing further study' but it is not included in DSM-IV. The behaviour must have been directed towards more than one person and not solely for the purpose of sexual arousal. At least four of the following are required:

has used physical cruelty or violence for the purpose of establishing dominance in a relationship . . .; humiliates or demeans people in the presence of others; has treated or disciplined someone under his or her control unusually harshly, e.g. a child, student, prisoner, or patient; is amused by, or takes pleasure in, the psychological or physical suffering of others (including animals); has lied for the purpose of harming or inflicting pain on others . . .; gets other people to do what he or she wants by frightening them (through intimidation or even terror); restricts the autonomy of people with whom he or she has a close relationship, e.g. will not let spouse leave the house unaccompanied . . .; and is fascinated by violence, weapons, martial arts, injury, or torture.

Clinical features

There is generally a pattern of cruelty and/or violence which establishes dominance in relationships, and escalating violence may result from the victim trying to assert him or herself, but not all persons with this disorder are physically violent. Various behaviours, including verbal intimidation, show a lack of respect for others, although this pattern may only involve those people who can be subjugated or dominated. Such victims are often humiliated in the presence of others, or, in the case of children (or others under his or her control) discipline may be excessive. For example, a teacher may insist that a student spends many hours in detention at school for a minor offence. The person often restricts the autonomy of those who are dominated, for example, by not allowing family members out of the house for social occasions, and gets others to do what he or she wants by frightening them. In severe cases, the person may enjoy producing physical or psychological pain or suffering in others or in animals.

Fiester & Gay (1991) have reported on 235 adults who had been accused of child abuse and found that 12 (5%) met the criteria for sadistic PD. These individuals were functioning well in some areas, as eight were in regular work and many were capable of remorse and sadness. Eight were men and only two were considered to have another DSM-III-R PD (narcissistic and antisocial). Nine gave histories of childhood physical abuse, often with sexual or emotional abuse and neglect. In eight there was a history of early loss of a parent or sibling by death or separation. The behaviour of this group included demeaning verbal abuse, threats to kill, beating, murder and abuse of spouse. There was a reluctance to acknowledge problems and to receive help or treatment unless it was imposed.

The other main source of data is a survey of forensic psychiatrists by Spitzer *et al.* (1991). Almost all cases described were male; there was a frequent history of childhood abuse (emotional, physical and sexual) and parental loss in 52%. Also, there was evidence that the diagnostic criteria for sadistic PD were relatively sensitive and specific. Sensitivity is the frequency of individual criteria in cases of the disorder, and ranged from 65% to 94%, while specificity (the frequency of the absence of the criteria in non-cases) varied between 93% and 99%. Forty-seven per cent had co-occurring narcissistic PD and 67% had co-occurring antisocial PD, but 20% had neither. (Other PDs were not evaluated.) Twenty-seven per cent had a depressive disorder and 61% a history of substance abuse. It was concluded that the disorder may not be rare in forensic settings and that the prevalences of a history of emotional, physical and sexual abuse (90%, 76% and 41% respectively), were much higher than in general population studies, indicating an intergenerational transmission of violence.

Several other studies, reviewed by Fiester & Gay (1991), gave varying prevalence rates (2.5–33%) in various populations, as assessed by different methods. The highest prevalence, 33%, was in a group of 21 sex offenders, mostly in prison. However, there are particular difficulties in assessing this disorder unless there is independent information, as the person must admit to various behaviours that are especially socially unacceptable.

A few studies have compared the performance of the various DSM-III-R criteria in relation to the sadistic PD diagnosis (Fiester & Gay, 1991); the sixth criterion ('gets other people to do what he or she wants by frightening them') had the highest correlation with the diagnosis, while the lowest correlations were with criteria 3 and 7 ('has treated or disciplined someone under his or her control unusually harshly . . .' and 'restricts the autonomy of people . . .').

Presentation to medical services

In general, individuals with sadistic PD do not recognize their behaviour as abnormal or problematic, and do not present to medical services unless this is instigated following a court appearance, perhaps after being charged with child or spouse abuse. But such people may also come to medical attention because of associated substance use disorders, self-injury or pressure from family and employers.

Associated features

Several studies have noted that sadistic PD often co-occurs with other PDs, in particular narcissistic and antisocial PDs, but also with other PDs (Fiester & Gay, 1991). In a study of 12 individuals with sadistic PD, two had alcohol dependence, four a history of mixed substance abuse, and one had current substance abuse. Spitzer *et al.* (1991) found that 27% of 113 subjects had a co-occurring depressive syndrome and 61% had substance abuse. The disorder is far more common in males than females.

Current status

It is uncertain whether it will be useful to separate sadistic PD from antisocial PD. But although PDs with predominant and severe features of sadistic PD are rare presentations to the general psychiatrist, these attributes are more common in forensic practice. It is possible that this category represents a PD with a characteristic childhood history of abuse and parental loss, but which, in comparison with antisocial PD, has a history of less childhood conduct disorder and adult criminality outside the context of the sadistic behaviour. A better understanding of any causal relationships between adverse childhood events and subsequent sadistic PD may have implications for the development of preventative interventions when child abuse is identified.

Depressive personality (or personality disorder) and allied disorders

Main features

The main features of 'depressive personality' (which is not a category that is found in the DSM-III-R or ICD-10) are 'excessive negative and pessimistic beliefs about oneself and other people' that are apparent from early adult life (Hirschfeld & Shea, 1992). These are associated with pervasive dissatisfaction, low self-esteem, feelings of inadequacy and worthlessness, and, for most of the time, a persistent unhappiness. Also, such individuals appear critical and negativistic. Depressive PD is a criteria set 'provided for further study' in DSM-IV.

Clinical origins

Kraepelin (1921) described a depressive temperament, which he considered was mainly caused by genetic predisposition, characterized by 'a permanent, gloomy, emotional stress in all the experiences of life', and Phillips *et al.* (1990) have noted that this concept emphasized 'persistent gloominess, joylessness, anxiety and a predominantly depressed and despairing mood'. Such individuals were also 'serious, burdened, guilt-ridden, self-reproaching, clinging, and lacking in self-confidence'. Schneider (1959) termed a similar disorder as 'depressive psychopathy', which also involved a persistent sense of gloom together with the following characteristics: gloomy, pessimistic, serious and incapable of enjoyment or relaxation; quiet; sceptical; worrying; duty-bound; and self-doubting.

Subsequently, Akiskal's work (Akiskal, 1983; Akiskal, Hirschfeld & Yerevanian, 1983), on patients with both PD and chronic depressive disorders, led him to subdivide such 'characterologic depressions' into two sub-types: 'sub-affective dysthymia' and 'character-spectrum disorder', and it is the former that appears to correspond closely to the earlier descriptions.

The psychoanalytic literature has provided a different perspective, in which aspects of personality are considered to be determined by environmental interactions during development. These traits then predispose the individual to some types of depressive disorder. It has been suggested that relevant experiences include generally adverse circumstances, poor parenting, and childhood loss or bereavement, and that relevant traits include dependency, obsessionality, low self-esteem with helplessness, guilt, and difficulty expressing anger (Phillips *et al.*, 1990). However, theories of environmental and genetic influences on depressive personality features are not incompatible, as PDs are multidetermined, involving biological, cultural and social variables.

The concept of depressive personality was included in the heterogeneous category of 'Depressive neurosis' in DSM-II in 1968, and Spitzer, Endicott & Woodruff (1977) defined the subtype of depressive neurosis that corresponded to depressive personality, i.e. 'individuals who for at least the past 2 years have been bothered by depressed mood much of the time, with periods of normal mood lasting from a few hours to a few days ... there is usually no clear onset ...'. It should be noted that antidepressants were increasingly being shown to be useful in the treatment of many patients with chronic, relatively mild depressions, so that interest was developing in the subtypes of this heterogeneous group of disorders (Klerman, Endicott & Spitzer, 1979).

The consideration of the relationship of personality, PDs and depressive disorders is complicated by the heterogeneity of depressive disorders in respect of both clinical features and causation. However, various classifications of depressive syndromes have attempted to obtain aetiologically homogeneous patient groups.

When considering this confusing area it can be helpful to bear in mind that there appear to be three main interacting categories of aetiological factors. The first is 'endogenous' (or 'biological') aetiology related to episodes of depression, which involves hypothetical abnormal brain functioning, for example, related to a genetically-determined vulnerability. The resulting depression may appear 'out of the blue', but even if the disorder is precipitated by life-events, the nature or severity of the symptoms may be clearly out of the context of the patient's personality and environment, corresponding to the lay person's concept of disease. Of course, the definition of 'abnormal brain function' is a complex process, akin to the definition of hypertension. But, although an arbitrary line between normality and abnormality may have to be drawn at one point in the spectrum of hypertension, some cases of hypertension at the most abnormal end of the spectrum are clearly due to qualitatively distinct abnormal biological function, and there is good evidence that the same can be said for some cases of depression. The second category of aetiological factor for depressive disorders is past and present adverse environmental situations, which often interact with the third category, which is PDs.

All three categories may contribute to a depressive disorder in some patients. For example, certain PDs, such as borderline PD, have been shown to be associated with genetic factors (Kendler *et al.*, 1981; Baron *et al.*, 1985; Cadoret *et al.*, 1985; Gunderson & Elliott, 1985), and, in the case of a patient with borderline PD, environmental problems that may be the consequences of the maladaptive behaviour in this disorder can contribute to a depressed mood. This appears, at least in part, understandable as a response to environmental adversity.

Such a three-category model of the causation of depressive syndromes must, of course, be oversimplistic, but provides a framework for clinical practice. A particular syndrome of depression may be considered to be derived from one or a mixture of two or three of these aetiological categories, although one may predominate.

Most categorical systems of classification of depression are based on symptoms and these can sometimes correlate with aetiology, as 'endogenous' aetiology related to episodes of depression appears to be associated with several specified clinical features. These comprise the syndrome of so-called 'endogenous depression', although these phenomena are not invariably present as markers of endogenous aetiology. The identification of biological markers of endogenous aetiology, such as time from sleep onset to the first period of rapid eye movements, and the dexamethasone suppression test, have been used to improve patient selection for research studies, and further advances in this area are to be expected (Gunderson & Phillips, 1991).

One of the most enduring classifications of the features of depression involves just two categories, 'endogenous' (or psychotic) and 'neurotic' (or reactive) (Young *et al.*, 1986), and, despite its limitations, the clinical usefulness of this approach has stood the test of time. However, these terms are unsatisfactory. This classification is based on clinical description, and although the features of the endogenous syndrome can indicate that there is endogenous aetiology related to an episode of depression, endogenous aetiology does not invariably present with the specified symptoms. (This is evident from the features of some patients with regular and frequent mood changes in the context of bipolar manic-depressive disorder.) The term 'psychotic', if it is used as an alternative to endogenous, is also misleading because it infers the presence of delusions or hallucinations; however these are not always part of an endogenous syndrome, which rarely presents with all or even most of the various specified 'endogenous' features. Finally, the term 'reactive', as an alternative to 'neurotic', makes an aetiological claim that is not always justified; while the nature and severity of 'neurotic depression' can often seem understandable (or meaningful) as a reaction of that individual to events, endogenous aetiology may also contribute to the development of a syndrome of 'neurotic depression', which would be reflected by, for example, a degree of severity or chronicity that seems incompletely understandable on the basis of personality and environment.

Many studies have examined the clinical features associated with the endogenous syndrome, which can be identified relatively reliably in patients with bipolar manic-depressive disorder; these include marked agitation or psychomotor retardation with slowed thoughts and actions; absence of mood reactivity to pleasant circumstances with a loss of interest in pleasurable activity; self-reproach; early morning wakening; marked loss of appetite and weight; a distinct quality of mood that is unlike normal unhappiness; mood-congruent hallucinations and delusions; and repeated diurnal variation in mood with morning worsening (Nelson & Charney, 1981). (The last two features seem to be relatively specific markers of endogenous aetiology related to episodes of depression, while features such as early morning wakening are much less specific.) However, the number and severity of these features vary considerably and Parker *et al.* (1994) have provided evidence that signs of psychomotor disturbance are also relatively specific in defining a depression with significant endogenous aetiology. These signs usually involve facial and bodily immobility, delay in responding verbally, and impaired spontaneity of talk. In patients with features of the endogenous syndrome there is less likely to be an identifiable precipitating stress compared with those with a 'neurotic' syndrome, but there are exceptions, as it seems that life events can sometimes precipitate the biological processes underlying the endogenous syndrome.

'Neurotic' depression encompasses an heterogeneous group of clinical presentations that tend to be less severe than endogenous depressions, but again there are exceptions. Such syndromes consist of a varying and inadequately defined number of a long list of symptoms, including anxiety, phobias and somatic concomitants of anxiety, in addition to depressed mood. The presentations of most patients with a depressive disorder are within the category of neurotic depression, but progress has been made in identifying clinically valid subtypes that reflect differences in aetiology. For example, Akiskal (1983) identified four chronic subtypes of neurotic depression; the first, 'primary depression with residual chronicity', occurs in an individual with previously normal mood and appears to be a syndrome with endogenous aetiology that usually responds to antidepres-

Table 2.2 *Some categories of depressive disorders*

1. Based on presence or absence of a previous history of mania:
     Unipolar depression*
     Bipolar depression (i.e. with a history of mania)
2. DSM-III-R classification:
     (DSM-IV categories in brackets)
     Bipolar disorder (Bipolar I disorder) – mixed or depressed
     Major depression (Major depressive disorder)
     Dysthymia* (Dysthymic disorder)
     Cyclothymia (Cyclothymic disorder)
3. ICD-10 classification:
     Bipolar affective disorder
     Depressive episode (or recurrent depressive disorder)
       Mild
       Moderate
       Severe without psychotic symptoms
       Severe with psychotic symptoms
     Persistent mood disorders
       Cyclothymia
       Dysthymia*

Note: *Heterogeneous categories each of which can be considered to include the concept of depressive personality.

sants. The second subtype, 'subaffective dysthymia', is believed to have similar endogenous aetiology, but can appear to be a PD as it begins before the age of 25 and the patient may have seemed chronically depressed throughout adult life. Such people may present as quiet, passive, gloomy, self-critical and conscientious. It is claimed that this disorder also responds to antidepressant medication. The third sub-type is 'chronic secondary dysphoria', and is a chronic depressive disorder that seems understandable as a reaction to some other chronic psychiatric disorder or medical condition such as severe deformity (Winokur, Black & Nasrallah, 1988). Akiskal suggested that some of these patients respond to a monoamine oxidase inhibitor. Finally, there are the 'character-spectrum disorders', in which the patient is chronically depressed since childhood or adolescence in the context of various types of severe PD, for example with dependent, borderline or sociopathic traits, which are often associated with self-injury and antisocial behaviour. Akiskal claims that, in contrast to those with 'subaffective dysthymia', such patients do not usually respond significantly to antidepressant medication.

Other classifications of depression have been based on the presence or absence of another non-affective psychiatric disorder, of delusions (Coryell *et al.*, 1994), or of a history of mania, and the latter provides perhaps the simplest and most robust classification. This involves the division of depressive disorders into the two subtypes of unipolar and bipolar depression (Table 2.2). There is evidence that genetic predisposition is required for the development of disorders in the bipolar group, while unipolar depression 'is usually considered to encompass a variety of illnesses with different aetiologies and treatments; it is not clear whether hypotheses relating to personality and depression are relevant to all forms of depression or only to specific subtypes. Therefore, different findings from different studies of depressed patients may be hard to integrate because of diagnostic heterogeneity' (Hirschfeld & Shea, 1992). Table 2.2 also shows the main categories of depressive disorders in the major international classifications; the concept of depressive personality is subsumed in the broader categories of 'dysthymias' in both DSM-III-R and ICD-10. In DSM-III-R, another important category is 'major depression', partly defined on the basis of increased severity and episodic course, when compared with dysthymia, but Kendler *et al.* (1993c), in a twin study, found that, in women, there is an association between 'neuroticism' and liability to major depression and it is clear that PDs can be of aetiological importance in some cases of 'major depression'. DSM-III-R's dysthymia usually begins in childhood, adolescence, or early adult life and precedes any superimposed major depressive episodes, if any, by years (Akiskal, 1991). (The return to a mild or moderate chronic dysthymia following recovery from a superimposed major depressive episode has been termed a 'double-depressive' pattern.) Dysthymia is described by the DSM-III-R as 'a chronic disturbance of mood involving depressed mood (or possibly an irritable mood in children and adolescents), for most of the day, more days than not, for at least 2 years (1 year for children and adolescents)'. Similarly, the ICD-10 describes dysthymia as

a chronic depression of mood. . . . The balance between individual phases of mild depression and intervening periods of comparative normality is very variable. Sufferers usually have periods of days or weeks when they describe themselves as well, but most of the time (often for months at a time) they feel tired and depressed; everything is an effort and nothing is enjoyed . . . It usually begins early in adult life and lasts for at least several years, sometimes indefinitely. . . .

However, dysthymia is a wider concept than depressive personality; the latter should have an early onset, which is not essential for dysthymia, and be more stable than some disorders that attract the dysthymia diagnosis.

Cyclothymia is also a category in both these classifications and has been reviewed by Howland & Thase (1993); in DSM-III-R this refers to 'a chronic mood disturbance . . . involving numerous hypomanic episodes and numerous periods of depressed mood or loss of interest or pleasure of insufficient severity or duration to meet the criteria for a major depression or a manic episode'. ICD-10 describes a similar disorder with 'a persistent instability of mood, involving numerous periods of mild depression and mild elation. This instability usually develops early in adult life and pursues a chronic course, although at times the mood may be normal and stable for months at a time'. This category has also been called 'affective personality disorder', 'cycloid personality' and 'cyclothymic personality', but is now considered to be a relatively mild variant of bipolar affective disorder (manic-depressive disorder), and not a PD. There is an increased prevalence of cyclothymia in relatives of patients with bipolar affective disorder, and some cyclothymic individuals will eventually develop bipolar affective disorder or recurrent depressive disorder (using ICD-10 terminology).

Both cyclothymia and borderline PD are associated with unstable mood and impulsivity, but cyclothymic patients, who may be misdiagnosed as having borderline PD, may show a greater response to treatment with lithium. Although it has been suggested that cyclothymia may have a specific association with borderline PD (Levitt *et al.*, 1990), this is not established.

Main definitions

Hirschfeld & Shea (1992) have proposed the following criteria for depressive PD: 'tendency to dysphoria, dejection, gloominess, cheerlessness, joylessness; prominent self-concepts of inadequacy, worthlessness and low self-esteem; critical, blaming, derogatory and punitive toward oneself, and prone to guilt; brooding and given to worry; negativistic, critical and judgemental towards others; and pessimistic'. Subsequently, the DSM-IV Work Group on Personality Disorders proposed that the core feature is excessive, negative, pessimistic beliefs about oneself and other people, as indicated by at least five of the following: usual mood is dominated by dejection, gloominess, unhappiness, cheerlessness, joylessness; prominent self-concept centres around beliefs of inadequacy, worthlessness, and low self-esteem; is critical, blaming, derogatory, and punitive toward oneself; is brooding and given to worry; is negativistic, critical, and judgmental towards others; is pessimistic; and is prone to feeling guilt, remorse. These must not occur exclusively during major depressive episodes (Hirschfeld & Holzer, 1994). These features form the research criteria for depressive PD in DSM-IV as a criteria set 'provided for further study'.

Table 2.3 *Categories of relationship between personality disorder (PD) and depressive disorders*

1. Personality traits that predispose to the development of depressive disorders
2. Personality traits that may be the consequence of depressive disorders
3. Personality traits that modify the symptom pattern, course and outcome of depressive disorders
4. 'Depressive PD' refers to:
    (a) some examples of DSM-III-R's 'dysthymia'
    (b) some examples of ICD-10's 'dysthymia'
    (c) 'subaffective dysthymia'
    (d) some examples of the 'general neurotic syndrome'
   Hypothesis: some examples of 'depressive PD' (e.g. patients with subaffective dysthymia) are variants of bipolar affective disorder
5. 'Character-spectrum disorder,' similar to:
    (a) 'depressive-spectrum disease'
    (b) 'hysteroid dysphoria'
   Hypothesis: this category of depression is mainly a psychological reaction to complications of behaviour related to PDs, in particular borderline PD

Clinical features

Depressive PD reflects one type of association between PD and depressed mood, and there are five main relationships that have been identified. These are shown in Table 2.3 (Phillips *et al.*, 1990; Hirschfeld & Shea, 1992).

Firstly, personality traits may predispose to the development of a depressive disorder (Klerman & Hirschfeld, 1988) and claims have been made in this respect for excessive dependency; an excessive need for reassurance, support and attention; and high reward dependence, harm avoidance and novelty seeking (Hirschfeld & Shea, 1992; Svrakic, Przybeck & Cloninger, 1992). In a prospective study of antenatal subjects, high interpersonal sensitivity appeared to be a risk factor of subsequent depression 6 months after childbirth (Boyce *et al.*, 1991).

Secondly, maladaptive changes in personality may follow as a consequence of a depressive disorder. For example, in a recent review, Akiskal (1991) identified the syndrome of 'residual major depression', in which patients with an unremarkable premorbid adjustment develop residual chronicity after one or more depressive episodes, which do not remit fully. He noted that the course of an unipolar depressive illness beginning after the age of 50 is often protracted, and secondary personality changes can involve pessimism, passivity, a sense of resignation, generalized fear of inability to cope, adherence to rigid routines and inhibited communication. Also, more serious maladaptive behaviour may follow, involving unstable relationships, promiscuous behaviour, and substance abuse. This syndrome should be distinguished from 'anxious or atypical depression', which is another chronic depressive disorder and involves mild to moderate anxiety and depression with fatigue (Akiskal, 1991). These disorders are conceptualized as secondary to anxiety disorders although other PD features may co-occur by chance. Clinical features in patients (who are typically young) include fatigue, low self-confidence, feeling worse in the evening, insomnia, oversleeping in the morning and overeating.

Thirdly, personality may have a pathoplastic effect on the symptom pattern, course and outcome of depressive disorders. Obsessive-compulsive traits or PD may contribute to the development of pronounced morbid worry and preoccupation with guilt, and obsessionality has been associated with poor outcome (Duggan, Lee & Murray, 1990), while features of histrionic PD may be associated with hostility, demanding or manipulative behaviour and complaints. Also, in a study of the relationship between PDs and treatment outcome in 239 outpatients, those with PD had a significantly worse outcome in terms of social functioning and residual symptoms of depression (Shea *et al.*, 1990). But although a clinician's attention is usually directed towards maladaptive aspects of a patient's personality, the presence of adaptive features (i.e. a person's strengths of character) are also likely to exert pathoplastic effects. Another long-term study has shown that personality variables can influence outcome of depressive disorders (Andrews *et al.*, 1990).

The fourth category of relationship between PD and depressive disorders involves the concept of 'depressive PD', which corresponds to various descriptions, including 'dysthymia' and Akiskal's 'sub-affective dysthymia' (Phillips *et al.*, 1990). The latter has been associated with a favourable response to antidepressant drugs and sometimes with the following: development of hypomania; shortened REM latency which is a characteristic of severe primary major depression; family history of unipolar or bipolar affective disorder; unremarkable developmental history; relatively good social outcome; equal sex distribution; and indeterminate onset (usually before age 25). Rihmer (1990) reported that such patients had abnormal results on the dexamethasone suppression test, which are also associated with severe primary major depression. Associated personality traits were similar to those described by Schneider (see above), i.e. gloomy, pessimistic, serious, incapable of enjoyment or relaxation; quiet, passive, indecisive; sceptical, hypercritical, complaining; worrying, brooding; duty-bound, conscientious, self-disciplining; self-doubting, self-critical, self-reproaching, self-derogatory; and preoccupied with inadequacy, failure, and negative events to the point of morbid enjoyment of one's failures. Although such individuals were generally introverted, with minimal social life, they could pursue a limited range of interests.

The relationship between depressive PD and the 'general neurotic syndrome' (GNS) as described by Tyrer *et al.* (1992), is uncertain, but there appears to be some overlap. The GNS is a combination of anxiety and depression, with features of avoidant, obsessive-compulsive and dependent PDs. It also involves excessive timidity, poor self-esteem, avoidance of anxiety-provoking situations and excessive dependence on others.

The fifth and final category of relationship between PD and depressive disorders involves 'character-spectrum disorder', which has been associated with the following: irritability; relatively poor response to antidepressant medication; normal REM latency; normal dexamethasone suppression; family history of alcoholism and sociopathy; childhood parental loss, separation or divorce; poor social outcome; greater prevalence among females; onset in childhood or adolescence; and polysubstance or alcohol abuse (Akiskal, Rosenthal & Haykal, 1980). The associated personality traits are variable but a mixture of dependent, histrionic, antisocial and borderline PD features is usually found, and there is more social and mood instability than is found with subaffective dysthymia. It has been suggested that character-spectrum disorder involves a mood disorder that is secondary to the complications of an heterogeneous mixture of PDs, in particular borderline PD, whereas depressed mood is an integral part of the various subtypes of depressive PD.

Although borderline PD with depression can be considered as just one type of character-spectrum disorder, many claims that patients with borderline PD have a high prevalence of depression have led to particular attention to this association. Such depression tends to show features specific to co-occurrence with borderline PD, i.e. complaints of chronic emptiness and feelings of loneliness (Grinker, Werble & Drye, 1968). (The term 'hysteroid dysphoria', which refers to repeated episodes of depressed mood in response to relationship difficulties, is often associated with borderline PD.) However, Gunderson & Phillips (1991) concluded that the relationship between borderline PD and depression is probably non-specific, as some other PDs are as likely, or more likely, to be associated with depressive symptoms, in particular obsessive-compulsive, avoidant and dependent PDs. Although depression with borderline PD may respond to some degree to tricyclic antidepressants in a minority of patients, both hysteroid dysphoria and depression with borderline PD may respond preferentially to MAOI (monoamine oxidase inhibitor) antidepressants, in particular tranylcypromine (Dowson, 1987). However, other drugs, such as phenothiazine, fluoxetine, lithium and carbamazepine, have also been shown to have some effect on depressive symptoms with borderline PD, and it has been suggested that the effects of these drugs may be mediated by a reduction in behavioural dyscontrol (impulsivity) rather than by a change in mood. Gunderson & Phillips (1991) concluded that the affective symptoms of patients with borderline PD may respond as well to antipsychotic drugs as to antidepressants, and while this does not imply that antidepressants do not have a role in the treatment of depression with borderline PD, their effect 'is not likely to be as specific or profound as in uncomplicated depressions'. However, some patients with borderline PD appear to have, by chance, co-occurring bipolar disorder or major depression with episodic endogenous aetiology.

'Character spectrum disorder' is very similar to Winokur's concept of 'depressive-spectrum disease', which was defined by the presence of unipolar depression with a history of alcoholism and/or antisocial personality in first-degree relatives, while, in contrast, 'pure depressive disease' showed no such family history. Compared with the latter, depressive-spectrum disease was associated with earlier age of onset, female gender, personality problems and difficulties (particularly more frequent divorce and separation), lifelong irritability, and more variable symptoms. Other studies have reported similar findings (Akiskal, 1991), but unlike Winokur's claim of a favourable outcome for character-spectrum disorder, recent studies have found that depressed patients with PDs appear to have a worse outcome (Hirschfeld & Shea, 1992).

Character-spectrum disorder also appears to incorporate 'hysteroid dysphoria' (Liebowitz & Klein, 1979) in which women are usually affected and there are repeated episodes of depressed mood as a consequence of feeling rejected within close relationships. Such individuals are over-reliant on approval, attention or praise, and show an extreme intolerance to personal rejection. They have been called 'attention junkies'. Mood reactivity is preserved, and fatigue is a common complaint together with overeating and oversleeping.

Although, in general, character-spectrum disorder appears to be less responsive than other main categories of depressive disorder to antidepressants, lithium or both, certain subtypes of this heterogeneous category and certain individual patients may benefit from medication. For example, phenelzine has been claimed to be useful in 'hysteroid dysphoria' (Kayser *et al.*, 1985), and Akiskal (1991) suggested that many of the character-spectrum disorders may eventually respond to future new antidepressant medications.

Character-spectrum disorder seems to be associated mainly with DSM-III-R's cluster B PDs, which include borderline PD, but other PDs are also common in depressed patients (i.e. those with DSM-III-R's major depression or dysthymia), for example obsessive-compulsive, passive-aggressive, schizoid, schizotypal, paranoid and dependent PDs (Alnaes & Torgersen, 1988a, b, 1991). In patients with major depression ($n = 197$), with dysthymia ($n = 62$) and with both disorders ($n = 32$), at least one PD was found in 50%, 52% and 69% of the sample respectively, and the most common were avoidant and dependent PDs (Sanderson *et al.*, 1992).

Presentation to medical services

DSM-III-R dysthymia (which can be considered to include depressive PD) is common in clinical practice and appears to be more prevalent in females, while character-spectrum disorder involves depressive features in the context of various PDs and may present with social and relationship problems, substance abuse and self-harm episodes.

Associated features

Depressive PD can sometimes be associated with a good response to antidepressant medication, while the heterogeneous group of character-spectrum disorders are generally less responsive to drug treatments. However, there are claims that some individuals with character-spectrum disorder, for example with hysteroid dysphoria, respond to medication, in particular MAOIs (Tyrer, Casey & Gall, 1983).

Current status

The concept of depressive PD remains controversial and this term is not featured in the main international classifications, although in DSM-IV it is a criteria set 'provided for further study'. There is evidence to support such a category (Widiger, 1989), such as reports in relation to the similar concept of sub-affective dysthymia, involving young adults with chronic depression and maladaptive personality traits (other than antisocial and borderline features), who appear to respond to antidepressant medication. Such individuals may have a variant of bipolar manic-depressive disorder, mediated by genetic predisposition, and many patients who would have been previously diagnosed as having a PD can be reclassified as having a form of chronic reversible depression. This has led to successful treatment with antidepressant medication and the claim that 'physicians should therefore attempt vigorous pharmacological interventions with most forms of chronic depression ... psychotherapy alone proves inadequate for many of these patients' (Akiskal, 1991). In addition, Hirschfeld & Holzer (1994) claimed that the results of the DSM-IV Mood Disorders Field Trial show that the DSM-IV criteria for depressive PD (previously described) identifies a group of patients many of whom do not receive other diagnoses involving depressive symptoms.

Organic personality disorder

Main features and clinical origins

This category is found in the ICD-10 classification and refers to an alteration of personality and behaviour that 'can be a residual or concomitant disorder of brain disease, damage, or dysfunction' and involves 'a significant alteration of the habitual patterns of premorbid behaviour', particularly in relation to the expression of emotions, needs and impulses.

Main definitions and clinical features

In addition to a history or other evidence of brain disease, damage or dysfunction, the ICD-10 requires two or more of the following criteria to be met:

consistently reduced ability to persevere with goal-directed activities, especially those involving longer periods of time and postponed gratification; altered emotional behaviour, characterised by emotional lability, shallow and unwarranted cheerfulness (euphoria, inappropriate jocularity), and easy change to irritability or short-lived outbursts of anger and aggression – in some instances apathy may be a more prominent feature; expressions of needs and impulses without consideration of consequences or social convention (the patient may engage in dissocial acts, such as stealing, inappropriate sexual advances, or voracious eating, or may exhibit disregard for personal hygiene); cognitive disturbance, in the form of suspiciousness or paranoid ideation, and/or excessive preoccupation with a single, usually abstract, theme (e.g. religion, right and wrong); marked alteration of the rate and flow of language production with features such as circumstantiality, over-inclusiveness ...; and altered sexual behaviour ...'.

Some of these features, for example emotional lability and lack of consideration of consequences, have been part of the so-called frontal lobe syndrome, but these and other features of organic PD can also occur with lesions to other parts of the brain.

Welch & Bear (1990) have reviewed many of the wide range of personality changes that can occur as a result of organic (i.e. identifiable) brain disorders. A variety of disorders need to be considered if there is an unexplained appearance of 'personality disorder', and these include temporal lobe epilepsy, tumours, Huntington's disease, Parkinson's disease, multiple sclerosis, AIDs encephalopathy and the effects of neurotoxins. For example, some reports have linked apparent obsessive-compulsive PD with temporal lobe epilepsy, paranoid and aggressive behaviour with Huntington's or Parkinson's diseases, and social withdrawal and indecisiveness with AIDS encephalopathy. A 'pseudo-psychopathic syndrome', with disinhibited, impulsive and socially inappropriate behaviour, is associated with orbital-medial frontal lobe damage, while a 'pseudodepressive syndrome', with lack of spontaneity, apathy and indifference is related to dorsolateral frontal lobe lesions.

Enduring personality change after psychiatric illness

Main features and clinical origins

The ICD-10 includes this category to describe apparent personality changes due to the experience of a severe psychiatric illness. These involve such features as excessive dependence, reduced interests and social isolation.

Main definition and clinical features

There should be no evidence of a similar pre-existing PD, although previous personality vulnerability may be a predisposing factor. ICD-10 specifies the following range of clinical features:

excessive dependence on and a demanding attitude towards others; conviction of being changed or stigmatised by preceding illness, leading to an inability to form and maintain close and confiding personal relationships and to social isolation; passivity, reduced interests, and diminished involvement in leisure activities; persistent complaints of being ill, which may be associated with hypochondriacal claims and illness behaviour; dysphoric or labile mood, not due to the presence of a current mental disorder or antecedent mental disorder with residual affective symptoms; and significant impairment in social and occupational functioning compared with the premorbid situation.

3

Personality disorders: less specific clinical presentations and epidemiology

J.H. DOWSON

Personality disorder not otherwise specified (DSM-III-R and DSM IV) or mixed and other personality disorders (ICD-10)

Main features and definitions

The DSM-III-R and DSM-IV category of 'personality disorder – not otherwise specified' refers to any disorder of personality that cannot be classified as one or more specific PDs, for example, features of one or more PDs that do not meet the full criteria for any one PD, yet cause significant impairment in social or occupational functioning, or subjective distress.

The ICD-10 category 'mixed and other personality disorders' is similar but also includes the disorders of patients who have several PDs but without a predominant set of symptoms. The latter would be expected to be the most prevalent PD diagnosis in psychiatric practice, as many studies have shown frequent co-occurrence of two or more PDs in various patient populations.

Clinical features

Most studies of PDs have found that at least 50% of patients with PD had two or more PDs (Oldham *et al.*, 1992); for instance Nurnberg *et al.* (1991) found 82% of patients with borderline PD had at least one additional PD diagnosis from another DSM-III-R PD cluster. Although the term 'co-morbidity' has generally been used to denote co-existing disorders that have distinct causes, the term 'co-occurrence' is more appropriate in relation to PDs, as it does not have any aetiological implications.

In a study of 106 applicants for long-term treatment of severe PD (Oldham *et al.*, 1992), which used structured interviews for PD assessment, statistically significant associations were found involving six pairs of PDs, namely histrionic and borderline, histrionic and narcissistic, narcissistic and antisocial, narcissistic and passive-aggressive, avoidant and schizotypal, and avoidant and dependent. It was concluded that frequent and consistent patterns of co-occurrence had been shown.

Many other studies have reported that co-occurrence is common, as evaluated by various methods in many clinical and non-clinical populations (Dowson, 1992*b*). Zimmerman & Coryell (1989) assessed DSM-III PDs with an interview method in a non-patient sample of 797 relatives of patients and controls; about 17% had at least one PD diagnosis and, of these subjects, about 25% had more than one. The most prevalent PDs were mixed, passive-aggressive, antisocial, histrionic and schizotypal PDs. With the increasing attention given to borderline PD as defined by DSM-III and DSM-III-R, several studies have examined its co-occurrence with other PDs (Grueneich, 1992). It appears that the most frequently-reported association has been with histrionic PD, but co-occurrence has also been found with other PDs including schizotypal, antisocial, dependent and passive-aggressive. Also, several studies have provided evidence in support of relationships between co-occurring PDs which reflect the three PD 'clusters' defined by DSM-III-R (Dowson & Berrios, 1991).

Associated features

The co-occurrence of PDs and non-PD psychiatric disorders may involve significant associations; for example, Nestadt *et al.* (1991) evaluated 810 randomly-selected non-patients in respect of DSM-III compulsive and antisocial PDs, generalized anxiety disorder, alcohol-related disorders and simple phobia, and found that generalized anxiety disorder and simple phobia were associated with obsessive-compulsive PD features, while alcohol-related disorders (and a reduced occurrence of generalized anxiety disorder) were associated with antisocial PD features.

Such associations can be investigated from the perspective of the non-PD disorder by using the latter as the starting point to define a patient population whose PD status is then determined. In the rest of this chapter this approach will be used in an examination of the PD characteristics of patient groups selected on the basis of other disorders.

Depressive disorders and personality disorders

There have been several claims that borderline PD is common among patients with DSM-III-R's 'major depression' (Alnaes & Torgersen, 1990), together with reports of the co-occurrence of major depression and several other PDs. Sato, Sakado & Sato (1993*a*, *b*), in a study of 4-month outcome in 96 outpatients with major depression, noted that while any co-occurring PD worsened outcome, this was particularly found for schizoid PD and other 'cluster A' PD features. Also, Marin *et al.* (1993), in a study comparing PD in patients with 'dysthymia' and episodic 'major depression', found a PD diagnosis in 51% and 42% respectively. The most common PDs in the dysthymia group were avoidant and NOS (not otherwise specified) PDs, while the most common PDs in the major depression group were borderline and NOS PDs. Joyce, Mulder & Cloninger (1994*b*), reporting a group of 84 patients with major depression treated with antidepressants, found that temperament (as measured by the Tridimensional Personality Questionnaire) accounted for 35% of the variance in treatment outcome, while clinical variables predicted only 5%. In relation to DSM-III 'dysthymic disorder', there were more co-occurrences with avoidant, self-defeating, dependent and borderline PDs, compared with a non-dysthymic patient group (Markowitz *et al.*, 1992).

Some of the associations between PD and certain types of depressive disorder have been described (see depressive personality, Chapter 2), and one of the main conclusions of clinical importance was that some young people with chronic depressive disorders with apparent PD, who have tended to be dismissed as pharmacologically untreatable, can respond to antidepressant medications. It is also important for the clinician to be aware that a non-PD psychiatric disorder, such as a recurrent depressive or manic episode, can lead to an exaggeration of PD psychopathology that may disguise the co-occurring episodic disorder. For example, a patient with some antisocial PD features and a mild manic illness may become considerably more antisocial during the course of the manic episode. The antisocial behaviour may be the predominant feature and, if the person has shown some previous antisocial tendencies, it may not be recognized that an additional disorder is present, namely a treatable manic illness. Another example would be a person with some histrionic and dependent PD features who develops a depressive episode, when his or her behaviour may become childish, demanding and manipulative; if this behaviour predominates, the additional diagnosis of an episodic depressive disorder may be missed.

Suicide and personality disorders

Suicide and other forms of violent death or self-injury have been investigated in relation to their associations with PD, and it should be noted that one of the DSM-III-R criteria for borderline PD is 'recurrent suicidal threats, gestures, or behaviour, or self-mutilating behaviour'.

Several large long-term studies have reported a link between persistent antisocial behaviour and excess mortality. In a follow-up of 500 psychiatric outpatients, unnatural death was associated with antisocial PD as well as with affective disorders, substance abuse and homosexuality, and in a retrospective study of 1056 antisocial Swedish adolescents who had been admitted to 'probationary schools', it was found that 13% of the boys and 10% of the girls had died over a 17-year period. Eighty-eight per cent of the dead boys and 77% of the dead girls had died sudden violent deaths by accident, suicide, death from uncertain causes, murder/manslaughter, or alcohol/drug abuse (Martin, 1986). Similar associations were reported in a prospective follow-up study of 50 465 Swedish conscripts. There were 247 completed suicides during 13 years' follow-up and strong predictors of suicide were early indications of antisocial PD (poor emotional control, deviant behaviour, substance abuse, contact with a child welfare authority or the police, and lack of friends), together with adverse social background (Allebeck, Allgulander & Fisher, 1988). This study also showed that, as well as PD, diagnoses of neurotic disorder or drug dependence at conscription were associated with a significantly increased risk for future suicide (Allebeck & Allgulander, 1990*a*, *b*), although a subsequent period of psychiatric inpatient care was the strongest predictor of suicide.

An approach from a different perspective compared the criminal history of 181 suicides and matched controls: although the difference in the frequency of a history of a criminal record (16% of the suicides and 11% of the controls) was not significant, there was a significant difference in the nature of the offences, as a greater number (more than half) of the offences committed by criminal suicides involved violations of the road traffic laws (Modestin & Emmenegger, 1986). In a study of adolescent suicides in Finland (44 males and 9 females), a history of antisocial behaviour was found in 43%. Separation from parents, and alcohol abuse and violence in the home, had been common in the males, who had shown more alcohol abuse and co-occurring mental disorders compared with those without antisocial behaviour (Marttunen *et al.*, 1994).

Retrospective studies have examined the association between borderline PD and suicide. A study of 58 consecutive suicides by adolescents and young adults (aged 15 to 19) in an urban community, reported borderline PD in 33% (which was the principal diagnosis in 28%), with antisocial PD in 14% (Runeson & Beskow, 1991). Also, a comparison of individuals with borderline PD who committed suicide, with a control group with borderline

PD, found that the suicide group had more frequent childhood loss, lack of treatment contact before hospitalization, longer hospitalization and more frequent discharges for violating a treatment contract (Kjelsberg, Eikeseth & Dahl, 1991).

Self-harm and personality disorders

Repetition of self-harm behaviour is common, with reports of 10–15% of patients being involved in further episodes within a year, and this is associated with a higher risk of completed suicide. But although several risk factors for suicide are known, such as previous self-harm, previous psychiatric treatment, personality disorder (in particular antisocial and borderline PDs), alcohol and drug abuse, unemployment and lower social class, accurate prediction is difficult for the individual patient.

'Self-harm' is an heterogeneous group of behaviours, and several subtypes have been identified, i.e. self-poisoning, self-wounding (which is usually of low lethality), self-mutilation (involving serious injury, usually in the context of a non-PD psychiatric disorder), and the person who makes 'a highly lethal suicide attempt', for example, 'one deep and dangerous cut' (Tantam & Whittaker, 1992). Self-wounding is associated with borderline PD and with a history of sexual or physical abuse; episodes are usually of low lethality, are often chronic and repetitive, are not typically associated with death-orientated thoughts and commonly involve multiple methods of self-injury (Russ, 1992). The patient usually carries out self-wounding behaviour when alone, often in response to a perceived rejection or loss and in a context of emotional arousal, i.e. with anxiety, tension, depression, anger or emptiness. Self-wounding behaviour is not aimed at mutilation or death and the motivation usually appears to be an attempt to influence others or relieve distress, in particular a feeling of tension. The most typical form of self-wounding appears to be wrist-cutting involving superficial wounds, but burning or hitting oneself is also common. However there is a continuum of behaviours, which can progress to severe self-mutilation. Favazza & Conterio (1989) reported 240 women who regularly wounded or mutilated themselves (although more men than women do it), in whom cutting was the commonest method, in 72%. Other behaviours included skin burning in 35%, hitting or punching parts of the body in 30%, interfering with wound healing in 22%, scratching in 22%, hair pulling in 10%, and breaking bones in 8%. The wrists were involved in 74%, the legs in 44%, the abdomen in 25%, the head in 23%, the chest in 18% and the genitalia in 8%. Implements included broken glass, needles, scissors, razor blades, knives, hammers and cigarettes. A study which compared a group of patients with PD and an history of self-wounding, with a control group without self-wounding but matched for PD, reported that the degree of self-wounding was significantly correlated with impulsivity, chronic anger and somatic symptoms of anxiety, and that the self-wounding group showed more severe PD, with greater aggression and antisocial behaviour. It has been suggested that self-wounding is related to underlying serotonergic dysfunction (Simeon *et al.*, 1992). Another study of self-wounding compared these behaviours with self-poisoning, and found that the former was more associated with youth, male sex, single status, PD, previous psychiatric inpatient status, use of alcohol at the time of the self-harm episode, alcohol problems, violence against others and violence received from relatives in the preceding 5 years, criminal record and unemployment (Robinson & Duffy, 1989).

Substance use disorders and personality disorders

Many studies have described high rates of PD in samples selected on the basis of substance use disorders, in particular involving antisocial, borderline and narcissistic PDs (Nace, 1989). In a study of alcoholic out-patients, 64% had PD, in particular paranoid PD (in 44%), antisocial PD (in 20%), avoidant PD (in 20%), passive-aggressive PD (in 18%) and borderline PD (in 16%) (Nurnberg, Rifkin & Doddi, 1993), and PD was associated with poorer outcome. Also, the trait of 'alexithymia' has been associated with substance abuse (and with post-traumatic stress disorder), involving an inability of the subject to identify a depressed mood, together with a concrete style of thinking (Wise, Mann & Shay, 1992). Also, in 501 patients seeking treatment for alcohol and other drug problems, the most common other 'lifetime' disorders in their past histories were antisocial PD, phobias, psychosexual dysfunctions and depressive disorders (Ross, Glaser & Germanson, 1992). Co-occurring PD can affect the symptom pattern of substance use disorders as well as treatment response and outcome; of 160 patients admitted to a private inpatient substance abuse programme, the 57% who had PDs differed from the rest in being more impulsive, isolated and depressed (Nace, Davis & Gaspari, 1991). Also, it has been noted that features of PD may occur secondary to (i.e. after) substance abuse, such as when antisocial behaviour results from efforts to obtain money for illicit drugs or alcohol, or when pre-existing mild personality vulnerability becomes more pronounced.

Cloninger and colleagues (1988) have made claims for two main subtypes of alcoholism, which differ in respect of alcohol-related symptoms, personality traits, ages of onset and patterns of inheritance. 'Type 1' alcoholism is associated with later onset, anxiety and dependent PD features, rapid development of tolerance, dependence on the anti-anxiety effects of alcohol, loss of control, bingeing on alcohol, difficulty stopping binges, guilt feelings and liver complications, while 'type 2' alcoholism is related to earlier onset and antisocial PD traits. In the type 2 pattern, alcohol is persistently sought for its euphoriant effects, there tends to be an inability to abstain (rather than bingeing), and various complications occur earlier; these include aggression and criminal involvement when drinking. Also the type 2 disorder appears to be associated with a higher incidence of familial alcoholism.

Although this classification appears to have identified various associations within patient groups and their relatives, some investigators have reported that these two symptom patterns may not be a satisfactory basis on which to divide alcoholism; for example, in a study of 360 male alcoholic patients in hospital, 91% satisfied criteria for both symptom clusters, and when the sample was divided on the basis of early or late onset of alcoholism (which is a variable that can contribute to the 'types 1 and 2' classification, i.e. ≤ 25 years associated with type 2, and ≥ 26 years associated with type 1), 96% of the early onset and 83% of the late onset subgroups still showed a history of both symptom clusters. It was considered that the 'types 1 and 2' classification mainly reflects age of onset of problem drinking, at least in hospital settings (Penick *et al.*, 1988). A similar conclusion resulted from a study which applied Cloninger's subtypes to alcoholic women (Glenn & Nixon, 1991). These subjects were also divided into early and late onset groups (≤ 25 and ≥ 26 years), and group membership did not correlate with the symptomatology of types 1 and 2 as predicted. Most of the women were positive for both types on the basis of symptoms, and this study also suggested that the criteria for grouping patients with alcoholism should be based on age of symptom onset, regardless of symptom type.

In a study which grouped patients on the basis of age of alcoholism onset, those with onset before their 20th birthday had a significantly higher incidence of paternal alcoholism (Buydens-Branchey, Branchey & Noumair, 1989), and patterns of inheritance appear to make a valid contribution to the criteria for the classification of alcoholism. Bohman *et al.* (1987) examined the inheritance of alcohol abuse and PD in 862 men and 913 women adopted by non-relatives, and found that both male and female adoptees were at increased risk of developing alcohol abuse if their biological, but not their adoptive, parents were alcoholic. Three disorders appeared to be associated in biologically related individuals, namely alcohol abuse, somatoform disorders in women and antisocial behaviour in men, and evidence for both genetic and environmental risk factors for alcoholism were found. One of the associations could be explained by a common vulnerability that was expressed as antisocial, violent and criminal behaviour with recurrent alcohol abuse in males, but as frequent somatic complaints (somatoform disorders) in females.

Despite the difficulties in separating some patient populations with alcoholism into subgroups based on types 1 and 2, various features of these subtypes have been related to outcome variables. In a 2-year outpatient treatment programme, all those with an early stable improvement were type 1 alcoholics, while most who improved during the later part of treatment were type 2 (Ojehagen & Berglund, 1986a). Also, in a 20-year follow-up of 84 male alcoholics, those of type 2 showed a relatively high frequency of sporadic abuse and a lower frequency of abstinence and social drinking (Nordstrom & Berglund, 1987).

Many studies have reported on the frequent associations between alcoholism and antisocial PD. In a study of 260 men starting inpatient treatment, those with antisocial PD were distinguished by an earlier onset of alcoholism, involvement with illegal drugs and more problems with control of drinking (Yates, Petty & Brown, 1988), while in another study of 241 alcoholic men, also in hospital (Penick et al., 1988), the most frequent co-occurring disorders were depressive disorders, antisocial PD and drug abuse. Also, a 1-year follow-up study of 266 patients with alcoholism found that, for both men and women, having an additional diagnosis of antisocial PD or drug abuse was associated with a poorer outcome (Rounsaville et al., 1987),

The prevalence of antisocial PD in patients with alcoholism is less in females than in males, but a survey of 50 women attending an alcohol-treatment unit found a high frequency of other behaviours that are often related to PD; about half had taken an overdose, or described a history of impulsive physical violence, or had had a period of promiscuity, while about 25% had an history of self-wounding, and at least 16% had had an eating disorder (Evans & Lacey, 1992).

PDs other than antisocial PD have been claimed to be related to the outcome of alcohol abuse. Griggs & Tyrer (1981) reported that outcome was better for those with schizoid PD than for those with antisocial or no PD, although another study came to the opposite conclusion (Zivich, 1981).

With regard to the abuse of other substances, a study of 76 outpatients who abused cocaine and 'crack' found antisocial PD in 21%, but also passive-aggressive PD in 21%, borderline PD in 18% and self-defeating PD in 18% (Kleinman *et al.*, 1990). Subtypes of cocaine abusers have been suggested by Weiss & Mirin (1986), and include patients with antisocial PD who use cocaine as part of an overall pattern of antisocial behaviour, in contrast to those with narcissistic and borderline PDs who use cocaine for social prestige and to bolster self-esteem. In a comparison of cocaine users and opioid addicts, cocaine users showed lower rates of borderline and antisocial PD features (Malow *et al.*, 1989). Antisocial PD has also been reported to commonly co-occur with chronic solvent abuse (Dinwiddie, Zorumski & Rubin, 1987).

Intravenous drug abuse is of particular importance, as it is associated with HIV transmission. In a study of 273 intravenous drug abusers, who were examined by a structured interview (Brooner *et al.*, 1992), antisocial PD that included a history of childhood conduct disorder was present in 44%, while another 24% met only the criteria for antisocial PD that related to adult life. The former group had a more pervasive and serious pattern of adult antisocial behaviour, and it was suggested that the antisocial behaviour of those who met only the adult criteria for antisocial PD have a late-onset and less severe form of PD. Associations of the injection of illicit drugs in relation to PD was investigated in a study of 92 intravenous drug users who were compared with three other groups: a drug-free group, a group that used cannabis, and a group that had used illicit drugs other than cannabis but had never injected (Dinwiddie, Reich & Cloninger, 1992). It was found that the main difference between the drug users who injected and those that did not was the much higher prevalence (68%) of antisocial PD among the intravenous drug users, and it appeared that this was not just a secondary effect of drug-related antisocial behaviour. Another study of intravenous users showed that those with antisocial PD reported significantly higher rates of sharing of injection-equipment, and of the number of people involved with sharing, than those without antisocial PD (Brooner *et al.*, 1990). There is also evidence that relatively high scores on borderline and antisocial PD features is associated with multiple substance dependence. However, needle-sharing is also influenced by social relationships and gender (Barnard, 1993), and women injectors may be at greater risk of HIV transmission than males. Perkins *et al.* (1993) found that PD was common in the HIV-positive population, and that those with PD had a reduced ability to cope with the threat of AIDS.

Somatization disorder and personality disorders

The features of DSM-III-R's 'somatization disorder' are 'recurrent and multiple somatic complaints, of several years' duration, for which medical attention has been sought, but that apparently are not due to any physical disorder. The disorder begins before the age of 30 and has a chronic but fluctuating course'. It is mainly diagnosed in women and estimates of lifetime prevalence rates have varied between 0.2 and 2%. DSM-III-R also notes that

the male relatives of females with this disorder show an increased risk of antisocial personality disorder and psychoactive substance use disorders. Adoption studies indicate that both genetic and environmental factors contribute to the risk of this group of disorders, because both biologic and adoptive parents with any of the disorders increase the risk of antisocial personality disorders, psychoactive substance use disorders and somatization disorder.

Therefore, somatization disorder has been considered as a female equivalent to antisocial PD in men, both sharing a similar genetic substrate. In a study of 25 women with somatization disorder and matched patient controls with depressive or anxiety disorders, the prevalence of PDs among the former group was 72% compared with 36% among controls. Dependent and histrionic PD features were among those that occurred significantly more often (Stern, Murphy & Bass, 1993).

Somatization disorder (which is also known as Briquet's syndrome) has also been considered to be a variation of DSM-III-R's 'conversion disorder' (or 'hysterical neurosis, conversion type'), which involves 'an alteration or loss of physical functioning that suggests physical disorder, but that instead is apparently an expression of a psychological conflict or need. The symptoms of the disturbance are not intentionally produced and, after appropriate investigation, cannot be explained by any physical disorder or known pathophysiologic mechanism' (American Psychiatric Association, 1987). Examples of conversion symptoms can include apparent paralysis, blindness and co-ordination disturbances. PD, in particular histrionic PD, has been associated with somatization disorder and conversion disorder, and has been suggested as a predisposing factor, but histrionic and other DSM-III-R 'cluster B' PDs are not invariably present. Chandrasekaran, Goswami & Sivakumar (1994), in a follow-up study of 'hysterical neurosis' found that premorbid 'hysterical personality' predicted poor outcome.

The association of PD with the related condition of DSM-III-R 'dissociative disorders' (or 'hysterical neuroses, dissociative type') is less certain.
In dissociative disorders there is a change in the way identity, memory, and
conscious awareness are experienced and integrated. If identity is mainly
affected, the person's usual identity can be temporarily 'forgotten' (i.e. is
not available to conscious awareness), and, in an extreme variant of this
disorder, a new identity (or more than one new identities) may be evident.
The latter variant has been called 'multiple personality disorder' but this is
not grouped with the other PDs as it more closely resembles other
dissociative disorders. 'Multiple personality disorder' 'involves two or
more distinct "personalities", sometimes with unique memories, behaviours and social relationships. Such "personalities" can be aware of the
others but this is not invariable as the 'personality' that presents for
treatment may have little or no awareness of the existence of the other
"personalities"' (American Psychiatric Association, 1987). But concepts
and diagnosis in relation to multiple personality disorder are confusing and
controversial (Piper, 1994). Usually most 'personalities' of multiple personality disorder report lost periods of time or periodic confusion about past
experience of time. Sometimes one or more of the 'personalities' shows
features of another disorder, such as borderline PD, but 'it is unclear
whether these represent coexisting disorders or merely associated features
of multiple personality disorder' (American Psychiatric Association, 1987).
This syndrome appears to have been diagnosed from 3 to 9 times more
frequently in females, and complications include self-wounding, violence
and substance use disorder. In such cases a PD may co-occur by chance,
and the existence of specific predisposing PD features is uncertain. However, as histrionic PD appears to be more frequently associated with
somatization disorder compared with the other PDs, this PD, together with
related 'cluster B' PDs, may also be a predisposing factor for the related
dissociative disorders. Other, more common, dissociative disorders include
a 'psychogenic fugue', i.e. 'a sudden, unexpected travel away from home or
customary work locale with assumption of a new identity and an inability
to recall one's previous identity', and 'psychogenic amnesia', i.e. 'a sudden
inability to recall important personal information' (American Psychiatric
Association, 1987). Another related syndrome is 'factitious illness' or
'Munchausen's syndrome', in which physical symptoms and signs of illness
are fabricated; for example, a cut may not heal because the individual
repeatedly opens the wound. While deliberate malingering can occur,
dissociative states may reduce awareness of the individual's actions in

factitious illness, and co-occurring PD may act as a non-specific predisposing factor. A variant of this disorder is factitious illness 'by proxy' involving, for example, a parent fabricating the disorder in a child (Sims, 1992).

In addition to an apparent association between histrionic PD and somatization disorder, there has been accumulating evidence for an association between somatization disorder, conversion disorder and antisocial PD (Lilienfeld *et al.*, 1986). Guze, Woodruff & Clayton (1971*a*) found an increased prevalence of conversion symptoms associated with antisocial PD, while Guze, Woodruff & Clayton (1971*b*) compared 30 women with a form of 'hysterical' disorder (i.e. conversion or dissociative) with 33 women with anxiety neurosis, and found a higher rate of childhood delinquency in the former. Also, Cloninger & Guze's study of 66 female felons (1970) reported that 40% of those with antisocial PD had received an additional diagnosis of an hysterical disorder. Follow-up studies have also provided evidence for such an association; Robins (1966) found that of 76 girls referred to a child guidance clinic for antisocial behaviour, 20 subsequently developed an adult hysterical disorder, compared with no cases in a control group. Family studies have also shown that antisocial PD and somatization disorder are related; for example, Woerner & Guze (1968) found a high prevalence of antisocial PD among the first-degree relatives of subjects with somatization disorder, while Guze, Wolfgram & McKinney (1967) reported a high frequency of somatization disorder among the female relatives of male criminals. Also, somatization disorder and antisocial PD are often seen among the parents of hyperactive children. Lilienfeld *et al.* (1986) reported the association of antisocial PD, histrionic PD and somatization disorder within individuals and within families in 250 patients; the strongest relationship was between antisocial and histrionic PDs in different individuals. In this study, a high prevalence of antisocial PD was found in the families of patients with somatization disorder but not in the families of patients with histrionic PD, and it was suggested that somatization disorder in women and antisocial PD in men may represent gender-related variants based on similar causal factors.

If histrionic PD and somatization disorder co-occur, the demanding, dramatic behaviour of histrionic PD will focus attention on any unexplained somatic symptoms. This would be expected to increase the likelihood that somatization disorder will be diagnosed, as patients are likely to return relatively often for medical consultations (Morrison, 1989).

Anxiety disorders and personality disorders

The main categories of anxiety disorders in DSM-III-R and DSM-IV are panic disorder (with or without agoraphobia), agoraphobia, social phobia, specific phobia and generalized anxiety disorder.

In a review of the role of personality in anxiety disorders, Papp *et al.* (1990) concluded that PDs are more common in patients with anxiety disorders than in the general untreated population, although the significance and nature of the associations are uncertain; for instance, it is often unclear whether the apparent PD features are premorbid, or the result of the chronic experience of anxiety. Sanderson *et al.* (1994) studied a group of 347 patients with anxiety disorders and found that 35% had at least one PD. PD was rare with simple phobia, and the most common PDs were those of 'cluster C', in particular avoidant and obsessive-compulsive PDs.

It might be expected that there are relationships between anxiety disorders and schizotypal, borderline and avoidant PDs, as all these PDs have criteria related to anxiety. Schizotypal PD can involve excessive social anxiety, borderline PD criteria include affective instability which may involve anxiety, and avoidant PD is associated with fear of negative evaluation. The ICD-10 category that corresponds to avoidant PD is termed 'anxious PD', which involves 'persistent and pervasive feelings of tension and apprehension ...', so that it has been argued that avoidant (or anxious) PD cannot be usefully distinguished from social phobia, a view that is supported by the finding that most patients with social phobia qualify for the diagnosis of avoidant PD (Schneier *et al.*, 1991). One model for the relationship between avoidant PD and anxiety disorders is that anxiety exaggerates the features of avoidant PD, so that the number and degree of the features of avoidant PD are positively correlated with the severity of anxiety, and this hypothesis was supported by the finding that avoidant PD scores fell in association with successful treatment of anxiety symptoms. But although certain avoidant PD features appeared to be highly correlated with an improvement in anxiety symptoms (i.e. they were 'state-dependent'), others showed little change (Noyes *et al.*, 1991).

Several studies have examined groups of patients with panic disorder and/or agoraphobia, and reported rates of co-occurring PDs which ranged from 27% to 58% (Pollack *et al.*, 1992). Patients with frequent panic attacks often have high anticipatory levels of anxiety, and seem dependent, avoidant and unassertive. Also, Hoffart *et al.* (1994) found that avoidant and dependent traits were related to symptom severity in patients with agoraphobia and panic disorder. Although some PD features, such as those of dependent PD, may become less marked if panic symptoms are successfully treated, others, such as those of histrionic PD, appear to be more resistant to change (Mavissakalian & Hamann, 1986). This suggests that some PD traits as measured by current methods are 'epiphenomena' of panic disorder, while others may represent a premorbid predisposition for panic disorder and agoraphobia. However, predisposing PD features may not all have a high degree of specificity; for example, in a study of 187 patients with panic disorder and 51 with obsessive-compulsive disorder, the most frequent PDs in the former group (avoidant, dependent, histrionic and borderline PDs) were also more frequent in those with obsessive-compulsive disorder (Mavissakalian, Hamann & Jones, 1990*a, b*). But it has been suggested that panic disorder and features of certain PDs may share causal factors (Mavissakalian, 1990), and it seems that behaviourally inhibited and anxious children are at increased risk of developing adult anxiety disorders. Complex interactions are possible, as childhood anxiety may be a factor in the development of certain PD features.

Papp and colleagues' review (1990) concluded that, in eight studies, about half the patients with panic and/or agoraphobia had one or more DSM-III-R 'cluster C' PDs, involving avoidant, dependent, obsessive-compulsive and passive-aggressive PDs. But other associated PDs have also been reported; for example, in a study of 55 outpatients with anxiety disorders, 13% had borderline PD, 11% histrionic PD, 11% passive-aggressive PD and 13% schizotypal PD (Alnaes & Torgersen, 1988*b*). Although this study found a relatively low co-occurrence with borderline PD, severe and chronic anxiety has been described as a characteristic feature of this disorder, and affective instablity is featured in its DSM-III-R criteria. Benjamin *et al.* (1989) compared groups of subjects on several measures of anxiety; the groups included 11 patients with discrete border-line PD, 31 normal subjects, and 16 with depressive disorders. Those with borderline PD did not appear to be more anxious than the other patient groups, but showed more hostility, interpersonal sensitivity and suspiciousness. It was suggested that marked mood changes, including anxiety, are mainly related to interpersonal contexts in those with borderline PD, while methods used to assess anxiety often relate to feelings that the patient has when alone or out of the interpersonal context. Outside interpersonal situations, those with borderline PD may experience mood changes such as non-specific arousal or agitation, which are not described as anxiety, but give rise to complaints such as being 'unreal', 'detached' or 'lost'. For those with borderline PD, even in an interpersonal context, the usual terminology of anxiety disorders may not be used; instead, a patient may say they are angry, misunderstood or criticized. This calls into question the definition of anxiety; if this is based on autonomic arousal, it may be that those with borderline PD would often show high scores, but the usual assessment methods may not identify the particular type of anxiety often experienced by many patients with borderline PD.

Several studies have indicated that co-occurring PD can adversely affect the response to treatment, course and outcome of anxiety disorders, as well as of other syndromes such as major depression and obsessive-compulsive disorder (Brooks *et al.*, 1991; Reich & Green, 1991). In a study of the effect of borderline PD on outcome in 110 outpatients with anxiety disorders or (non-major) depressive disorders, borderline PD was present in 20%, and those patients with co-occurring anxiety disorder and borderline PD had the poorest outcome (Nurnberg, Raskin & Levine, 1989). It was noted that PD must be recognized as a potential source of variance in treatment studies of various disorders including anxiety disorders. A similar conclusion was reported in a study of 52 patients with panic disorder, in which the outcome of 8 weeks' treatment with benzodiazepines was negatively associated with antisocial, borderline, histrionic and narcissistic PDs (Reich, 1988). Also, the presence of a PD in a sample of 316 patients, many with anxiety disorders, significantly impaired the outcome of treatment with phenelzine (Tyrer *et al.*, 1983). (Obsessive-compulsive PD was the most prevalent PD diagnosis in this study.)

Schizophrenia and personality disorders

Eugen Bleuler (1911) introduced the term 'schizophrenia' in his book *Dementia Praecox or the Group of Schizophrenias*, although he noted 'For the sake of convenience, I use the singular, although it is apparent that the group includes several diseases'. Dalén & Hays (1990) have pointed out that subsequent authors have tended to 'vacilitate between assumptions of homogeneity and heterogeneity', and that 'there is general agreement about the importance of genetic factors in schizophrenia but no evidence shows that genes are equally important in all cases'.

The division of schizophrenia into subtypes, together with their relationships with unipolar depressions, bipolar affective disorders and schizoaffective disorders, remains unclear. Crow (1986) has suggested that schizophrenia and affective disorders are related to a genetic continuum, while Cloninger *et al.* (1985) claimed 'a point of rarity' between symptoms of schizophrenia and other psychiatric disorders. A review by Pope & Lipinsky (1978) considered that 'schizophrenics of the good prognosis category show typically two to three times as much familial affective illness as schizophrenia; poor prognosis groups show a two to three fold difference in the opposite direction'. Such claims support the view of Murray & O'Callaghan (1991) that 'the appropriate genetic distinction is not between schizophrenia and affective psychosis, but rather between acute schizophrenia, schizoaffective disorder and affective psychoses on the one hand and chronic schizophrenia and schizotypal personality on the other'.

The influential definitions of schizophrenia in the DSM-III-R and ICD-10 each produces a relatively broad category which incorporates the more chronic disorders, so that most research has been based on heterogeneous patient groups. Broadly-defined schizophrenia has been shown to be associated with a higher-than-expected history of obstetric complications (which is itself associated with earlier onset of schizophrenia, male gender and chronic course), of minor physical abnormalities (postulated to indicate abnormal development during the second trimester of foetal life and itself associated with earlier onset, male gender and cognitive impairment), and of childhood behavioural abnormalities. The latter include poor social adjustment and premorbid schizoid or schizotypal features. Patients with schizophrenia and a history of such childhood abnormalities are associated with an early onset of illness, male gender, a family history of schizophrenia or a history of obstetric complications. (The findings in relation to gender and schizophrenia have been reviewed by Goldstein & Tsuang, 1990.)

Murray & O'Callaghan (1991) have reviewed the evidence for the identification of a 'neurodevelopmental' or 'congenital' subtype of schizophrenia resulting from a genetic defect (associated with smaller temporal lobe structures and neuropathological changes in the hippocampus) or from an early adverse effect on brain development in foetal or neonatal life, perhaps due to obstetric complications or maternal influenza. It was suggested that this neurodevelopmental subtype is particularly likely to show social impairment in childhood, such as unusual patterns of thought and communication as early as the age of 5, together with abnormal premorbid personality in adolescence. It was also hypothesized that some other subtypes of schizophrenia are genetically related to some affective disorders.

Bleuler (1911) was the first to describe features reminiscent of schizophrenia in some relatives of patients with schizophrenia, and the convincing evidence for an association between schizoid (and schizotypal) PD features and schizophrenia in genetically related families has been reviewed in Chapter 2, together with the evidence for the association between premorbid schizoid (and schizotypal) PD and the subsequent development of schizophrenia. Also, Dalkin *et al.* (1994) found that premorbid explosive and paranoid traits were commoner in patients with schizophrenia than in patients with other non-organic psychoses, and these features were associated with later onset of schizophrenia.

Obsessive-compulsive disorder and personality disorders

Obsessive-compulsive disorder (OCD) has a lifetime prevalence of about 2.5% (Karno, Golding & Sorenson, 1988). It is a disorder with maladaptive recurrent or persistent thoughts (obsessions), with or without repetitive or rigidly-patterned behaviours (compulsions) (Dowson, 1977). When severe, this disabling disorder usually follows a chronic course with exacerbations, and is associated with secondary anxiety and depression.

In the account of obsessive-compulsive PD in Chapter 2, it was noted that there have been many claims that obsessive-compulsive PD is associated with OCD. But despite the similarity of the terms, 'the majority of patients with OCD do not meet criteria for obsessive-compulsive PD' (Pfohl & Blum, 1991), although compared with normal controls, patients with OCD are more likely to have a PD (Black *et al.*, 1993). These are the conclusions of most of the studies that have reported on retrospective evaluation of PD in groups identified by the presence of OCD, although Rasmussen & Tsuang (1986) found that 55% of 44 outpatients with OCD met DSM-III criteria for compulsive PD. Joffe, Swinson & Regan (1988) compared PD in 23 patients with OCD and in a matched group with major depressive disorder, and found no significant difference between the two patient groups in respect of the frequency or type of PD as assessed by the self-report Millon Clinical Multiaxial Inventory. In the OCD group, a mixed PD (i.e. with features of more than one PD) was the most common finding; avoidant and passive-aggressive PDs were found in 44%, and dependent PD in 35%. Only 4% met criteria for obsessive-compulsive PD, while 17% had co-occurring schizotypal PD. An investigation with another self-report instrument (the PDQ) also failed to provide evidence of a specific association between obsessive-compulsive PD and OCD, and the 21 patients with OCD had more DSM-III-R 'cluster B' PDs than a 'normal' control group (Black *et al.*, 1989). Also, two groups of patients with OCD and panic disorder respectively, had a similar PD profile, with avoidant, dependent, histrionic and borderline PDs as the most frequent (Mavissakalian *et al.*, 1990*a*), and Sciuto *et al.* (1991), in another study of two diagnostic groups based on OCD and panic disorder, also concluded that no specific PD was associated with either group.

The various studies that have addressed this issue have used various assessment methods, mainly involving self-report questionnaires, and the patient groups have been selected in different ways. Baer *et al.* (1990) have provided one of the few reports based on a structured interview for DSM-III PDs, which was used to assess 96 patients with OCD; 52% met criteria for at least one PD, and mixed, dependent and histrionic PDs were the most frequent. Obsessive-compulsive PD was diagnosed in only 6% of patients, most of whom had an early childhood onset of OCD, which made the distinction between PD and OCD difficult, while schizotypal PD was found in 5%.

OCD appears to respond to drug treatments, such as some antidepressants, and also to behavioural treatments, such as 'flooding' and 'response prevention'. However, not all patients improve; in a 2-year follow-up study, 20% failed to show a treatment response, while many of the others continued to show some symptoms and periodic exacerbations. Several variables have been claimed to be related to outcome, such as depressive symptomatology, lack of insight that some obsessional thoughts are not realistic, and the presence of PD, in particular features of schizotypal PD (Stanley, Turner & Borden, 1990).

Two retrospective studies have indicated that when schizotypal PD co-occurs with OCD, this is a significant predictor of poor treatment response to both drugs and behavioural treatment methods (Jenike *et al.*, 1986; Minichiello, Baer & Jenike, 1987). Jenike and colleagues reported schizotypal PD (retrospectively assessed) in 33% of their sample with OCD, while Stanley *et al.* (1990) studied 25 patients with OCD with the Structured Clinical Interview for DSM-III-R PDs and found that 28% had schizotypal features, although only 8% met criteria for schizotypal PD. Co-occurring schizotypal PD features may identify a subgroup of OCD patients with relatively severe social maladjustment, delusional experiences and a history of abnormal visual experiences such as perceptual distortions. Such patients may be relatively treatment-resistant, although some of the apparent schizotypal features (such as delusional ideas) in OCD may be part of the OCD itself and improve with treatment of the OCD.

Eating disorders and personality disorders

The main distinction between subtypes of psychogenic eating disorders has been between anorexia nervosa (AN) in patients who have maintained a low weight by a restrictive diet, perhaps with excessive exercise (who are known as 'restricters' or 'dieters'), and AN in patients who have shown various combinations and patterns of bulimia with binge-eating, self-induced vomiting and laxative abuse (who have been classed as 'vomiters and purgers', 'bulimics', 'bulimic anorectics', 'low-weight bulimics' or 'non-restricters'). It has also been suggested that a distinct subtype of bulimia is bulimia nervosa (BN), which is associated with relatively small deviations from normal weight (i.e. 'normal-weight bulimia'), and low-weight bulimics may be more closely related to normal-weight bulimics than to restricters. Most studies of AN subtypes have involved bulimia as the distinguishing feature, although vomiting and purging have also been used (Dowson, 1992c).

It has been suggested that the nature and degree of co-occurring personality disorder (PD) can have major effects on the prognosis of eating disorders and should be an important factor in deciding treatment strategy (Rosenvinge & Mouland, 1990). Borderline PD has been reported to be common in patients with eating disorders (Gartner et al., 1989) and several studies have described a variety of PD psychopathology associated with bulimia, i.e. histrionic, borderline, schizoid, schizotypal, antisocial, narcissistic, obsessive-compulsive, avoidant, dependent and passive-aggressive PD features (Dowson, 1992c), although Pope et al. (1987) concluded that their results argued against a specific relationship between bulimia and borderline PD in patients with normal-weight bulimia. However, although the latter study found no difference in borderline PD ratings between patients with bulimia and another group with major depression, both these groups had higher borderline ratings than the non-patient control group. Also, a relatively high prevalence of obsessive-compulsive PD traits has been described in 'restricters', and it was suggested that this can be of aetiological significance (Beumont, George & Smart, 1976).

Several studies have reported personality differences between 'restricters' and patients with AN together with a history of bulimia or vomiting and purging. Beumont et al. (1976), using unstructured interviews, investigated 31 patients divided into 'dieters' and 'vomiters/purgers', although occasional vomiting did not disqualify a patient from the former group. Histrionic traits (considered as childish behaviour, affective instability, evanescent enthusiasm, dramatic exaggerations and the impression of emotional shallowness) were much more prevalent in the 'vomiters/ purgers', and obsessional traits (i.e. reliability, precision, scrupulousness, conscientiousness and love of order and discipline) and social withdrawal were more common in the 'dieters'. Casper et al. (1980) studied 105 inpatients with AN using the Minnesota Multiphasic Personality Inventory (MMPI) and found that frequency of bulimia was associated with various MMPI scale scores, including the psychopathic deviate scale. In contrast to the fasting (i.e. 'restricter') AN patients, those with bulimia were more extroverted and more likely to steal. Garfinkel, Moldofsky & Garner (1980) reported a series of 141 patients with AN who were divided into 'restricters' and 'bulimics' on the basis of recent history at the initial consultation, although some 'restricters' had a history of vomiting. Various intergroup differences were found, including an association between bulimia, premorbid obesity and family history of obesity. Also, the bulimic group were more outgoing, less isolated and more involved sexually. Their moods were more labile and they showed more impulsive behaviour such as self-harm (suicide attempts and self-mutilation), stealing and abuse of alcohol and street drugs. Piran, Lerner & Garfinkel (1988) described similar findings using the Diagnostic Interview for Borderline Patients as well as structured interviews: 60% of the 'restricters' received a diagnosis of avoidant PD, and the most common PD diagnosis in the 'bulimic' group (i.e. in those with AN and bulimia) was borderline PD in 55.3% compared with only 6.6% in the 'restricters'. However, the consensus in the above studies was not sustained by Gartner *et al.* (1989) in their report of DSM-III-R PD in 35 inpatients using a structured interview, as they found no evidence of significant PD differences between 'restricters' and those with 'low-weight bulimia', although the number of 'restricters' was small ($n = 6$). Therefore, although most reports that have compared subtypes of AN have found that 'low-weight bulimia' is associated with PD characteristics related to impulsive and harmful behaviour, this was not confirmed in the only study that used a standard structured interview method for the assessment of all the DSM-III-R PDs. But in a study of 55 patients with a history of AN, assessed by a modified version of the revised self-report Personality Diagnostic Questionnaire (PDQ-R), based on DSM-III-R PDs, 'vomiters' showed significantly higher scores than non-vomiters on self-report measures of borderline and antisocial PD criteria (Dowson, 1992*c*).

PD has been assessed by a structured interview for DSM-III PDs in a large sample of 210 women seeking treatment for AN ($n = 31$), BN ($n = 91$), or a mixed disorder ($n = 88$) (Herzog *et al.*, 1992), in which the prevalences of PDs were low compared with previously-reported similar samples. Twenty-seven per cent had at least one PD, and the most frequent was borderline PD in 9%. The highest prevalence of 'at least one PD' was found in the group with a mixed disorder at 39%, followed by 22% in the AN group and 21% in the BN group. There were higher rates of borderline PD in the mixed and BN groups than in the AN group, and higher rates of the 'anxious' PD cluster (i.e. DSM-III-R's 'Cluster C') in the AN and mixed group. Those patients with co-occurring PD had significantly slower recovery rates than those without PD, and the question of whether assessment of PDs can have predictive value for the long-term course and outcome of eating disorders is important, in view of the frequency of eating disorders and the cost of providing treatment regimes for the most severely affected. A high rate of eating disorders has also been found in a sample of 130 patients referred on the basis of PD to a therapeutic community (Dolan *et al.*, 1994).

Lacey (1984) has also found that, in patients with 'normal-weight BN', a poorer prognosis was associated with co-occurring PD, particularly if the PD was associated with alcohol abuse. This is in accord with the findings of Yates *et al.* (1990), who reported that while BN and some examples of alcohol abuse share intermittent behavioural loss of control of oral intake, a comparison of 30 women with BN, and 30 age-matched women with alcohol abuse, found that those with BN were less likely to have antisocial or borderline PD features. Also, Fahy, Eisler & Russell (1993) found that PD was related to poor treatment outcome with cognitive behavioural therapy for BN.

Sohlberg *et al.* (1989) reported that impulsivity was the strongest predictor of outcome in their study of patients with AN or BN, and that this variable accounted for 25% of the variance of AN symptoms at 2 to 3 years' follow-up, and for 14% at 4 to 6 years, as measured by the Eating Attitudes Test. Also, in a study of 30 patients followed for 4–5 years, the results suggested that borderline PD was predictive of poor eating disorder outcome (Wonderlich *et al.*, 1994). Sohlberg (1990) suggested that, for those patients with eating disorders and co-occurring PD, non-specific therapeutic efforts to help patients cope with stressful life events may result in measurably reduced eating disorder morbidity.

Increased use of health care facilities and personality disorders

Many of the behaviours associated with PDs would be expected to be reflected by an increased use of health care services and this was demonstrated by Reich *et al.* (1989) in a non-patient survey of 401 randomly selected subjects who showed a correlation between DSM-III 'cluster B' PD features and visits to the family doctor with symptoms of other psychiatric disorders. Also, Nestadt *et al.* (1990), in a study of DSM-III histrionic PD in a community sample, found that individuals with this disorder tend to use health care facilities more frequently than the rest of the population.

Complaints of chronic pain and personality disorders

The term 'idiopathic pain disorder' has been used when there is no clearly identifiable somatic disorder (Williams & Spitzer, 1982), while Blumer &

Heilbronn (1982) have suggested that this can be a feature of some depressive disorders. Von Knorring, Almay & Johansson (1987) have compared aspects of personality in patients with idiopathic pain disorder and other groups, including healthy volunteers, and reported that certain personality features were associated with idiopathic pain, including high scores on an 'inhibition of aggression' factor and low scores on impulsivity and suspicion.

It is likely that complaints of pain can be associated with various psychiatric disorders in addition to depressive disorders, such as anxiety states, conversion disorders and PDs. Jensen (1988) investigated chronic pain in 73 non-psychotic psychiatric outpatients and found that in the group with pain ($n = 54$), unskilled work status and a history of various psychiatric diagnoses including PD were significantly overrepresented, but it must not be assumed that idiopathic pain is always secondary to a psychiatric disorder.

Bowel disorders and personality disorders

Several studies have claimed associations between personality traits, PDs, and various bowel diseases but the interpretation of such findings is unclear. Chronic inflammatory bowel disease has been associated with introversion (Robertson *et al.*, 1989), while personality has been suggested as a possible risk factor in large bowel cancer (Kune *et al.*, 1991). In the latter study of 637 confirmed new cases of colorectal cancer and 714 controls, self-reported suppression of reactions that may offend others and the avoidance of conflict showed a significant difference between cases and controls.

Neuropsychological impairment and personality disorders

Malloy *et al.* (1990) have pointed out that those with antisocial PD may be at risk for the development of neuropsychological impairment due to alcohol or illicit drug abuse, and for a higher prevalence of head injury associated with alcohol abuse, violence and risk-taking behaviour. Also, Judd & Ruff (1993) have claimed that borderline PD is associated with neuropsychological dysfunction, involving visuospatial tasks.

Post-traumatic stress disorder (PTSD) and personality disorders

This syndrome includes depression, anxiety, sleep disorder, distressing memories and images, and irritability, and follows severe stressful life events, such as combat, natural disaster, criminal assault or accident (McCarroll *et al.*, 1993). Its medico-legal importance has been increasing, and it can be presented as a disorder that justifies claims for damages or as a mitigating factor for criminal behaviour.

Borderline PD, as well as a history of stressful life events and childhood maltreatment, are often found to co-occur with PTSD, although reasons for these associations are unclear. Famularo, Kinscherff & Fenton (1991) have suggested that PTSD in children can present with a syndrome that is similar to borderline PD in adults. Southwick, Yehuda & Giller (1993) found PDs to be common in combat veterans with PTSD, in particular borderline, obsessive-compulsive, avoidant and paranoid PDs.

Sierles *et al.* (1983) described 25 combat veterans in hospital for PTSD and found that the majority had at least one additional psychiatric disorder, in particular alcoholism, drug dependence, antisocial PD and somatization disorder. A more recent study of 189 male Vietnam veterans admitted to an inpatient treatment programme found that 72% had PTSD, and that this group was significantly associated with passive-aggressive, schizoid, avoidant and borderline PD features (Sherwood, Funari & Piekarski, 1990). As in the previous study, drug and alcohol abuse commonly co-occurred.

It is likely that co-occurrence of PDs, in particular borderline PD, may be a predisposing factor for the development of PTSD and can affect the course of the disorder (Gunderson & Sabo, 1993*b*).

Attention deficit hyperactivity disorder (ADHD) and personality disorders

Hyperactivity in children is an heterogeneous syndrome which has been termed 'hyperactive syndrome' or 'minimal brain dysfunction', as well as ADHD. It has been suggested that ADHD is a predisposing factor for the development of antisocial PD and criminality (Mannuzza *et al.*, 1989), and a review by Lie (1992) concluded that although 'hyperactives without conduct problems do not have an increased frequency of delinquency, ADHD in addition to another disorder indicates a more unfavourable prognosis than for each of these disorders separately'.

In another literature review, Biederman, Newcorn & Sprich (1991) came to the same conclusion, noting frequent co-occurrence of an history of ADHD with conduct disorder, borderline PD and other psychiatric disorders. In a prospective follow-up of 103 males with ADHD, Mannuzza *et al.* (1989) considered that their findings also supported the view that childhood ADHD is a risk factor for later criminality when co-occurring with other disorders. ADHD in adults has been reviewed (Editorial, 1994) in relation to a report that methylphenidate and d-amphetamine were associated with significant improvements in behaviour in adults with the diagnosis of ADHD (Matochik *et al.*, 1994). However, this is a controversial diagnosis in adults and is becoming increasingly frequent as a self-diagnosis in the setting of chronic difficulties.

Antisocial behaviours and personality disorders

West (1983) has noted that some antisocial behaviours are common among young males, and that unusually frequent or serious misbehaviour (as admitted in response to self-report questionnaires), is associated with having or subsequently obtaining a criminal conviction. Among males in the UK, the incidence of convictions falls after the age of 18, although the number of juvenile convictions, and a relatively young age at first conviction, predict a greater risk of a persisting record of convictions. In a community study of a sample of males from a region of London (West & Farrington, 1977), most of those with a history of criminal convictions had histories of at least four out of the following features: gambling, driving after drinking, immoderate smoking, sexual promiscuity, unstable work record, anti-establishment attitudes, involvement in acts of violence, unconstructive use of leisure, association with antisocial groups, use of prohibited drugs and having tattoos. But it has been argued that persistent delinquents, whose antisocial attitudes and behaviour are pervasive and frequent, are not just ordinary members of under-privileged groups in society but have a disorder (usually a PD) that would bring them into conflict with any society.

The relationship between PD and pathological gambling (which involves chronic and increasing inability to resist impulses to gamble, with disruption or damage to family, personal or vocational pursuits), has also been investigated. In a comparison between 19 male gamblers and controls, a number of differences in measures of personality were found, such as a higher total hostility score in gamblers (Roy *et al.*, 1989*a*). Also, there have been reports of biological correlates, involving abnormal functioning of the central noradrenergic system (Roy, De Jong & Linnoila, 1989*b*).

Other studies have identified groups of males with a history of involvement in spouse (or partner) abuse, and examined possible correlates. A literature review has suggested that there are associations with several PDs, and subtypes have been defined (Hamberger & Hastings, 1988). The most frequent co-occurring disorders in another study were sadistic, antisocial and borderline PDs (Hart, Dutton & Newlove, 1993). Not surprisingly, alcohol-abusing 'batterers' have been identified as a particularly difficult group to manage. Some batterers may be so dangerous that the provision of residential treatment programmes may be indicated.

Dangerous, violent or seriously irresponsible behaviour and personality disorders

Many examples of dangerous, violent or seriously irresponsible behaviour may involve both the police and health care services. Antisocial PD is partly defined by such behaviour that may start in childhood and is more common in men. Also, a study of 91 female offenders admitted for psychiatric assessment found that early age of onset of criminal behaviour was associated with adult PD (Brownstone & Swaminath, 1989).

Many examples of dangerous behaviour are unknown to police or medical services or may be called 'accidents'. A study of male alcoholics compared 57 who reported personal injury accidents with the 131 who did not; the former group had more severe alcoholism, an earlier onset of heavy drinking, and a higher prevalence of antisocial PD (Yates *et al.*, 1987). Also, in a study of several hundred male drivers referred by courts for a treatment programme for alcoholism, the 'heavy' drinker subgroup had more anti-social characteristics, a lower educational level and a greater tendency to drop out of treatment programmes (McGuire, 1980). In 1990 there were 46 300 deaths from motor vehicle accidents in the USA, accounting for 50% of all accidental deaths, and providing the fourth leading cause of death in the USA, above infections. Many of these deaths are likely to result from behaviour related to PDs.

Inadequate and abusive parenting and personality disorders

Evidence has been found for associations between antisocial PD in parents and psychiatric disorders in their children, which is likely to be mediated, at least in part, by bad parenting. Comparing child psychiatric clinic attenders with other groups, an excess of a history of psychiatric hospital referral among parents of behaviourally disturbed children has been noted, together with a significant excess of parental PD, especially antisocial PD. Also, it has been considered that parental behaviour, in particular marital discord and violence, is often an important cause of conduct disorder, particularly in boys (Wolff, 1983).

In a study of 54 mothers who had maltreated their children and 37 controls, the former group showed a greater prevalence of PD as well as mood disorder and alcohol abuse. Also, mothers who had maltreated their children were more likely to have a history of post-traumatic stress disorder (Famularo, Kinscherff & Fenton, 1992), while a highly abusive home environment has been associated with one or more of the triad of enuresis, firesetting and cruelty to animals (Prentky & Carter, 1984).

Sexual deviation disorders and personality disorders

Legal constraints on permissible sexual behaviour, and possible 'treatment' for those individuals with sexual deviation disorders, have to be considered when the well-being or rights of others are compromised (Berlin & Meinecke, 1981). It does not appear that there are specific associations between sexual deviation disorders and PD, but co-occurring PD, in particular antisocial PD, is likely to be a risk factor in contributing to the occurrence of criminal behaviour in the context of sexual deviation. However, a study of transsexuals found a greater prevalence of PDs, mainly within 'cluster B' compared with a control group (Bodlund *et al.*, 1993).

Epidemiology

Methodological problems

The literature provides a range of prevalence rates and age or sex distributions of the various PD syndromes, but this is to be expected in view of methodological problems in their assessment and the use of different selection criteria for groups of subjects. Morey & Ochoa (1989) compared the DSM-III-R PD ratings of 291 clinicians for recent patients seen by each (one patient per clinician), with their PD diagnoses based on global impression. It was found that there was only a modest correlation between the two procedures, producing a kappa of only 0.58 between the clinicians' own diagnoses of borderline PD based on clinical impression, and their diagnoses based on their own assessments of the individual DSM-III-R PD criteria. This indicated that, in routine practice, there is often a failure to systematically assess the individual DSM-III-R criteria, even though the DSM diagnostic categories may be used. A clinician may often obtain an initial impression of the most obvious feature of PD and then focus the rest of the assessment on one or two probable PD diagnoses. However, even though the DSM PD categories have often shown poor inter-rater reliability and stability, it is generally recognized that their features are

'highly prevalent in psychiatric settings and consume a significant proportion of mental health resources' (Mulder, 1991). Also, epidemiological
studies have shown a surprising consistency for many aspects of PDs in
clinical practice.

Gender and PD

DSM-III and DSM-III-R made various claims in relation to gender and PD
syndromes, which were not all based on experimental evidence; males were
considered to be more prone to develop paranoid, antisocial and obsessive-
compulsive PDs, while increased prevalences of histrionic, borderline and
dependent PDs were associated with females. The clearest evidence for any
of these claims exists for antisocial PD in males, but an association between
male gender and paranoid or obsessive-compulsive PDs has also been
supported, as has an association between female gender and borderline,
histrionic and dependent PDs. But the evidence is conflicting: the latter
associations with females were not found in a series of 298 outpatients
(Alnaes & Torgerson, 1988a) in which passive-aggressive, schizotypal and
narcissistic PDs were more prevalent among men; these findings had not
been predicted by DSM-III/DSM-III-R.

Prevalence rates of individual PDs

Estimates of the lifetime prevalence of DSM-III-R antisocial PD have
ranged from 0.5 to 3.5% in non-patient community samples, and this
disorder has been associated with male gender, younger age (less than 45
years), lower socioeconomic status and urban residence (Jordan *et al.*,
1989). For example, Swanson, Bland & Newman (1994) reported 104
subjects with antisocial PD out of 3258 randomly-selected adult household
Canadian residents; the overall lifetime prevalence rates for antisocial PD
were 6.5% for males and 0.8% for females. In those with antisocial PD, the
age at which conduct disorder appeared was usually under 10 and there was
an increased lifetime prevalence of co-occurrence with nearly every other
psychiatric disorder. Antisocial PD was most often found in the 25–34 year
age group, followed by the 18–24 age group.

For borderline PD, estimates of prevalences in non-patient community
samples and in the relatives of non-patients have been between 1 and 4%
(Loranger, Oldham & Tullis, 1982; Baron *et al.*, 1985; Maier *et al.*, 1992),
but for inpatient groups higher rates of between 15 and 25% have been

reported. In various studies it appears that two-thirds or more of subjects with this disorder have been female (Gunderson & Zanarini, 1987). In a study of 1583 inpatients there were no significant differences in the prevalences of borderline PD among racial groups classed as whites, blacks and hispanics (Castaneda & Franco, 1985).

Histrionic PD as defined by DSM-III criteria was found to have a prevalence of 2.1% in a non-patient community sample (Nestadt *et al.*, 1990); males and females were equally affected, and those with this syndrome tended to use health care facilities more frequently than others. Data from the same study indicated a prevalence for DSM-III compulsive PD (obsessive-compulsive PD) in 1.7%; male, white and employed subjects received this diagnosis more often than the complementary groups, and it was concluded that this PD is associated with a vulnerability for the development of anxiety disorder (Nestadt *et al.*, 1991).

Many studies have examined prevalence figures for at least one PD in non-patient community samples. Srole *et al.* (1962) reported 1660 adults, assessed by a self-report method, in whom 10% were considered to have 'probable PD', while more restrictive criteria have given rates below 4% (Weissman, Myers & Harding, 1978; Myers *et al.*, 1984). In the UK, 200 randomly chosen adults were assessed by a structured interview and PD was found in 13% (Casey & Tyrer, 1986). In this study 'explosive' and 'anankastic' categories were most common (6% and 3% respectively), which probably reflected borderline and obsessive-compulsive PDs. Summarizing the literature, Casey (1988) noted that a lifetime prevalence for PD of between 2 and 18% has been found depending on the method of assessment and the populations studied, and that PD is associated with young adult age and the male gender. Reich, Nduaguba & Yates' study (1988) of age and sex distribution of DSM-III PDs suggested that these generalizations conceal different relationships between age, sex and the various PD syndromes. This study found that the prevalences of schizoid, schizotypal and paranoid PDs did not show a change with age, while the number of features of antisocial, narcissistic, borderline and histrionic PDs (and to some extent the 'anxious' cluster C PDs) declined from younger to older groups. The highest levels of PD features in men were found between the ages of 18 and 30, while in women the highest levels were in the 31 to 40 age range. Although some studies found 'one or more' PDs to be more prevalent in inner-city areas, Blazer *et al.* (1985) did not find any urban–rural difference in the prevalence of antisocial PD. These authors studied groups in five parts of the USA and also found a decrease in 'one or more'

PDs with increasing age and a higher prevalence in men. There was also an association with poor educational attainment.

Maier *et al.* (1992) investigated DSM-III-R PDs by an interview assessment in 452 non-patient 'community' subjects who they considered to be a 'good approximation' of a representative sample of the population. Of the males, 9.6% (and of the females, 10.3%) had at least one PD; older subjects were less likely to have PD than younger subjects; mixed PDs (i.e. more than one PD) were found in 2.6% of females and 2.3% of males; obsessive-compulsive PD was the most prevalent PD in males, while dependent and passive-aggressive PD were the most frequent in females; only borderline PD showed a clear tendency to co-occur with other PDs; and dependent, passive-aggressive and histrionic PDs were more prevalent in females, while borderline and avoidant PDs showed a similar but less marked association. Obsessive-compulsive, schizotypal and antisocial PDs were found more often in males. Also, anxiety disorders were associated with avoidant PD, and affective disorders with borderline PD. It was noted that there was a low prevalence of antisocial PD and schizophrenia in the sample, so that other expected associations with these disorders could not be evaluated. It was suggested that associations between PDs, major depressive disorders and anxiety disorders may be less marked in non-patient samples, and that the low prevalence of antisocial PD represented a selection bias in this study.

These findings can be compared with those of Coryell & Zimmerman (1989), who also examined a non-patient sample, although DSM-III diagnoses were used. In this study, 9.2% of relatives of healthy controls had at least one PD; but this is likely to be an underestimate of the prevalence of PD in the general population as the sample was selected in relation to a healthy control group. Nevertheless, the prevalence of PD in the general population is similar in the two studies, despite the differences in methodology, and points to a frequency of about 10% for significantly maladaptive PD in adult samples of the population.

Zimmerman & Coryell (1989) also reported a large non-patient sample made up of 797 'normal' controls and of first-degree relatives of patients with a variety of psychiatric disorders; of those with a PD, about 25% had more than one, and the most prevalent diagnoses were mixed (3.6%), passive-aggressive (3.3%), antisocial (3.3%), histrionic (3.0%) and schizotypal PD (2.9%). Half the subjects with avoidant PD also met criteria for schizotypal PD. Paranoid, schizotypal, avoidant and borderline PDs most frequently co-occurred with other PDs, and schizoid and dependent PDs occurred relatively often in isolation.

PD in primary medical care settings

When an individual consults a primary care physician, he or she can be selected for assessment on this basis alone or because of the presence of 'conspicuous psychiatric morbidity'. Casey, Dillon & Tyrer (1984) used this latter criterion in their study of a sample of patients in urban general practice, in which the primary care physician rated PD as the primary (main) diagnosis in 8.9%; the corresponding prevalence diagnosed by a psychiatrist who made parallel ratings was 6.4%. But subsequent detailed assessment by a structured interview suggested that no less than 33.9% had at least one PD, in particular 'explosive' PD, which was diagnosed in 17%. This suggests that a more detailed assessment of PD in primary care would yield considerably more PDs than are apparent in routine assessments. It is likely that this hidden PD psychopathology is the starting point for many presenting symptoms in primary care settings (Casey & Tyrer, 1990).

PD in psychiatric inpatient and outpatient samples

In England and Wales in the mid 1980s, 7.6% of all psychiatric admissions had a diagnosis of PD with the ICD classification (Department of Health & Social Security, UK, 1985). This is likely to have been a considerable underestimate as any non-PD psychiatric disorder would usually have been recorded in preference to a co-occurring PD. The DSM-III and III-R have encouraged the recording of co-occuring diagnoses, and co-occurring PD has been identified in 40–50% of many inpatient psychiatric samples. PD is the sole diagnosis in a minority of inpatients, and more often a PD co-occurs with other psychiatric disorders; for example, Cutting and colleagues (1986) assessed a series of consecutive admissions with non-PD disorders to an urban psychiatric unit and found co-occurring PD in 44%. Mulder (1991) reported on admission trends for those with a principal (main) diagnosis of PD admitted to New Zealand psychiatric hospitals over a 7 year period. The most common diagnostic category was unspecified PD (45%), followed by dependent PD (12%). Other rates included antisocial PD (10%), histrionic PD (9%), explosive (i.e. similar to borderline) PD (6%), schizoid PD (5%), paranoid PD (3%) and obsessive-compulsive PD (2%). Antisocial PD was more common in men ($\times$ 3.2), as were paranoid, schizoid and explosive PDs, while histrionic PD was more frequently diagnosed in women. In general, the patients with PD were relatively young; 73% were less than 35 years and more than 40% were under 25. Also in relation to inpatients, Jackson *et al.* (1991) found that schizophrenia was associated with antisocial and schizotypal PDs, manic disorder with histrionic PD, and unipolar affective disorder with borderline, dependent and avoidant PDs. The nature of these relationships is unclear but it is likely that a subgroup of those with unipolar depressive disorder consists of subjects in whom the PD is a major causal factor for the subsequent development of mood disorder.

Groups of individuals from outpatient clinics in psychiatric services have been associated with lower rates for the prevalence of PD, compared with inpatients, but substantial rates of PD have been reported, often between 20–40% (Kass, Skodol & Charles, 1985; Morey, 1988). In an outpatient sample selected on the basis of a diagnosis of 'neurosis' (i.e. mainly anxiety disorders and subtypes of depressive disorders), Tyrer and colleagues (1983) found that 39% had PDs, in particular anankastic (obsessive-compulsive) and passive-dependent (dependent).

PD in forensic samples

For antisocial PD, various prevalence rates up to 70% have been reported in forensic samples (Gunn *et al.*, 1978).

PD in self-harm populations

A wide range of prevalences of PDs have been found in self-harm populations (Casey, 1988), in particular when the risk to life is judged to be relatively low (Pallis & Birtchnell, 1977). Relatively serious risk has been associated with obsessive-compulsive traits (Murthy, 1969) but this was not confirmed in a subsequent study (Pierce, 1977).

4

Longitudinal aspects of personality disorders

J.H. DOWSON

Introduction

The longitudinal perspective

The course of a disorder is examined by data collection at a minimum of two points in time, but an assessment on several occasions is required to identify a fluctuating course; if only two sets of data are available, their comparison is merely an outcome study. Many variables affect the course of PDs, including various interventions, other co-occurring disorders and secondary effects, such as a break-up of family relationships or the loss of employment.

The evaluation of the course of PDs is adversely affected by the complexity of PD assessment, so that even if a detailed evaluation has been carried out at one time-point, it may be difficult to obtain the subject's cooperation for further time-consuming interviews. Consequently, most longitudinal studies of PD have relied on relatively crude measures such as re-admission rates and suicide. Also, a high drop-out rate is a problem in any longitudinal study and, in relation to PD, has been associated with males and a diagnosis of antisocial PD.

Most PD traits appear to have a dimensional relationship with aspects of 'normal' personality in non-clinical populations, and it has been shown that several such traits show stability for the decades over the age of 30 (Zuckerman, 1991). In a study of 769 male volunteers aged 17–97, the factor structure of several aspects of personality was similar in different age groups (McCrae *et al.*, 1980) and a 9-year longitudinal study of 4942 subjects aged 25–74 provided further support for the view that some personality features are enduring; it appeared that, for most 'normal' personality traits, there is stability from the age of 30, which follows a period of significant change from adolescence for some attributes (Costa & McCrae, 1992).

While the literature on clinical or forensic samples with PDs also provides evidence for varying degrees of stability of some PD features, others have been shown to be subject to change. Such instability is of two main types, namely rapid short-term, and slow, linear long-term. Short-term changes in PD features are often in relation to life-crises or other co-occurring disorders, (in particular depression, anxiety disorders and substance abuse, Bronisch & Klerman, 1991), while slower long-term improvements in adaptation, which are characteristic of many individuals with features of borderline and antisocial PDs, can provide realistic hope in many young patients with seemingly intractable problems. Long-term improvements in adaptation have also been found in a non-patient sample in relation to antisocial and histrionic PD ratings, and it seems that those features of normal personality and PD which involve lability (i.e. rapid changeability) are particularly associated with age-related changes for the better (Tyrer & Seivewright, 1988*b*). Therefore, changes with age are most associated with features of DSM-III-R's 'cluster B' PDs, (and perhaps with passive-aggressive PD), in contrast with 'cluster A' PDs and obsessive-compulsive PD. The outcome of avoidant PD is unclear.

Longitudinal studies of PD have mainly involved borderline, antisocial and schizotypal PDs (Stone, 1993). These have generally reported on inpatient or prison samples, so that the results relate to relatively severe examples of these particular syndromes, and to individuals who usually have several co-occurring disorders. There have been relatively few long-term prospective studies, and while Robins (1978) found clear evidence of a link between childhood conduct disorder and adult antisocial PD, most long-term reports have been concerned with borderline PD (Perry, 1990).

Perry (1993) has reviewed 26 longitudinal studies, which were mostly related to inpatient samples and borderline PD. There was a bimodal distribution of follow-up periods, (between 2–4 years and 13–16 years), and only two studies had more than two sets of assessment data. Of the nine studies which looked at suicide in patients with borderline PD, there was a mean suicide rate of 6.1% after a mean follow-up of 7.2 years, and it was found that the highest risk period was in the year after 'index' admission at which the patient was identified for study. With regard to the stability of diagnoses, five studies found that a mean of 57% of those with borderline PD had retained the diagnosis after a mean follow-up of 8.7 years. Also, most subjects had 'significant symptoms and impairment in social functioning on follow-up'.

Associated variables

Longitudinal studies of PD need to evaluate a range of variables that affect and reflect course and outcome, other than the features of PD. Therefore, evaluation of the course of a PD should, if possible, consist of a variety of measurements at multiple points in time. Measurements should include global assessments, such as those involving occupational and social functioning, while repeated data sets can evaluate the rate of change, which can be an important characteristic of a PD that is not addressed in an outcome study. Of the variables that may influence course and outcome of PDs, some will co-occur by chance (e.g. a bereavement), some may share aetiological factors with the PD being studied (e.g. social isolation due to schizoid PD), while others may be secondary to aspects of PD (e.g. some mood disorders and substance abuse). Variables affecting the results of longitudinal studies include the patient's demographic characteristics, adverse environmental experiences, co-occurring disorders, the individual's positive or adaptive potential, and treatments or interventions.

Relevant demographic variables include age, age when first in contact with psychiatric services, sex, socioeconomic status of subject and parents, marital/relationship status, cultural background, position in sibship, twin status, being an adoptee and being born or raised without two parents in the household. An adverse environment and co-occurring disorders may have involved childhood abuse (physical, sexual or psychological), childhood mistreatment or neglect, loss events, stress, illicit substance abuse, a history of other psychiatric disorders such as eating disorders, childhood conduct disorder, physical disease, low intelligence and sexual disorders or difficulties. Positive or adaptive qualities are seldom considered in PD research, but are important variables in relation to course and outcome; Kolb (1982) has specified courage, flexibility, commitment, perseverance, responsibility, humour, empathy, trust, charm and likeability. Also, a very high IQ may be of some advantage, while talent, female beauty, social position and wealth appear to predict a relatively good outcome for borderline PD (Stone, 1990).

The evaluation of these variables is important for the further understanding of the range of causal factors that contribute to the development, course and outcome of PDs. Variables that are potentially amenable to intervention, such as the adverse care of children, are of particular interest.

Outcome measures

Longitudinal studies have mainly involved measures of aspects other than those directly related to PD characteristics (Perry, 1993). These include hospitalization, other interventions from medical services, global functioning, social and occupational functioning, general interests, marriage (or long-term live-in relationships), child rearing, symptoms of other psychiatric disorders and mortality.

Epidemiological data

Longitudinal data can be deduced from epidemiological studies of prevalence and incidence of PD features and associated variables in specified populations. For example, the prevalence of antisocial and borderline PDs in different age groups can indicate an improvement in these disorders with increasing age.

Methodological aspects

In addition to the formidable methodological problems in the 'cross-sectional' evaluation of PDs, longitudinal studies involving two or more assessments are subject to additional sources of error. For example, the criteria for PDs have been subject to frequent revision, available data in retrospective studies have often been inadequate, and social and cultural changes may have affected the pattern of the disorders. For instance, changing patterns of drug misuse have provided a variable background to the expression of antisocial PD traits. Also, the course of co-occurring psychiatric disorders has to be taken into account when evaluating the course of PDs; for example, agoraphobia with avoidant PD, depressive disorders with various PDs, and obsessive-compulsive disorder with obsessive-compulsive PD (Perry, 1993). Improvement or worsening of a co-occurring disorder may influence PD-related behaviour, while improvement in PD (such as the gradual improvement in adaptation found in many subjects with antisocial and borderline PD) can result in a corresponding change in the co-occurring disorders.

Because of the lack of a 'gold standard' for PD assessment, the use of more than one PD assessment method has been recommended to increase reliability. Discrepant findings may then be assessed further by additional methods (Perry, 1990).

It must be remembered that nearly all longitudinal studies involve groups who have presented to medical services, so that there is little knowledge about those who do not seek help. Some individuals with severe PD disorders who do not seek help may have a worse course and outcome compared with those who receive some intervention, although for others, not seeking help may reflect co-occurring positive attributes, with a better course and outcome.

Borderline personality disorder

Longitudinal studies of borderline PD

Most longitudinal studies of borderline PD have used inpatient samples, consisting of those who have usually been referred to psychiatric services in adolescence or the early 20s. Improvement was generally identified by 8–10 years after initial diagnosis, but a mean of 6.1% of patients (range 3–9%) had committed suicide by a mean of 7.2 years (range 1.75 to 16) (Stone, 1992; Perry, 1993). The risk was greatest in the year following index admission. After 10–30 years, the outcome for inpatient samples varied from 'very good' to 'suicide', but was generally favourable with about 60% of subjects functioning at least reasonably well with global outcome measures, despite many examples of residual mild psychiatric disorders. About a third of the well-functioning group, particularly women, had a very good outcome, with no symptoms and the eventual achievement of satisfying relationships (Stone, 1993). (In Stone's opinion, the outcome for outpatients with a borderline PD is at least as good, and perhaps better.) Five studies reviewed by Perry (1993) found that, after a mean of 8.7 years, 57% of patients still received the borderline PD diagnosis. The negative correlation between lengths of follow-up and percentage retaining the diagnosis suggested a linear model for at least a degree of remission that eventually disqualified the subject from the borderline PD diagnosis. Such a diagnosis is rarely made for patients over the age of 40. However, some patients may re-present to psychiatric services in their 40s, with depressive disorders following the break-up of close relationships that have taken the toll of borderline PD behaviour over many years.

Several studies have involved inpatients who received a diagnosis of borderline PD on the basis of the DSM or Gunderson's Diagnostic Interview for Borderlines (DIB) (Stone, 1992). For example, Stone and colleagues (Stone *et al.*, 1987; Stone, 1990) have reported longitudinal data on 96% of 206 patients with borderline PD (male: $n = 61$, female: $n = 145$), followed up for 10–25 years. These individuals were mainly of middle to upper-middle socioeconomic status in New York State. Ninety-one per cent were single and the average age at index admission was 22 (range 13–39). Fifty-two per cent were Jewish. The average length of hospital admission was 12.5 months. These patients were admitted to a unit of the New York Psychiatric Institute, which specialized in intensive, psychoanalytically orientated psychotherapy of adolescents and young adults, but individual and group sessions were also accompanied by drug treatments in most cases. The 206 subjects were drawn from a wider sample of 550 (the PI-500), 25.7% of whom were presenting with their first admissions. Of those traced, 8.5% had committed suicide after a mean of 16.5 years, which was similar to the rates for the PI-500 patients with schizophrenia and manic-depressive disorder. Stone has pointed out that this is equivalent to a rate of 616 per 100 000 of similar patients with borderline PD, which is 55 times more than the rate for Caucasians in the US general population. Therefore, borderline PD is likely to be an important causal factor in suicide for individuals in their 20s, and it must be noted that, between 1950 and 1975, there has been a considerable increase in the suicide rate for young adults in the second half of their 20s, i.e. from 11.9 to 25 per 100 000 for white US males, and from 5.1 to 8.0 in females (Solomon & Murphy, 1984). Other results from the New York State longitudinal study included the finding that the marriage rate was half the US average for the equivalent cultural group, and the rate for childbearing was about a quarter of average. The majority eventually lost the borderline PD diagnosis, but most of these subjects still qualified for other PD diagnoses, such as histrionic, avoidant and obsessive-compulsive PDs. After the index admission, the subsequent readmission rate was about one-third of the rate for those PI-500 subjects with schizophrenia. Another contrast with the schizophrenia group was that patients with borderline PD were more likely to have had a job and have achieved more occupational responsibility.

McGlashan (1986, 1993) has reported the follow-up of 81 patients who had received a diagnosis of borderline PD by DSM-III or Gunderson & Kolb's criteria (1978) at index admission to a private residential unit, Chestnut Lodge in Maryland, US. The average length of follow-up period was 15 years, with a range of 2–32. Initial diagnoses were made retrospectively, and most follow-up contacts were by telephone. Patients with borderline PD were compared with those with schizophrenia or affective disorder. Most of those with borderline PD were single females whose disorder had presented significant problems in late adolescence and worsened during their 20s. The index admission to Chestnut Lodge was usually after the age of 20 but there was generally a history of previous contacts with psychiatric services. There was usually at least moderate impairment in social, occupational and sexual adjustment.

Outcome was, in general, superior in relation to those groups with schizophrenia and bipolar affective disorder, and comparable to subjects with unipolar depressive disorder. At follow-up, most were living independently from parents or institutions and had reasonable work records. However, many had needed short 'crisis' hospital admissions, nearly half had subsequent outpatient psychotherapeutic support, and other psychiatric disorders were common, in particular depressive disorders and substance abuse. The subsequent pattern of relationships showed considerable variation; while one group avoided intimacy, others managed to achieve stable relationships. While the latter had sometimes achieved satisfactory sexual relationships, others had developed social relationships only, perhaps supplemented by partial intimacy. The degree of improvement was related to the duration of follow-up, when data for the first 9 years was compared with those for the period 10–19 years.

The remaining inpatient studies are those of Plakun *et al.* (1985), Kroll *et al.* (1985), Paris *et al.* (1987) and Links (1993). Paris and colleagues followed up 100 subjects for a mean of 15 years and found a similar rate of suicide (8.5%) to that reported by Stone and colleagues. Another finding that was comparable with similar studies was that 75% no longer qualified for the borderline PD diagnosis. Links reported a 7 year follow-up of 88 patients with borderline PD diagnosed by the DIB; of 57 who were DIB-positive initially, and reinterviewed, 52.5% were no longer DIB-positive, and males were more likely to refuse the follow-up interview.

Prognostic factors

Stone (1990) has identified several attributes which were associated with a relatively good prognosis, including cooperation with the self-help group Alcoholics Anonymous (when appropriate), the presence of obsessional personality traits with a capacity for self-discipline and work-orientation, unusual talent, very high intelligence and, in women, a high degree of 'attractiveness'. Also, anecdotal evidence suggested that both negative and positive chance events can affect the course of borderline PD, as subjects are very sensitive to environmental changes; for instance, a patient who unexpectedly survives a determined suicide attempt may never again carry out self-harm behaviour. Also, Plakun (1991), in a follow-up study of 33 inpatients for a mean of 14 years, found that a good outcome was associated with self-destructive acts during the index admission.

Poor outcome for inpatients with borderline PD has been particularly associated with a history of parental cruelty and also with childhood neglect, childhood sexual abuse (especially father–daughter incest) (Paris, Zweig-Frank & Guzder, 1993), and a history of fire-setting in childhood (Stone, 1993). Relevant aspects of more recent history that predict poor outcome include relatively long periods of inpatient management (around 10 months or more), rape, imprisonment and poor global functioning.

At index admission, poor prognostic features have been the presence of positive ratings for all eight DSM borderline PD criteria, co-occurring features of antisocial PD with marked irritability and anger, schizotypal PD features, being a male without a major affective disorder, severe features involving impulsivity or affective instability, low intelligence and being a male who discharges himself against medical advice (Links *et al.*, 1990; Links, 1993; McGlashan, 1993). Subsequent to index admission, continuing substance abuse has indicated poor outcome (Stone, 1993). This can be 'deceptively mild' in women (Stone, 1990) and requires careful evaluation.

Prognostic factors in relation to suicide deserve particular attention as, on the basis of one large series (Stone, 1990), a prediction can be made that '4 out of 10 hospitalized "eight-item" borderline PD patients, in their early 20s or younger, will commit suicide within 5 years ...'. ('Eight-item' patients are those who are rated positive on all eight DSM-III-R criteria.) This study found a similar risk of suicide in the follow-up period (37.5%) for patients with a combination of borderline PD, major affective disorder and alcoholism. Also, the rate was 19% in a subgroup with continuing alcohol abuse and was higher in those who refused to attend self-help groups. Co-occurring antisocial PD increased the risk of subsequent suicide by a factor of 3 compared with the risk for borderline PD alone. For the co-occurrence of borderline PD and 'major depression', the suicide risk was doubled for men only.

Other studies have reported similar findings; for instance Zilber *et al.* (1989) found that in a group with various PDs together with drug or alcohol abuse, the risk of suicide was 3 times (21%) that of a group with PD alone.

Suicide in patients with borderline PD has also been associated with previous imprisonment (in a white middle-class sample), more frequent childhood loss, lack of treatment before hospitalization, longer hospitalization, more frequent mandatory discharges by staff, previous self-harm and higher education (Kullgren, 1988; Paris *et al.*, 1989; Kjelsberg *et al.*, 1991).

Co-occurring psychiatric disorders

The co-occurrence of borderline PD with combinations of substance abuse, major depression and antisocial PD have been identified as indicators of poor prognosis.

Affective disorders (mainly depression) are common with borderline PD, and in five studies reviewed by Perry (1993) a mean prevalence rate for affective disorders of 42% was found during the follow-up periods reported. Such depressive disorders are aetiologically and clinically variable, and in one study about 10% developed a manic-depressive disorder (Stone, 1992). Also, borderline PD has been commonly reported in association with agoraphobia (Stone, 1990), while Coid's study of a forensic sample (1993*b*) showed an association between borderline PD and unspecified psychotic episodes as well as with mood disorders.

Other variables associated with course and outcome of borderline PD

Adverse childhood events

There is considerable evidence of a significant association between a variety of adverse childhood events or circumstances and the later development of borderline PD (Marziali, 1992). However, causal relationships are likely to be complex, as, although the psychological effects of adverse events may be of considerable importance, the behaviour of some children may contribute to their adverse environment, and their genetic vulnerability in relation to future PD may be shared by their living group if this includes their biological relatives.

A wide range of events have been associated with borderline PD, such as neglect (including emotional withdrawal by the caregivers), physical abuse, parental loss (by death or separation), poor quality of parenting, and various forms of sexual abuse, in particular father–daughter incest. It has been claimed that an history of sexual abuse carried out by a single individual is rare (Westen *et al.*, 1990) and that it is common in groups with borderline PD, i.e. 26–71% in various studies (Crowell *et al.*, 1993). However, it is also common in some other patient samples, and it has been considered that an important causal factor for some examples of borderline PD may be severe and repetitive abuse involving multiple traumas, rather than a specific type of adversity.

In adult psychiatry, 'post traumatic stress disorder' (PTSD) has been receiving increasing attention. This syndrome involves re-experiences of traumatic events, avoidance of some situations, reduced emotional responsiveness and increased arousal, and it has been suggested that these features may follow adverse events in childhood, in particular severe physical abuse and incest, and contribute to the later development of borderline PD (Stone, 1990).

Adverse events in adulthood

In addition to associations between borderline PD and childhood loss events, there is evidence of a relationship between severity of borderline PD features and rates for the recurrence of depressive disorders following stressful life events in adulthood (Perry *et al.*, 1992).

Duration of follow-up period

As has been previously noted, borderline PD tends to be associated with gradual improvement, and this is reflected by findings of a correlation between length of follow-up interval and scores on adaptive aspects of global outcome (Perry, 1993).

Gender

Borderline PD has been more commonly diagnosed in females. However, in males these features often co-occur with those of antisocial PD, and as this PD is more common in males, it may often be given diagnostic precedence. McGlashan (1993) in the Chestnut Lodge study, found that, at index admission, females were more likely to be married with better heterosexual adjustment, to be more depressed and be more prone to self-harm. In contrast, males were more antisocial and uncooperative. Subsequently, of those with relatively poor outcome, males were more likely to be involved with alcohol abuse and females with self-harm episodes.

In Coid's study (1992) of 243 patients detained in forensic psychiatric units, there was a higher prevalence of borderline PD in females than in males (i.e. 90% to 50%), although several co-occurring PDs was the usual finding.

Adverse childhood experiences have been suggested as causal factors for some examples of borderline PD, and as girls are more likely than boys to be sexually abused as children (Marziali, 1992), this may contribute to the apparently greater prevalence of borderline PD in females.

Implications of longitudinal data for the management of borderline PD

Although about a third of hospitalized patients with borderline PD have a poor long-term outcome, the outcome is very varied even for severe cases, ranging from complete remission to suicide. This must reflect the hetero-geneity of this disorder resulting from the variable interaction of a range of causal factors. Therefore, it is not surprising that there are considerable variations in what appears to be the appropriate management, while improvement can occur without any interventions from medical services.

Nevertheless, certain principles of management can be recognized from longitudinal studies (McGlashan, 1993). As the long-term outlook is generally fairly good, even in severe cases, patience and optimism are usually appropriate. Patients can be reassured that a significant (albeit gradual) improvement in their adjustment is possible, and in the meantime, the clinician can provide advice, support and protection in times of crisis. This often involves short-term admissions to a psychiatric unit to protect the patient from the harmful consequences of impulsive self-destructive behaviour with self-injury, suicidal attempts or substance abuse. For a small minority of patients, long-term asylum can seem appropriate, involving continuous or intermittent institutional residence for up to several years. It has been claimed that there is less danger of the negative effects of an institution for those with borderline PD, compared with patients with schizophrenia, and that the expected improvement in the 20s and early 30s holds out a realistic hope of eventual rehabilitation to independence from residential care.

For many patients, especially those who have pronounced problems with intimate relationships, a focus on developing their capacity for work is important. However, as individuals with borderline PD find it difficult to live alone, there is a tendency to seek intimate relationships which may regularly degenerate into an unstable hostile dependency. For those patients who cannot improve their adaptation in intimate relationships, some learn that they are able to cope better by avoidance. This may involve a compromise, with strong attachments to groups of people associated with work, religion, political parties or self-help organizations. Commitment to a cause rather than one (or a few) individuals may be successfully combined with relatively superficial relationships that can be sustained. Longitudinal studies of inpatients with borderline PD have indicated that men are less likely to get married than women, but, for both sexes, divorce or separation is common. The principle that a patient should 'control the distance' of a relationship to avoid a degree of intimacy that cannot be sustained, extends to the relationships with medical services. Provision of treatment and support often needs to be on a flexible, 'as required' basis, which is under the patient's control as far as is possible and reasonable. A further principle is that a treatment 'package' should be designed in relation to the individual patient.

A psychiatric service can plan its provision on the basis that the majority of the most severely affected patients with borderline PD will require short periods of hospitalization and flexible outpatient support for up to several years, although, within this group, a few subjects appear to need long-term residential care or intensive outpatient psychotherapy. The general pattern of appropriate service delivery may change at different stages of the disorder. In middle age, when many patients will no longer qualify for the borderline PD diagnosis, a more sustained psychotherapeutic approach may be indicated for the depressive symptoms that can follow the break-up of a long-standing, stormy but supportive relationship.

Longitudinal studies of borderline PD can provide, from the public health perspective, ideas for reducing the suicide rate in young adults, to which this disorder contributes. A serious degree of childhood physical and sexual abuse, which has been implicated as a probable causal factor for some individuals with borderline PD, might be reduced by measures such as improvements in social work services, in child-care provision and in community recreational facilities. Also, as various studies have concluded that self-help groups for those who abuse drugs and alcohol can have a favourable impact on the course of these behaviours, the encouragement of these organizations might also be expected to result in less maladaptive behaviour, including suicide, shown by those with PD.

Antisocial personality disorder

Longitudinal studies of antisocial PD

Overview

DSM-III-R's category of 'antisocial PD' relies heavily on an history of specified antisocial acts and identifies individuals who show considerable heterogeneity, while Hare's criteria (1991) lay more emphasis on traits that affect personal relationships. These include lack of remorse or guilt, callousness, lack of empathy and failure to accept responsibility for one's own actions. Such attributes can be considered as 'core' traits for antisocial PD (psychopathy), although they are not prominent in many patients who would qualify for the DSM-III-R diagnosis. Also, subjects can have pronounced 'core' traits without an history of unlawful behaviour, although there is a clear association between the 'core' traits and overtly criminal or violent behaviour. For instance, Hare (1991) found that scores on his rating instrument, the PCL-R, were associated with the degree of violent and aggressive behaviour in prison settings.

The broad category of DSM-III-R's antisocial PD has to be evaluated in the context of a high level of 'sub-cultural delinquency' in some geographical areas and socio-cultural groups. West & Farrington's community survey of males of low socioeconomic status in part of London (1977) found that, at age 17, about 20% had a criminal record and that this had risen to 33% by age 24. But although the incidence of convictions fell considerably with increasing age over the age of 18, a minority showed a pattern of repeated convictions, which persisted into adult life. This group had a younger age at first conviction, a larger number of convictions up to the age of 18 and showed antisocial behaviour in a wide range of contexts. Such individuals can be considered to have a PD, and are often unpopular with their peers, tending to stand out even within a group in which lawbreaking is common. Despite the heterogeneity of the characteristics of antisocial individuals, and the various criteria sets for diagnosis of 'antisocial PD', recurrent or persistent antisocial behaviour has been validated as a successful marker for PD by both genetic and longitudinal studies. The demonstration of genetic factors associated with antisocial PD has been considered to be 'convincing' (Dahl, 1993), as has the association between childhood conduct disorder and adult antisocial PD.

Longitudinal studies that link childhood conduct disorder and adult antisocial PD have also found that conduct disorder tends to be associated with adverse and disordered family settings, involving violent and inconsistent patterns of child-rearing and increased criminality (Coid, 1993a). This is consistent with a model of causation that involves a variable interaction of genetic factors, other biological variables and social environment. But although most of those with the adult features of antisocial PD give a history of significant childhood conduct disorder, (a minority do not show problem-behaviour until mid or late adolescence), most children with conduct disorder do not become adults with antisocial PD (Crowell *et al.*, 1993). However, for most seriously antisocial adults, antisocial behaviour generally becomes apparent before the age of 10 (West, 1983).

As would be expected in relation to an heterogeneous disorder, the course of adults with serious antisocial behaviour shows considerable variation. One of the main defining characteristics of a 'disease' is increased mortality, and this is found in relation to antisocial PD, mediated by increased rates of suicide, accidental death, substance abuse and being a victim of violence (Martin, 1986). Hare *et al.* (1988) have claimed that those individuals with predominant 'core' features of psychopathy tend to show a persistently high level of criminal activity in their early adult years but that this decreases sharply after the age of about 40. However, this change is less marked in relation to violent crimes, and, in some forensic studies, about

20% of those with antisocial PD in early adult life still meet criteria at the age of 45 (Coid, 1993*a*). Nevertheless, it is encouraging that even in samples selected on the basis of serious criminal activity, with a typical history of childhood conduct disorder, most show considerable improvement during middle age.

Studies related to epidemiology

Information about the course of a disorder can often be deduced from epidemiological data, for instance when prevalence is related to age. In a catchment area study in three US sites (Robins *et al.*, 1984), the mean lifetime prevalence rate for antisocial PD was 2.6% (range 2.1–3.4) with the male:female ratio as 4.5:0.8. The diagnosis was relatively high in the 25–44 age group and was associated with early drop-out from education and inner-city populations. A similar lifetime prevalence of 2.5% was reported in another study of six US sites (Regier *et al.*, 1988) and of 3.1% in New Zealand (4.2% in males and 0.5% in females) (Wells *et al.*, 1989).

Robins *et al.* (1991), in another epidemiological study, found that only 47% of subjects with a diagnosis of antisocial PD had arrest records, while only 37% of a group who had been arrested met DSM-III criteria for antisocial PD. Also, 51.6% of those who originally received the antisocial PD diagnosis did not receive the diagnosis after follow-up at one year, which may have been related to those subjects with substance abuse at the initial contact whose behaviour had improved after a period of abstinence. In Canada, Bland *et al.* (1988) found lifetime prevalence rates for antisocial PD of 3.7% (6.5% in males, 0.8% in females), and this diagnosis was associated with the 18–34 age group and lack of sustained intimate relationships. However, lower rates have been reported in Taiwan (Hwe, Yeh & Chang, 1989) and in two US cities (Zimmerman & Coryell, 1990). In the latter study, this was probably due to an underestimate with a self-report questionnaire assessment.

In prison populations, prevalence rates for antisocial PD have varied from 39–76%, but of male prisoners whose behaviour caused serious problems in the UK, 86% received this diagnosis (Coid, 1991, 1992). Also, the pattern of violence has been found to be different between groups of prisoners with and without antisocial PD. This diagnosis was associated with bout drinking, violence directed more towards males, unknown victims, feelings of revenge, callousness and displays of aggression. In contrast, in a group without antisocial PD, violence tended to be associated with emotional arousal, domestic argument and directed to female victims who were known to their assailants.

Studies of childhood conduct disorder

The best-known study of the outcome of conduct disorder, especially theft and aggression, is that of Robins (1966), who followed up children referred to a child guidance clinic for up to 30 years. There was a significant increase in the subsequent development of antisocial PD in comparison with a group who had been referred for other problems.

Studies of non-clinical and non-forensic populations

Allebeck *et al.* (1988) and Allebeck & Allgulander (1990*b*) reported a prospective 13 year follow-up study of 50465 Swedish conscripts, which examined personality and behavioural predictions of suicide in young men. It appeared that several early indications of antisocial PD were strongly predictive of the 247 suicides that occurred, i.e. poor emotional control, substance abuse, contact with the police or child welfare authorities and lack of friends. However, a subsequent psychiatric diagnosis in inpatient care (in particular schizophrenia), was the strongest predictor of suicide.

Studies in psychiatric and offender populations

Various studies have reported different proportions of 'transient delinquents' and 'continuous antisocials', although many individuals do not easily fit either of these broad categories.

Studies of hospitalized adolescents or young adults with PD (McGlashan, 1986; Stone, 1993) have shown that some of the males and most of the adolescent females with less serious antisocial behaviour subsequently made a good adjustment in their late 20s or 30s, despite often leaving the unit against advice. The 'continuous antisocial' tended to show criminal behaviour at an earlier age.

While the eventual outlook is 'fair to good' for many individuals with antisocial PD who present as young adults to psychiatric services, there is little evidence of benefit from short-term treatment programmes. Gabbard & Coyne (1987) claimed that out of 33 patients with antisocial PD, 19 were 'completely unresponsive' to treatment.

The 'transient delinquents' show improvement relatively quickly, i.e. within a decade, but improvement has also been described in more severe and 'continuous' samples, often in the fifth decade. The sample described by Tong & McKay (1959) consisted of 587 patients discharged from an English maximum security hospital; it was found that 171 committed further offences but that these generally involved a reduction in violence. Therefore, even in such a severely affected group, a substantial number appeared to improve (Whiteley, 1970). In a sample of male prisoners with an antisocial PD diagnosis, 87% retained the diagnosis after 3 years and 72% at 9 years (Guze, 1976).

De Jong *et al.* (1992) followed up 348 male criminals who received a forensic psychiatric assessment after committing manslaughter, attempted manslaughter, or arson, at a mean age of 31 (SD 11.5); follow-up data were obtained from the criminal registry of Finland for periods following release ranging from 1 to 115 months with a mean of 41.4 months. While antisocial PD was associated with both violent and non-violent recidivism, violent recidivism in the groups that had killed or attempted to kill was associated with the degree of impulsivity of the original crime. High impulsivity was indicated by an unknown victim, no significant provocation, no premeditation and lack of motivation for financial gain. In the arsonists' group, a history of a suicide attempt was the strongest predictor of future violence.

It has also been found that prisoners with antisocial PD have a greater incidence of parole violation and further offences after release.

As has been stated, criminal convictions mainly occur in males before the age of 20. Most offenders do not continue their criminal behaviour beyond their early 20s and, in various samples of offenders, around 5% are responsible for a disproportionate amount of crime (Wolfgang *et al.*, 1972; Blumstein & Cohen, 1979). For the minority who engage in persistent criminality for much of their adult life, various stages have been identified although progression is not inevitable (Coid, 1993*a*). For this minority, a common pattern between the ages of 10 and 18 involves theft (in particular car theft) and burglary, often in the company of other adolescents, while thrill-seeking and status within the peer group are frequent motivations. The late 20s may coincide with a change for the better, but if the criminality persists, the seriousness of the crimes may increase although they are generally less numerous. Although improvement is still possible, usually in the 40s, a few will continue with criminal activity throughout their active adult life and it has been estimated that such individuals constitute a lifetime prevalence of 0.5% of the US population.

Prognostic factors

In general, age and intelligence are inversely related to future violence for those with antisocial PD (Klassen & O'Connor, 1988). It has been noted that definitions of antisocial PD differ in their reliance on the nature of interpersonal relationships involving the 'core' features of psychopathy, and on specified antisocial acts, and it is clear that the best predictor of future antisocial behaviour is not the degree of the 'core' features, but the extent of previous antisocial behaviour (De Jong *et al.*, 1992). For instance, in prison samples, Hare (1991) has shown that scores for specified antisocial behaviour using the PCL-R assessment schedule are related to revocation of parole or re-offending to a greater extent than scores related to the 'core' features.

Other 'poor prognosis' variables for re-offending have included the impulsivity of the original crime (in relation to males convicted of man-slaughter or attempted manslaughter), previous suicide attempts (in male arsonists), the degree of severity of offences, persistent lying and conning behaviour, and early onset of childhood conduct disorder (Stone, 1993).

When evaluating characteristics of childhood conduct disorder, the number and range of antisocial behaviours has been found to be more predictive of adult behaviour than environmental influences (Robins, 1978).

Other predictors of violence have included various cognitive deficits, poor social and coping skills, and alcohol and drug abuse. Aspects of various biological characteristics have also been claimed to be predictive of violence, involving levels of a metabolite of serotonin in the cerebrospinal fluid, the EEG, heart rate, skin conductance characteristics, and mild hypoglycaemia (Virkkunen *et al.*, 1989), although the latter was not confirmed (De Jong *et al.*, 1992).

Co-occurring psychiatric disorders

Antisocial PD significantly co-occurs with other PDs and other psychiatric disorders, which influence course and outcome in longitudinal studies.

In a sample of 243 subjects in special hospitals and prisons with the legal category (in England and Wales) of 'psychopathic disorder', 86% of the male prisoners had antisocial PD and 67% paranoid PD (the latter was present in 45% of those with antisocial PD) (Coid, 1991, 1992). Only two subjects with antisocial PD had this as the only PD diagnosis, and common associations were with paranoid, narcissistic, borderline and passive-aggressive PDs. The paranoid features were of particular note as they seemed to reflect a subgroup who were extremely suspicious and intolerant. Violence in such individuals could be easily triggered even by a hint of criticism. In two studies of female prisoners and patients with 'psycho-pathic disorder', who also had co-occurring borderline PD (Coid *et al.*, 1992; Coid, 1993*a*), the severity of mood disorder led to the suggestion that this should be considered as an affective disorder in its own right. Anxiety, irritability, depression and tension were associated with certain destructive behaviours which provided symptom-relief. This pattern usually appeared around puberty.

A history of other psychiatric disorders was also common in the sample of 243 subjects in English maximum security hospitals and prisons (Coid, 1993*a*), i.e. major depression in 50%, alcoholism in 35% and drug abuse in 27%. Other co-occurring disorders included sexual deviation (in particular sadism), sadistic masturbatory fantasies of rape and homicide, and compulsive homicidal urges which, if carried out, produced a sense of power, pleasure and non-sexual excitement. Pyromania and kleptomania were more common in females.

Other studies have reported that antisocial PD is also associated with somatization disorder, involving frequent bodily symptoms and complaints (Tyrer & Seivewright, 1988*b*).

Other variables associated with course and outcome of antisocial PD

Adverse childhood events

Many studies have reported associations between adverse childhood experiences and antisocial PD; Robins (1978) has suggested that the following factors may be of causal relevance in some individuals: the child placed out of the family, severe poverty, an absent parent, and antisocial behaviour by parents or caretakers. Zanarini *et al.* (1989) have noted an association between antisocial PD and separation from parents for a month or more, and claimed that harsh and rejecting parenting can also be causally implicated. Child-rearing practices involving harsh or inconsistent discipline and lack of rewards may be of particular importance as causal variables for antisocial PD in vulnerable individuals. This may involve undesirable behaviour not being consistently challenged, while good behaviour remains unacknowledged and unrewarded.

Loss events

There is some evidence that features of antisocial PD can make an individual more vulnerable to depressive symptoms after stressful life events (Perry *et al.*, 1992).

Duration of follow-up period

Although the heterogeneity of antisocial PD has been repeatedly noted, it is clear that the incidence of offending decreases with age, although the rate and timing varies between different offender subgroups. The eventual fate of the 'core' attributes of antisocial PD involving interpersonal relationships is unclear, and it may be that they are often not significantly modified with time, even though the individual has developed a more socialized behaviour pattern.

Gender

Cloninger & Gottesman (1987), reviewing genetic and family studies, concluded that while genetic factors for the development of antisocial PD are similar in men and women, the lower incidence in women is due to a higher threshold for expression. Therefore, if a woman is to develop the overt antisocial behaviour associated with antisocial PD, there may have to be a greater degree of genetic vulnerability and/or a more adverse environment, and there is evidence that when men and women with antisocial PD are compared, the women have the more disturbed childhood environments (Coid, 1993*a*). Cloninger (1978) has suggested that mild antisocial PD in women may sometimes present as somatization disorder, and there is an increased prevalence of antisocial PD and somatization disorder in the relatives of subjects with either syndrome.

Childhood conduct disorder in males usually has an earlier onset than in females, when it becomes apparent around puberty (Robins, 1986). Also, males tend to have more traffic offences, a criminal record and more promiscuity, while women are more likely to be involved with domestic violence. Compared with males, women with antisocial PD who had been previously assessed at a child guidance clinic had lower intelligence, a history of increased institutionalization, parents who were more often chronically unemployed and fathers who were more often alcoholic or antisocial.

Implications of longitudinal data for the management of antisocial PD

The evidence that has indicated that an adverse childhood can be an important, although variable, causal factor for antisocial behaviour, suggests that educational, social and economic measures aimed at improving child-rearing practices may have beneficial effects. In adult life, the long-term nature of the antisocial behaviour pattern in the recidivistic subgroup is not satisfactorily managed by a series of custodial sentences. A logical approach to an individual who repeatedly offends would be to provide longer periods of external controls but of a variable nature. While some individuals may require long terms of imprisonment, others might be provided with sufficient external constraints by careful monitoring or by a flexible system involving day, night or weekend attendance at designated centres, with the sanction of custodial provision for relatively short periods if lapses occur.

Individuals with antisocial PD have been generally considered to respond poorly to various forms of medium- or long-term psychotherapy, unless there is a co-existing depressive disorder (Perry, 1990). However, many of these patients can be assisted in a crisis by advice, counselling, psychotropic medication and short psychiatric admissions in relation to self-harm or substance abuse. It is often necessary to impose firm conditions on such contacts with medical services. In a few cases it may be appropriate to consider recommending a placement for up to a year in a residential setting (therapeutic community) involving individual and group psychotherapy.

Other personality disorders: longitudinal studies

'Cluster B' PDs (antisocial, borderline, narcissistic and histrionic PDs)

Most longitudinal data for specified PDs relate to antisocial and borderline PD, but narcissistic PD features are often associated with these (and other) PD syndromes (McGlashan & Heinssen, 1989). Plakun (1989) found that a group of inpatients with predominant narcissistic PD fared worse than a comparison group with borderline PD in respect of general level of functioning and readmission rates. It has been noted that a combination of borderline, antisocial and narcissistic PD features have a particularly poor prognosis (Stone, 1993).

'Cluster A' PDs (paranoid, schizoid, and schizotypal PDs)

Patients with paranoid and schizoid PDs tend not to seek help or to cooperate with follow-up, so that outcome data are sparse. Although there is some information for schizotypal PD, various definitions and assessment methods make interpretation difficult. McGlashan (1986) found that an inpatient group with schizotypal PD had a worse outcome compared with a borderline PD group, while patients who had a mixture of the two syndromes occupied an intermediate position. In the PI-500 series, 12 subjects had a combination of schizotypal and borderline PD, and of the ten traced, only three were self-supporting, while in a study of 97 patients attending a day unit, followed up for 3 years, schizotypal PD had the worst outcome compared with borderline PD and 'cluster C' PD groups (Stone, 1993).

'Cluster C' PDs (avoidant, dependent, obsessive-compulsive and passive-aggressive PDs)

Patients with 'cluster C' PDs tend to appear anxious or fearful, as do those with self-defeating and depressive PDs.

Patients with these PD features often have other disorders such as anxiety disorders, agoraphobia, depressive disorders and obsessive-compulsive disorder. While, in general, many patients with these features can be helped by psychotherapeutic measures, severe passive-aggressive behaviour has been considered to be very resistant to intervention. But in a study of patients with PDs at a day unit followed up for 3 years, those with 'cluster C' PDs had the best global outcome, which included reduced features of co-occurring disorders (Stone, 1993).

Effects of interventions for personality disorders – general trends shown by longitudinal studies

It appears that various forms of individual psychotherapy for PDs produce the best results for those with 'cluster C' (anxious and fearful) PDs, while the more focussed and specific cognitive-behavioural psychotherapeutic strategies are best for 'cluster B' PDs (Stone, 1993).

In a study of 357 patients with psychiatric disorders in primary care, 301 were followed up after 3 years (Casey & Tyrer, 1990). There had been significantly more PD psychopathology in those who could not be traced, and a diagnosis of PD had been made in 24% of those who were followed up. In this subgroup there had been a greater referral rate to psychiatric services and, of those admitted to hospital for psychiatric disorders, the subgroup with PD had more and longer admissions.

It is clear that PD is present in many patients who receive various forms of psychotherapy. Smith *et al.* (1980), in a review of 475 studies, concluded that the psychotherapies had been beneficial, but that efficacy had not been clearly associated with specific characteristics of treatment. Key outcome variables were the presence of positive or adaptive personality traits, such as motivation in relation to appropriate goals, candour, introspection, and a willingness to accept responsibility for one's own actions. Woollcott

(1985) has noted the prognostic importance of likeability; this is reduced if the patient is hostile, irritable and angry, so that the degree of anger in an individual with PD may be an important outcome variable.

Studies related to gender and sexual orientation

Gender and 'normal' personality

Gender differences in normal personality development have been described, for instance that young girls appear to be less selfish and aggressive than boys, but although these differences persist into adolescence, they have been reported to disappear by early adult life (Cohn, 1991). This suggests that adolescent girls achieve developmental stages, such as a capacity for moral judgement and empathy, earlier than boys, but that differences then decline with increasing age as males 'catch up'.

Gender and PD – the longitudinal perspective

Antisocial PD has a considerably higher incidence in men, while borderline PD is diagnosed more frequently in women. There are also gender differences in age of onset of PDs and related behaviour; for instance, males generally present with childhood conduct disorder at an earlier age than females, whose disordered behaviour is often apparent around puberty (Coid, 1993a). Also, in a prison sample of 25% of all women serving a prison sentence in England and Wales, women showed a higher rate of PD than a comparison group of male sentenced prisoners (18% versus 10%) (Maden, Swinton & Gunn, 1994).

Gender can be associated with various behaviours related to PDs. For patients with borderline PD in the PI-500 series (Stone, 1990), male patients married less often, found a better niche for themselves in relation to work or hobbies, and coped better with being alone. In contrast, females were more likely to become married, to relate better heterosexually, and to have more depression and self-harm. Also, they were more likely to develop an eating disorder, which occurred in about 17%.

Bardenstein & McGlashan (1988) also noted that females with borderline PD were subsequently more likely than men to get married, and, at follow-up, females reported more stressful events, and more feelings of worthlessness and guilt. In mid-life, females more often showed a decline in overall functioning and became chronically depressed in their 40s. In contrast, men were more likely to leave hospital against medical advice and obtain a forensic history. Males tended to show more alcohol abuse, while females engaged in more self-harm (McGlashan, 1993).

In relation to antisocial PD, it has already been noted that there is a gender-related difference in the age of onset of childhood conduct disorder. Also, women with antisocial PD generally report a more disturbed child-hood environment than men (Coid, 1993*a*). Gender also affects the pattern of antisocial behaviour, with female gender associated with less physical violence and more arson.

PD and gender-related variables – the longitudinal perspective

An interesting feature of reports of the PI-500 series (Stone, 1990) was that there had been a courageous attempt to rate the physical attractiveness of its female patients with borderline PD! In general, extreme attractiveness was a good prognostic indicator, together with unusual creative talent. For those who had a poor outcome despite a high rating on attractiveness, there seemed to be an association with previous sexual contact involving a first-degree male relative.

Other features that have been associated with aspects of outcome of borderline PD included having children born out of marriage and com-plaints of a premenstrual syndrome, when the features of borderline PD appeared to be intermittent and related to premenstrual mood changes.

Homosexuality and PD – the longitudinal perspective

Twelve per cent of 118 men with borderline PD in the PI-500 series had features of homosexual orientation such as homosexual fantasies, homo-sexual activity, and problems with gender identity (Stone, 1990). This appears to be a greater prevalence than in the general population, for which rates of up to 5% have been claimed for male homosexuality. The rate for female homosexuality in the PI-500, which was 1% in the borderline group, approximately mirrored that of the general population.

Perhaps the difficulties that some men can experience in relation to homosexual orientation can be a non-specific causal factor in the develop-ment of their patterns of PD behaviour, on the basis that any parallel problems can lower the threshold for the expression of behaviour related to PDs.

Longitudinal studies related to childhood precursors of personality disorders

Overview

The literature on childhood precursors of PD is mainly concerned with conduct disorders, attention deficit hyperactivity disorder (ADHD) and schizoid or schizotypal disorder. Also, there has been a renewed interest in the importance of a relatively small number (3–5) of basic temperaments (Cloninger, 1986), which appear to be identifiable in very early childhood, and are largely due to genetic factors. But while the importance of genetic inheritance for the development of personality and PD has become established by many research findings, it is also clear that adverse environmental events and interactions between specific or non-specific genetic or biological vulnerability and the environment, together with protective factors, are all important in the development of PDs. For instance, relatively low intelligence was a poor prognostic factor for the later development of antisocial PD in women, in a child guidance clinic sample (Coid, 1993*a*).

The landmarks of the literature are the associations between childhood conduct disorder (and/or ADHD) and the development of antisocial PD, and between solitariness, rigidity and hypersensitivity in children and the later diagnosis of schizoid PD (Wolff & Chick, 1980).

Both 'conduct disorder' and 'antisocial PD' are broad concepts, and the former has been defined as behaviour which violates the rights of others or social norms. It has been estimated that between 4–10% of children develop some significant degree of conduct disorder, and of those who receive this diagnosis in a medical setting, up to 40% have been reported to show serious behavioural problems in adulthood (Robins, 1978; Rutter & Giller, 1983). Aggression is often the most troublesome feature of conduct disorder and may present in different ways; younger children usually show arguments or tantrums, and these may develop into defiance and opposition. Later still, examples of aggression can include arson, theft, truancy, vandalism and substance abuse.

Early predictors of PD

Renewed interest in a small number of broad 'temperaments' has been stimulated by studies in infants and very young children, which have linked early behavioural patterns with later personality and PD features.

A community sample of 976 infants and children were first assessed (at 'T1') between the ages of 1 and 10, and followed up on two occasions, i.e. at 'T2' ($n = 778$, age 9–19) and 'T3' ($n = 776$, age 11–21). At T1, the assessment consisted of structured interviews with the mothers, which focussed on aspects of conduct problems, depression, anxiety and immaturity. Later assessments also involved interviews with the subjects. Conduct problems at T1 were related to subsequent maladaptive patterns of behaviour in adolescence, although for children under the age of 5, this was only found for girls, and related to subsequent 'cluster B' and 'C' disorders (Bernstein, 1993).

Another area of longitudinal research in relation to personality has been shyness, which has been investigated by rating the reaction and degree of behavioural restraint of very young children to unfamiliar stimuli (Kagan *et al.*, 1988). Two groups were identified at the extremes of reaction (i.e. showing 'restraint', with fear and avoidance, or showing unconcern and approach), and by the age of 7 the 'restraint' group were generally much less talkative and interactive, and more socially avoidant with unfamiliar people. It was suggested that the relevant differences in the underlying biological substrate may involve the threshold of arousal to novel stimuli.

Conduct disorder and PD

DSM-III-R notes that the essential feature of childhood conduct disorder is 'a persistent pattern of conduct in which the basic rights of others and major age-appropriate societal norms or rules are violated', while the ICD-10 specifies 'a repetitive and persistent pattern of dissocial, aggressive or defiant conduct'. The DSM-III-R criteria for conduct disorder in children form part of the criteria for antisocial PD.

Various subtypes of conduct disorder may have a predictive value, such as when behaviour is confined to the family context, the presence or absence of good integration with the peer group, and when problem behaviour is restricted to 'oppositional defiant disorder', for which DSM-III-R provides nine criteria, including 'often loses temper', and 'often argues with adults'.

In a community sample of 19 482 subjects interviewed in the NIMH Epidemiologic Catchment Area Program (Robins & Price, 1991), a history of childhood conduct disorder was associated with increased prevalence of a range of psychiatric disorders, including antisocial PD but also mania and schizophrenia.

Course and outcome of conduct disorder varies considerably, mainly in relation to criteria used and the characteristic of the sample (Lofgren *et al.*,

1991). However, most childen who receive a medical diagnosis of conduct disorder have a favourable outcome, even though Robins' classical study (1966) of 406 children referred to a child guidance clinic for behaviour such as theft and aggression found that this group went on to develop a higher rate of antisocial PD than did a comparison group of 118 referred for other reasons. After a follow-up of up to 30 years, 75% of men and 40% of women had been arrested for non-traffic offences. Childhood factors which predicted repeated adult antisocial behaviour were a variety of types of conduct disorder, many episodes, and behaviour involving strangers rather than school and home. Of the 76 girls in this study, about 20% went on to develop a disorder similar to histrionic PD. In a more severely affected sample of 55 adolescent girls in a locked unit for conduct disorder, follow-up for between 2–4 years gave a generally poor outcome (Zoccolillo & Rogers, 1991); 6% had died and about half had re-offended.

The Kauai longitudinal study of 698 children on this Hawaiian island has provided further evidence of the interaction of biological and environmental causal factors for the development of adult antisocial behaviour (Werner, 1985; Dolan & Coid, 1993).

ADHD (attention-deficit hyperactivity disorder) and PD

ADHD is defined by DSM-III-R by the presence of at least eight out of 14 behavioural characteristics, with an onset before the age of 7. The equivalent syndrome in ICD-10 is 'hyperkinetic disorders', which is a term chosen to avoid assumptions about aetiology; early onset is also claimed to be found with the latter, usually within the first 5 years, and the main feature is excessive motor activity. However, diagnosis is more readily made after the age of 5 in the early school years. ADHD occurs in around 3% of children, but is much more frequent in boys, i.e. × 6–9 in clinic samples, and × 3 in community samples.

In both classifications, the core features of the hyperactivity syndrome are overactivity and marked inattention, associated with impaired ability to complete tasks. Overactivity may involve restlessness, difficulty in remaining seated, excessive talking, frequent running and jumping, excessive fidgeting, and difficulty in playing quietly, while inattention is reflected by distractibility, rapid loss of interest, a failure to listen or to complete tasks, frequent changing from one activity or task to another, and a tendency to lose objects. However, as these features are most obvious when sustained attention is required, behaviour may seem normal in a relatively structured situation such as a clinical assessment. Also, impulsivity is a common feature, shown by frequent interruptions and intrusions to others, careless and poor schoolwork, and not taking turns or not following the rules of games. This often makes the subject unpopular with both peers and teachers. Recklessness is another feature that is commonly described, involving lack of foresight as to dangerous consequences of actions, together with behaviour which is 'accident-prone'. Finally, cognitive impairment and motor clumsiness have also been considered as part of this variable syndrome.

Almost as important as the features of the syndrome itself, is the common co-occurrence of several other apparently related disorders, particularly conduct disorder (which may have a later onset in childhood), but also 'oppositional defiant disorder' (Rey, 1993), 'specific development disorders (e.g. learning disability)', 'Tourette's syndrome', 'encopresis' and 'enuresis'. Secondary complications include low self-esteem, lability of mood with temper, depression and anxiety, a low frustration tolerance and academic underachievement.

While relatively mild overactivity and inattention are common in conduct disorder, it appears that it is important, in relation to adult outcome, to distinguish subjects with ADHD alone from those who also qualify for the co-occurring diagnosis of conduct disorder. When both disorders are present, the ICD-10 provides the diagnosis of 'hyperkinetic conduct disorder'.

The literature on ADHD has to be interpreted in the light of the characteristics of each sample reported, in particular the origin, and the degree of co-occurrence of conduct disorder. In general, the DSM-III-R claims that about one third of those from clinic samples will eventually retain some aspects of the syndrome in adult life, and there is evidence to support the validity of the diagnosis of ADHD in adults (Biedermen *et al.*, 1993). A general trend to improvement has been claimed by Klein & Mannuzza (1991), who found that one third of their sample showed remission of ADHD by mid-adolescence, and most showed reduced impairment by late adolescence. Also, Weiss (1985) found that most hyperactive children grow up without showing serious adult disorder, although about half continued to show one or more features in adolescence and early adulthood, and there was an increased risk of antisocial PD. Various adult outcomes of ADHD are possible, including: firstly, normality; secondly, significant problems with concentration, social difficulties, problems with emotional control and maladaptive impulsivity; and, thirdly, serious problems involving antisocial PD and substance abuse (Hechtman, 1991). Of the variables that influence outcome, probably the most important is co-occurring conduct disorder, which is related to the development of antisocial PD, but other factors related to poor outcome include living in an environment with a high crime rate, low measured intelligence, psychiatric disorder in parents (particularly PD), criminality in parents, loss of parents (particularly with divorce), large family, periods 'in care', violent abuse, inconsistent discipline, low socioeconomic status, and a lack of structured environment. In contrast, there are protective factors such as relatively high intelligence, adaptive personality features, a supportive family, an extended family, and a law-abiding social environment.

Mannuzza *et al.* (1991, 1993) followed up 101 young adult males, who had been previously diagnosed as hyperactive in childhood, for a mean of 16 years, and found higher-than-expected rates of ADHD features, antisocial PD and substance abuse, while a number of studies have distinguished between the outcomes of subgroups of hyperactive children based on the co-occurrence or absence of conduct disorder. For instance, a 4-year follow-up study compared 34 boys with 'pure' ADHD with 42 hyperactive boys who were also aggressive and more unsocialized (August *et al.*, 1983); it was found that the latter group, whose parents showed more PD and alcoholism, remained relatively antisocial, while inattention and impulsivity continued to be the main problems in the former group. In a recent review, Lie (1992) concluded that hyperactive children without co-occurring conduct problems do not have a significant risk for future delinquency or antisocial PD, but that if ADHD is accompanied by conduct disorder, there is a worse outcome compared with conduct disorder alone. It seems that some remnants of ADHD can be found in early adult life in about a third of children with ADHD who are followed up, and that there is a significant association between ADHD and conduct disorder, i.e. their co-occurrence is not just due to chance. This was indicated in a study of 283 male adoptees (Cadoret & Stewart, 1991), when it was found that a history of criminality in a biological parent was associated with an increased incidence in ADHD in their offspring.

Several studies have provided evidence that medication can benefit children and adults with ADHD.

Schizoid features in childhood and PD

Schizoid PD in childhood, as described by Wolff (1991), was noted to be more common in boys, and to consist of features such as unusually solitary behaviour, poor social conformity and emotional outbursts. Relative social isolation was found to persist into early adult life.

Other childhood-related variables associated with PD

Many aspects of an adverse childhood environment have been shown to be associated with PDs in adults, in particular with antisocial and borderline PD. But such relationships are complex and it is important not to assume a simple cause-and-effect model. Poor parenting may be related to parental genetic predispositions that may also be present in the child, while complex interactions between genetic, other biological, and environmental variables are likely to be involved, including the subject's behaviour influencing his or her environment.

Various aspects of experience can be subsumed under the heading of an 'adverse childhood environment'. Robins (1978), in a child guidance sample, found that girls who later had a diagnosis of antisocial PD had more institutional care, more fathers with alcoholism or antisocial behaviour, and more parents who were chronically unemployed. Other studies have confirmed associations between childhood conduct disorder and disordered family backgrounds including increased parental criminality, violence, neglect, death or absence of a parent, and erratic practices of child-rearing.

Physical abuse, including neglect, violence and sexual abuse, is of particular concern, and has been estimated to be of significance in about 1% of children in the US (Raczek, 1992). There is a clear association between physical abuse in childhood and the later development of aggressive, antisocial and criminal behaviour, with some children becoming school truants, teenage parents, delinquents, criminals and, in turn, parents who give physical abuse to the next generation. However, some children who are subject to physical abuse become shy, socially inhibited and suspicious, and may present in adulthood with low self-esteem and a pattern of failure. Also, it has been suggested that overprotection and humiliation may be related to subsequent development of avoidant PD.

Associations between PD and childhood environment can be approached from the adult perspective by examining the histories of patients with PD. Herman *et al.* (1989) found that 81% of a sample of patients with borderline PD had a history of severely adverse childhood events, such as physical abuse and witnessing serious violence, while Nig *et al.* (1989) claimed that a history of sexual abuse was associated with relatively severe borderline PD features. In a study of 50 servicemen referred for psychiatric evaluation (Raczek, 1992) there was, once again, an association between PDs (mainly antisocial and borderline) and a history of physical abuse, but it was noted that some individuals with avoidant or paranoid PD features also gave such a history, while some seemed relatively unscathed by such traumas.

The evidence does not suggest that certain childhood experiences are necessary for the development of a particular PD, or that the effects of sexual abuse are readily predictable in an individual. It has been pointed out that some children can be remarkably resilient in the face of serious childhood adversity. As causal factors for a particular PD syndrome are multiple, interactive and variable, it is not surprising that research has shown a variety of outcomes that are correlated with a range of causal variables (Crowell *et al.*, 1993).

Implications for management and prevention of PD from longitudinal studies of childhood precursors of PD

As antisocial and borderline PD are the PDs that produce the most apparent problems to society and medical services, these syndromes have attracted considerable attention. But it will be necessary to increase our knowledge of adverse and optimal childhood environments in relation to all PDs, as well as to well-adjusted personalities. This area of research is likely to be of particular importance during periods of rapid social change, for instance involving an increase in the number of one-parent families.

Even with present knowledge, it is possible to make recommendation for social policy in relation to antisocial PD and related behaviours. Measures to limit or prevent physical or psychological adversity in child-rearing are clearly important, and might involve the provision of more day-care and nursery education to pre-school children, particularly for families with identified problems. It is also important to realize that causal factors for serious conduct disorder in children are likely to be variable. In some cases, when a child's upbringing and parental background is unremarkable, it is likely that genetic or other biological factors are relatively important. For such a child, the emphasis may have to be on the management of the disorder by the provision of an appropriate limit-setting and supportive environment, while for others, who have experienced a seriously adverse environment, a more intensive psychotherapeutic approach may have more potential.

The recognition of children who are 'at risk' for adult PD provides an opportunity for educational, social and clinical services to target such groups for special help, in particular, children with both conduct disorder and ADHD. Ideally, a range of options for living and schooling should be available, so that an individually orientated approach can be attempted. What can be achieved in a special school unit with a small number of children may be impossible in the normal school system if one or more children with serious conduct disorder are part of large classes. Children and adolescents with behavioural problems may also benefit from help that focusses on social skills training, learning how to control impulsiveness, and the encouragement of self-esteem by trying to identify and reward desirable behaviour.

Longitudinal studies of personality disorders related to suicide and mortality

Some patient groups selected on the basis of PDs have shown a higher mortality than groups with affective disorders, for both inpatient and outpatient samples (Tyrer & Seivewright, 1988*b*). This was mainly due to suicide and accidents.

Patients with borderline PD have a particularly high risk of mortality within the 5 years after contact with psychiatric services. As previously noted, a review of nine studies of borderline PD found that a mean of 6.1% had committed suicide over a mean follow-up of 7.2 years, and the greatest risk appeared to be during the first 2 years after an hospital admission (Perry, 1993). This contrasts with a group with passive-aggressive PD of whom 1.3% had committed suicide by 11 years. In relation to antisocial PD, Martin *et al.* (1982) found that 2% of female felons had died at a follow-up after 6 years, and Guze (1976) reported that 3% of male felons had died violently by 9 years. This indicates that suicide is a more common outcome for severe borderline PD than for antisocial PD.

Another approach to the relationship between PD and mortality is to identify the characteristics of a group identified by suicide or other causes of death mediated by behaviour. For instance, when 62 suicides aged between 15 and 24, who had been previously admitted to hospital for self-harm, were compared with a group previously admitted but still alive, the diagnoses of PDs and substance abuse were significantly associated with the former group.

Studies of the effects of personality disorders on course and outcome of other psychiatric disorders

Overview

It has often been reported that the co-occurrence of PD is associated with a poor outcome and response to treatment of various other psychiatric disorders (Andreoli, Gressot & Aapro, 1989; Reich & Green, 1991).

Sometimes this may reflect the importance of the PD as a precursor and causal factor for the other disorder in question, for instance in relation to some cases of depressive disorders and substance abuse, but a chance co-occurrence of a PD may affect recovery from an unrelated disorder, such as brain damage or mania.

Substance abuse with PD (including alcohol-related syndromes)

Penick *et al.* (1988) have reported that the most frequent co-occurring diagnoses shown by 241 inpatient men with alcoholism were depressive disorders, antisocial PD and substance abuse, while other studies have classified alcoholism on the basis of the presence or absence of co-occurring disorders (Schuckit, 1985; Yates *et al.*, 1988; Liskow *et al.*, 1990; Powell *et al.*, 1992). Co-occurrence of antisocial PD and substance abuse had a worse outcome compared with substance abuse alone (Schuckit, 1985), but not all studies have found that such co-occurrence can predict outcome (Powell *et al.*, 1992).

Yates *et al.* (1988), in a study of 260 inpatient men with alcoholism, found that co-occurring antisocial PD was related to earlier onset of alcoholism and additional abuse of other substances, while Inman *et al.* (1985), in another inpatient study, noted that borderline PD was associated with a short duration of treatment. Another PD-related variable associated with substance abuse was found by Malloy *et al.* (1990), who reported that in 30 substance abusers with antisocial PD, there were more neuropsychological deficits compared with a control group without this PD. The explanation was assumed to be related to an earlier onset and increased severity of past alcohol intake, together with an increased incidence of head injury. In a 5-year follow-up study of subjects with repeated self-harm episodes, degree of repetition was related to a combination of PD and substance abuse, particularly alcoholism (Krarup *et al.*, 1991).

Other outcome studies of alcoholism, or other forms of substance abuse, have found that a relatively poor prognosis was associated with co-occurrence of schizoid PD (Zivich, 1981), relatively heavy drinking in a programme for those convicted of driving offences (McGuire, 1980), and drop-out rate from a residential treatment programme (Pekarik *et al.*, 1986). But in contrast to the above finding in relation to schizoid PD, there have been reports which indicate that this disorder can be associated with a better prognosis for substance abuse than when antisocial PD co-occurs (Griggs & Tyrer, 1981).

Many studies have focussed on the abuse of drugs other than alcohol.

Twenty-seven per cent of a sample of opiate addicts had co-occurring antisocial PD (Rounsaville *et al.*, 1986), and about one third of 298 cocaine abusers had a history of ADHD and conduct disorder (Carroll & Rounsaville, 1993). Of this latter subgroup, 78% were male and 47% had antisocial PD. When these subjects were compared with those without a history of ADHD, those with ADHD and conduct disorder had presented for treatment at a younger age, had an earlier onset and showed a more severe cocaine abuse. It was suggested that this form of substance abuse could, in some cases, be viewed as self-medication for residual ADHD features.

Studies of intravenous drug abusers are of increasing importance due to the spread of HIV, and the co-occurrence of intravenous drug administration with antisocial PD has been shown to be associated with increased risk of HIV transmission due to more needle sharing (Brooner *et al.*, 1993). In addition, antisocial PD has been associated with more sexual contacts (Gill *et al.*, 1992).

It is difficult to generalize from follow-up studies of substance abusers because of selection bias for the samples and high drop-out rates. However, of 60 subjects who presented to a London drug clinic in the 1970s, who were followed up for 10 years, 11 had died (Gordon, 1983). Of the rest, 75% had been abstinent for 5 years and 25% were still addicted. The latter group was associated with early parental loss, poor academic achievement, criminal conviction before the onset of substance abuse and longer terms of imprisonment, suggesting a relationship with antisocial PD. This wide disparity of outcome, with high mortality, has been shown in other studies (Edwards & Goldie, 1987; Gill *et al.*, 1992), and appears to be strongly related to the nature of co-occurring PDs.

As counselling and other forms of psychotherapy are in limited supply, it is important to deploy such resources to their best advantage. Woody *et al.* (1985), in a study involving 110 opiate addicts, concluded that co-occurrence of antisocial PD alone (i.e. without a depressive syndrome) predicted poor outcome with psychotherapy, but that if depression was present, psychotherapy appeared to be beneficial despite a history of criminal activity.

Depressive disorders with PD

The literature on the effects of PD on the course of depressive disorders is particularly difficult to interpret because of the variable range of relevant biological and environmental causal factors for both these categories of psychiatric disorder. However, it is clear that PD is common in patients with depressive syndromes, and can often influence response to treatment and outcome. Tyrer *et al.* (1983) have reported that about 40% of 313 psychiatric outpatients (many with depressive syndromes) appeared to have a PD diagnosis, and similar prevalences for co-occurring PDs have been reported for anxiety states. Merikangas, Wicki & Angst (1994) have stressed the importance of using the course of the disorder as a classification criterion for depressive disorders.

Andrews *et al.* (1990), in a 15-year follow-up study of depressive syndromes divided into 'endogenous' and 'neurotic', claimed that co-occurring PDs appeared to account for 20% of the outcome variance in the neurotic group but only 2% in the endogenous group. These results can be explained if it is assumed that this simple classificatory system produces an 'endogenous' group in which genetically mediated biological vulnerability to episodic depressive disorder is more marked, and a 'neurotic' group in which PDs are more prevalent.

Shea *et al.* (1990) described the outcome for 239 out-patients with a diagnosis of DSM-III-R's 'major depression' in the NIMH 'treatment of depression' programme. PDs were identified in 74% of the sample and these patients had a worse outcome in terms of social functioning and the degree of residual depressive symptoms. The results were similar in relation to the three DSM-III-R PD clusters and frequent PD co-occurrence was noted.

Several other studies have linked PD with poor outcome in depressed patients (Tyrer & Seivewright, 1988*b*; Duggan *et al.*, 1990; Perry, 1990; Reich, 1990*c*) and with poor response to antidepressant medication (Sato *et al.*, 1993*a, b*; Tyrer *et al.*, 1983). Also, Perry (1990) found that if depressive disorders co-occurred with borderline or antisocial PD, this was associated with relatively high recurrence rates compared with control groups with depressive disorders without PD, and that co-occurring borderline PD was related to a longer duration of depressive episodes compared with anti-social PD. Although Zimmerman, Coryell & Pfohl (1986) found that PD did not impair response to ECT in some severely depressed patients, PD was related to more frequent relapse.

When two groups of inpatients with 'major depression', with and without PD, were compared after a week in hospital without drug treatment, the presence of PD was associated with an improvement in symptoms (Mazure *et al.*, 1990). This suggests that the non-PD group in this study consisted of subjects whose depressive disorder was less respon-sive to a supportive environment, perhaps because of a higher prevalence of genetically-mediated biological causal factors. But the results of a particular study may not be relevant to groups of patients selected on a different basis (Tyrer *et al.*, 1993).

Schizophrenia with PD

It is difficult to differentiate an insidious onset of schizophrenia from a premorbid schizoid (or schizotypal) PD, but it has been claimed that such a premorbid PD is an indicator of poor prognosis (Tyrer & Seivewright, 1988*b*). However, any co-occurring PD is likely to have an adverse effect on the prognosis for schizophrenia.

Anxiety disorders with PD

In general, co-occurring PD has been found to be related to poor prognosis for anxiety disorders. In a study of 165 agoraphobic patients, 90% had at least one PD, most commonly avoidant and dependent PDs, and those with avoidant PD had the worst outcome (Chambless *et al.*, 1992). Hoffart & Martinsen (1993) reported a similar finding for avoidant PD in relation to panic disorder and agoraphobia, and to unipolar depression. Also, Reich (1988) found that for 52 patients with panic disorder who were treated for 8 weeks with anxiolytics, a poor outcome was related to PDs, in particular, antisocial, histrionic, narcissistic and avoidant PDs. However, Marchand & Wapler (1993) did not find that PD predicted the responses to cognitive behaviour therapy for agoraphobia and panic disorder.

Obsessive-compulsive disorder (OCD) with PD

PD was found to be related to outcome in 55 patients with OCD treated with clomipramine (Baer *et al.*, 1992). The co-occurrence of a 'cluster A' PD (paranoid, schizoid or schizotypal PD) was associated with a more severe syndrome, while a worse outcome was related to schizotypal, borderline and avoidant PDs, to the total number of PD diagnoses and to one or more 'cluster A' PDs.

Eating disorders with PD

Co-occurring PD has been shown to predict outcome for eating disorders, in particular for bulimia nervosa. For example, Sansone & Fine (1992), in a 3-year follow-up, found that the degree of borderline PD features was related to greater global distress, less life satisfaction and less perceived improvement in eating disorder symptoms. Also, Johnson *et al.* (1990), in a 1-year follow-up of borderline and non-borderline PD groups of patients with bulimia nervosa, found that the non-borderline group had a better symptomatic outcome. Alcohol abuse is another indicator of poor prognosis (Lacey, 1984; Rossiter *et al.*, 1993). However, these data relate to relatively short-term outcomes that do not take into account the gradual improvement in borderline PD over longer periods.

Stone *et al.* (1987), in a 10-year follow-up study, found that eating disorders with co-occurring borderline PD did not have a worse outcome compared with borderline PD alone, measured by a Global Assessment Scale score, and that severe obsessive-compulsive PD traits with anorexia nervosa may be associated with the worst outcomes.

Implications for the management of psychiatric disorders with co-occurring PD

It is clear that co-occurrence of PDs with other psychiatric disorders is common, and has implications for management and outcome, in particular for the common syndromes of substance abuse and depressive disorders. It is, therefore, most important to assess PD status in patients with all psychiatric disorders.

5

Assessment of personality disorders

J.H. DOWSON

Nature of personality disorders

The ingredients of PDs consist of higher mental activity such as attitudes, beliefs, motivations and feelings, and associated overt behaviour. However, only the overt behaviour, which includes speech, is available for investigation. Behaviour related to PDs has three characteristics: a varying degree of repetition, which means that future behaviour can be predicted; some degree of generalizability in which specified behaviour is shown in a range of situations; and some impairment or distress. But even relatively uncomplicated behaviours, such as driving recklessly, are subject to variability when repeated, and precise specification of behaviour is difficult.

A trait, such as sociability, is the most commonly used basic unit to describe and define PDs, and consists of a group of related behaviours. But each trait is also a theoretical entity which involves relationships between aspects of higher mental activity. In the main current definitions of PDs, traits vary in the number of related behaviours, in the degree of reliance on specified behaviours and on the nature of associated aspects of higher mental activity, such as motivation. The trait approach to PD also involves higher-order theoretical entities, in which several traits are combined to form a smaller number of broader dimensions, while lower-order or 'fine-grain' examples of specified behaviour have been included in definitions of some features of PDs. A trait has been considered as a summary of consistencies of behaviour, reflecting the individual's characteristics, the situation and the individual–situation interaction, so that a PD will always, to some degree, reflect the individual's environment.

An approach to PD assessment also depends on concepts of the relationships between PDs, normal personality and other psychiatric disorders. Paranoid and schizotypal PDs may be relatively discrete and related to schizophrenia (Grove & Tellegen, 1991; Livesley, 1991), while most PD traits appear to be on a severity-related continuum with higher mental activity and behaviour shown by the normal population (Cloninger, 1987a; Schroeder & Livesley, 1991). For such traits a dimensional approach to assessment would seem to be indicated.

Classification of personality disorders

PD assessment has to be evaluated in the context of the main classificatory systems, which are based on polythetic sets of defining criteria, each requiring a minimum number of positive ratings. But such a system is not necessarily ideally suited for all the purposes of classification, which include description of behavioural phenomena, distinguishing between PDs, or differentiating PDs from other mental disorders. Different criteria might be employed for different purposes; for instance the presence or absence of a clear desire for affection and acceptance would be expected to discriminate between avoidant and schizoid PDs.

Despite their shortcomings, categorical 'all-or-none' PD diagnoses, made on the basis of a minimum number of positive criteria, have been in widespread use for many years, suggesting that such an approach has some value. But although a categorical PD diagnosis can convey a considerable amount of information, the disadvantages of the main classification systems have been frequently described. For instance, for each criterion, and for each PD, the threshold between disorder and normality is often arbitrary and difficult to assess. Also, an 'all-or-none' rating generally loses information, although it has been argued that determining a clinically relevant threshold is more useful than measuring the degree of a characteristic (Widiger, 1992). Other problems with the DSM-III-R system for PDs have included overlap between features in the various PD syndromes, the time required to assess over 100 criteria, and the heterogeneity of each of the individual PDs due to the polythetic system. Also, this type of classification makes no allowance for the occurrence of very severely maladaptive examples of a limited number of criteria, which are insufficient to produce a PD diagnosis. Possible modifications to the DSM-III-R system include the provision of essential core criteria, weighted criteria and a greater use of exclusion criteria, perhaps involving the presence of normal personality features.

'Core' criteria can be considered as those which are either necessary or sufficient for a categorical diagnosis (Reich, 1992). In the case of borderline PD, Hurt *et al.* (1990) have claimed, on the basis of statistical analysis of previous studies, that there are three core dimensions, i.e. disorders of identity, mood and impulsivity. However, although relatively few criteria would be needed for diagnosis on this basis, a smaller number of criteria may not do justice to the descriptive function of a classification. A variant of the concept of core criteria consists of the identification of combinations of two or more criteria, which have particular diagnostic significance when both are rated positive. For example, Reich (1992) found that a combination of unstable and intense relationships, intense uncontrolled anger and physically self-damaging acts, had high values for both positive and negative predictive power for diagnoses which were based on all the borderline PD criteria.

If some of a group of individuals have received the diagnosis of borderline PD on the basis of the DSM-III-R criteria, the positive predictive power of each criterion is the number of positive ratings in the subgroup with borderline PD, divided by the number of positive ratings in the entire group. Similarly, the negative predictive power of each criterion is the number of negative ratings in those individuals who did not have a borderline PD diagnosis divided by the number of negative ratings in the entire group (Skodol *et al.*, 1988). These ratios are one means by which each individual criterion, or a combination of criteria, can be evaluated, when two groups of subjects are being compared.

Fundamental changes in the assessment of PD for clinical and research purposes have been suggested, in particular the use of dimensional ratings for many PD features and for the severity of impairment. The theoretical advantages are clear: this is more consistent with research findings related to the identification of most PD features in both normal and clinical populations; more information is retained; reliability of assessment should increase; and arbitrary boundaries between normality and disorder are avoided. A dimensional approach to PD assessment could also include other traits and higher-order traits derived from the study of normal personality; for example, the following five dimensions: neuroticism (with persistent or recurrent anxiety, anger and depression), extraversion, openness to experience, agreeableness and conscientiousness (Costa & McCrae, 1992). (The main adjectives defining these dimensions were calm/worrying, reserved/affectionate, down to earth/imaginative, ruthless/soft-hearted, and negligent/conscientious.) Also, the following eight dimensions of personality functioning have been described (Frances, 1982): managerial, responsible, cooperative, docile, self-effacing, rebellious, aggressive and competitive. Each can present to an intense and maladaptive degree and this model has two characteristics that appear to be relevant in any system of description and classification: some features are more likely to be associated than others, while other features are negatively correlated, for instance, responsibility and rebelliousness.

Livesley (1991) has attempted to identify a dimensional classificatory system for PDs based on clinical observations and considered that 'the personality characteristics of general-population subjects differ from those of patients with personality disorder only in degree'. Factor analysis of self-report ratings of a range of items gave 18 dimensions involving affective instability, anxiety, compulsivity, conduct problems, diffidence, identity disturbance, insecure attachment, interpersonal disesteem, intimacy problems, narcissism, passive oppositionality, perceptual-cognitive distortion, rejection, restricted expression, self-harm, social avoidance, stimulus seeking and suspiciousness. These gave four higher-order dimensions involving generalized behavioural instability ('psychopathic entitlement' with poor impulse control, poor socialization and need for stimulation); social withdrawal or avoidance; dependence; and compulsivity (with orderliness, conscientiousness, preoccupation with detail and a need to be active) (Schroeder & Livesley, 1991). In relation to PDs, there have been other descriptions involving four main dimensions; for example, Walton & Presly's (1973) similar descriptions of hysterical personality, social avoidance, submissiveness, and obsessional/schizoid characteristics. Tyrer & Alexander (1979) also reported four similar major PD dimensions, involving sociopathy, schizoid features, passive-dependence and anankastic (obsessional) features.

Cloninger (1987a) has described a method for description and classification of both normal personality and PD, based on a theory that there are three dimensions of stimulus-response characteristics, namely 'novelty seeking', 'harm avoidance' and 'reward dependence'. The interactions of varying degrees of these dimensions are hypothesized to explain the various clinical presentations of PD. 'Novelty seeking' involves frequent exploratory activity with active avoidance of monotony; 'harm avoidance' is a tendency to show marked response to aversive stimuli, including the avoidance of novel stimuli; while 'reward dependence' is a tendency to show marked response to rewarding stimuli, including approval and support. This model is compatible with some categories based on clinical data; for instance, antisocial PD can be considered to be a consequence of high novelty seeking, while excessive dependence could result from high degrees of harm avoidance and reward dependence.

Another concept which has been used in the context of the classification of PD is the 'ideal type'. This refers to a theoretical approach to the nature of, and relationships between, various PD traits, and can be considered as a hypothesis that gives a meaningful account of suggested relationships between various PD characteristics. Therefore it provides a framework to understand an individual patient (Livesley, 1991). An 'ideal type' might be provided by a selected case vignette that is considered to have general significance, although the presumed relationships between the features are not based on empirical data.

Information sources

Data for PD assessment can be obtained from three main sources: the patient, informants and observation in clinical settings over varying periods. There is evidence that some PDs are associated with a higher prevalence of the same or related disorders in first degree relatives, and with some biological variables, so that assessment may also include family history and physiological data (Reich, 1992).

Non-methodological variables that influence assessment

The evaluation of repeated behaviour is influenced not only by variables associated with the methods used, including sample selection, but also by several non-methodological variables, such as environmental changes and the presence of other mental disorders. The latter would include a premenstrual syndrome that can be associated with the intermittent appearance or exaggeration of relevant PD behaviour.

Features of PD can show apparent remission associated with improvements in any co-occurring mental disorders such as anxiety and depression (McMahon, Flynn & Davidson, 1985; Reich *et al.*, 1987a; Joffe & Regan, 1988; Boyce *et al.*, 1989; Endicott & Shea, 1989; Mavissakalian, Hamann & Jones, 1990b; Stuart *et al.*, 1992), although certain features of antisocial or narcissistic PD may become more pronounced if a co-occurring depressive syndrome improves (Stankovic *et al.*, 1992). Peselow *et al.* (1994) applied a structured interview for PD during a period when the subjects' mood was depressed and after recovery, and found that PD features from clusters A and C tended to decrease after successful recovery from depression, in contrast to features of cluster B. Also, any specified PD may interact with other co-occurring PDs or other mental disorders, with subthreshold PD features and with normal PD characteristics.

In addition, the manifestations of many PDs, such as antisocial and borderline PDs, change gradually over time. Such changes may be related to social class, which requires matching in comparative studies.

Assessment: an overview

PD assessment routinely involves a clinician's 'present or absent' rating for the predominant PD features in the history and presentation, based on a relatively unstructured interview and data from various informants. Such 'routine clinical assessment' will be considered in a subsequent section of this chapter. The interview with the patient should cover the main areas of maladaptive behaviour relevant to PDs: antisocial behaviour, dependence on others, problems in sustaining relationships, and attitudes towards other people (Tyrer, 1989). It must be noted that some patients with PD refuse to cooperate in any assessment method that involves any structured procedure; in such cases, methods involving the clinician's ratings are required.

There are three main types of assessment methodology: structured interviews, self-report questionnaires, and consensus ratings (or diagnoses) from various sources. This last type includes the 'LEAD standard', i.e. 'longitudinal expert evaluation using all available data' (Spitzer, 1983), which is based on information from patient assessments, past records, informants and observations over a period of inpatient or outpatient contact. The final ratings or diagnoses are based on a consensus of several experienced clinicians. The reliability of assessment is likely to be increased by the use of more than one assessment method. Informants are often important for PD assessment, in particular where the patient has another mental disorder such as a depressive syndrome or substance abuse.

Zimmerman (1994), in a review of research methods, noted that inter-rater reliability coefficients for the same interview, using standardized interviews, is usually good, in contrast to poor reliability in relation to unstandardized clinical assessments. As might be expected, test–retest reliability coefficients are generally lower than those for joint-ratings of the same interview, and decrease with increasing time between interviews. Some PDs, such as antisocial PD, are less affected than other PDs by the test–retest interval, while co-occurring disorders such as depressed mood tend to influence the results of PD assessment by both self-report question-naires and structured interview. Assessment is further complicated by a tendency for subjects to report less psychopathology at subsequent inter-views. Also, reliability of PD assessment would be expected to vary depending on the selection criteria of the sample, for example it is likely to increase if a sample of subjects with PD are selected on the basis of severity.

Information from the patient, from both interviews or self-report questionnaires, may be associated with inaccuracies and 'response-bias'.

But, although the questions that form part of interviews and questionnaires usually have 'face validity', and are mainly designed to elicit a true response, a question may still be useful if it produces a consistent response, whether or not it is true.

There have been several indirect approaches to PD assessment, but these have made little or no contribution to influential psychiatric research. Several such methods, such as the Thematic Apperception Test (TAT), the Rorschach inkblot test, and sentence completion tasks, present the patient with stimuli that have ambiguous meanings. The patient's subsequent response would be expected to reflect aspects of his/her higher mental functioning. The TAT was originally introduced as a measure of personality, and consisted of a series of cards, each with a picture of a situation. The patient was then asked to comment on what the situation might be. The rationale for this had been described thus:

the test is based upon the well recognized fact that when a person interprets an ambiguous social situation he is apt to expose his own personality as much as the phenomenon to which he is attending. Absorbed in his attempt to explain the objective occurrence, he becomes naively unconscious of himself and of the scrutiny of others and, therefore, defensively less vigilant.

But although this is likely to be true, the evaluation and rating of the responses present considerable problems.

Another focus for the assessment of PD is the cognitive aspect of personality. Although current DSM-IV and ICD-10 criteria include some motivations and attitudes, such phenomena have been insufficiently addressed in the clinical literature. For example, an evaluation of repeated acts of violence might explore the personal meaning of the violent acts to the offender (Blackburn, 1989).

The disadvantages of the DSM-III-R and DSM-IV PD classifications will affect any assessment method based on this system, and a frequent problem has been that an individual has often received several co-occurring DSM-III-R PD diagnoses that are cumbersome in clinical practice.

Perry (1992) has reviewed nine studies which compared two or more assessment methods for DSM-III-R PD diagnoses, administered to the same group of subjects. Reliability was low, with a median kappa of only 0.25. Agreement was lower between self-report questionnaire and structured interview than between two interview methods, and comparing dimensional scores for the different methods made little difference. The depressing conclusion was that, despite the good inter-rater reliability of the various assessment methods (although there was a lack of test–retest reliability data for longer periods than a few months), PD diagnoses were not significantly comparable across methods. However, agreement may improve in more severely ill populations (Reich, 1992).

It has been argued that the LEAD procedure, in particular if this involves a period of observation and multidisciplinary clinical conferences in an inpatient unit, is the best validity standard available with which to compare other methods of PD assessment. This procedure was compared with two structured interviews, and confirmed that diagnoses such as antisocial and schizoid PDs, which depend mainly on readily-identified behaviour, are relatively reliable between assessment methods. In contrast, passive-aggressive, self-defeating and narcissistic PDs were diagnosed much less often with structured interviews (Skodal *et al.*, 1990).

Methodological variables

Many relevant methodological variables affecting PD assessment have been studied, especially in relation to procedures involving structured interviews or self-report questionnaires. Such variables include the patient's perception of confidentiality, the relationship of the clinician or researcher with the subject, the duration of the period to be assessed, the wording of the questions and various types of response-bias (Goldberg, 1972). The 'true/false' (or 'yes/no') format has been commonly used, despite problems with arbitrary thresholds and loss of information, but if a more complex rating scale is used, other types of response-bias and different scoring methods need to be considered. These include an estimate on a scale with fixed points or on a scale with a continuous line, or the selection of alternative adjectives to describe higher mental activity or behaviour. It appears that the optimum number of positions on a scale should not generally exceed six. Also, if there are three or more points on an interval rating scale, unwarranted assumptions may be made about the distance between pairs of points, as the distances between the points is difficult to quantify in terms of each PD variable being measured, and may vary in clinical significance between different PD criteria. If several criteria are being rated, it is possible to weight the score for those considered to be essential to the diagnosis or of relative clinical importance, or to transform scores. When there are three or more points on a rating scale, various types of response-bias need to be taken into account, such as 'end-bias', 'middle-bias', or a tendency to mark the left or right side of the scale. Methods to counteract such problems include changing the pathological response side of the scale to the left or right in a random manner, and to score a 4-point scale as 0011 instead of 0123. A 4-point scale would be expected to avoid a central-tendency bias (Streiner & Norman, 1989).

When considering the wording of interview questions or questionnaires, commonly understood words need to be chosen and the item should avoid ambiguity, value-laden words, implied criticism and negative wording. For example, 'I sometimes steal' might become 'I can't help stealing sometimes'. A self-report method with a degree of reliability and validity requires an underlying PD classification that covers both the cognitive and overt behavioural aspects of a given trait. Also, when the presence of relevant behaviour is being assessed, it is best to enquire about a range of examples, and the underlying motivation may need to be evaluated; for instance, behaviour related to anger may be in response to very different PD traits such as sensitivity to criticism or fear of abandonment, while having no close relationships may reflect a lack of motivation or, in the case of avoidant PD, anxiety together with an underlying desire for social contact (Shea, 1992).

Response-bias may affect assessment procedures, for instance a 'yes' (or agreement) bias, a 'no' bias, a tendency to answer in a way that reflects social desirability, and the 'hello–goodbye' effect. The latter consists of a tendency to over-report problems at the start of a clinical contact and the opposite bias at its conclusion. Specific PD psychopathology may also affect response-bias, for instance, exaggerated answers may be associated with histrionic, narcissistic, self-defeating and dependent PD features. An additional problem with any response-bias is that it may vary depending on the content of the question. Social class is an additional variable which may contribute towards a response-bias, as there is an association between low socio-economic status and general dissatisfaction. A particular PD trait may be associated with a response-bias, for instance, a person with obsessive-compulsive PD traits may be very meticulous and tidy but does not rate him/herself in this way because of his/her impossibly high standards. Also, individual patients may have an idiosyncratic bias, and individual response-bias may be partly determined by the person's use of various psychological defence mechanisms such as denial. Assessment of response-bias can be attempted with additional questions which are directed to characteristics such as exaggeration, acquiescence, denial and lying.

Although self-report questions form the basis of both structured interviews and self-report questionnaires (SRQs), structured interviews may have advantages over SRQs, as an experienced interviewer can omit inappropriate questions, make a judgement as to the subject's concent-

Table 5.1 *Structured interviews for the assessment of personality disorders (PDs)*

Assessment target		Interview method
DSM-III or DSM-III-R PDs	SCID-II	(Structured Clinical Interview for DSM-III-R Personality Disorder)
	PDE	(Personality Disorder Examination)
	SIDP-R	(Structured Interview for DSM-III-R Personality Disorders)
	DIPD	(Diagnostic Interview for Personality Disorders)
	PIQ-II	(Personality Interview Questionnaire II)
24 personality dimensions and ICD PD categories	PAS	(Personality Assessment Schedule)
ICD-10 PD categories	SAP	(Standardized Assessment of Personality) – for informants only
18 subscales based on psychoanalytic theory	KAPP	(Karolinska Psychodynamic Profile)

ration, cooperation and understanding of the questions, and can often encourage compliance. Also, some subjects refuse to cooperate in questionnaire assessments, and their use and understanding of the spoken word is often better than the written word. But SRQs may have significant advantages for cooperative subjects: interviewer variables are reduced and the application of a SRQ is a simple and cheap procedure that can be applied to large samples in research studies. At present, SRQs are not recommended for use in making categorical PD diagnoses in clinical settings, but they can be used to compare groups of patients in research studies and as screening instruments to identify areas for further evaluation at interview.

Structured interviews

'Structured interview' is a term that incorporates 'semistructured' procedures in which 'probes' (i.e. further questions) can be added based on the interviewer's clinical judgement. But as an interview can never be completely structured in respect to interviewer behaviour, the term 'semistructured' is more accurate even for the set questions. Such interviews can be divided into those based on a comprehensive range of PD characteristics defined by various classificatory systems (Table 5.1), and those directed towards a relatively narrow range of specific features of PDs (Table 5.2). Most interviews involve the patient (or subject), although some have

Table 5.2 *Structured interviews for the assessment of specific features of personality disorders (PDs)*

Assessment target	Interview method
'Borderline' personality disorder based on various concepts	DIB (Diagnostic Interview for Borderlines) Kernberg's Structured Interview SBP (Schedule for Borderline Personalities) BDP scale (The Borderline Personality Disorder scale)
DSM-III-R Schizotypal PD and related features	SIS (The Structured Interview for Schizotypy) SSP (The Schedule for Schizotypal Personalities) Symptom Schedule for the Diagnosis of Borderline Schizophrenia
Narcissistic PD based on various concepts	DIN (The Diagnostic Interview for Narcissism)
Self-harm and aggression	SAS (The Suicide and Aggression Survey)
Social dysfunction	APFA (Adult Personality Functioning Assessment)

complementary informants' versions. However, the Standardized Assessment of Personality (SAP, Mann *et al.*, 1981) is used only with informants.

SCID-II

The Structured Clinical Interview for DSM-III-R personality disorder (Spitzer *et al.*, 1987) has 120 items and involves a 60–90 minute interview between clinician and subject. It is based on the DSM-III-R classification and is designed to be used in conjunction with the SCID-I instrument (i.e. related to the DSM-III-R axis I), which evaluates any co-occurring mental disorders.

The items cover each PD in turn and each DSM-III-R criterion is evaluated by a specified question (or questions) and subsequent specified probes. But the clinician can also probe further and clarify, using his/her judgement before rating each item on a 4-point scale: 'inadequate information', 'negative', 'subthreshold' and 'threshold'. One disadvantage of presenting all criteria for each PD in sequence is a risk of a 'halo effect', when subsequent ratings are influenced by prior positive ratings for the same PD (Widiger & Frances, 1987). A unique feature of the SCID-II

(which is also available as a computerized version) is the option to precede
the interview by a self-report questionnaire covering the same items.
Although such questionnaires have been shown to produce false positives
in comparison with interview ratings, there are very few false negatives, so
that the prior use of the questionnaire can identify a subset of items for
further evaluation at interview, while the others are omitted. The consequent saving of time should encourage its use in routine clinical practice as
well as in research (Reich, 1992).

PDE

The Personality Disorder Examination (PDE) (Loranger *et al.*, 1987;
Reich, 1989) can provide diagnoses and dimensional scores for each of the
DSM-III-R PDs, although the DSM-III-R structure is reorganized so that
items are presented in a sequence under six sections: work, self, interpersonal relations, affects, reality testing and impulse control. Each section
begins with open-ended questions and additional items relate to behaviour
at interview. The time required is usually up to 2 hours and there is a parallel
version for informants. At the beginning, the subject is told 'the questions I
am going to ask concern what you are like most of the time. I'm interested in
what has been typical of you throughout your adult life, and not just
recently. But if you have changed and your answers might have been
different at some time in the past, be sure to let me know'. Each of the 128
items is scored on a 3-point scale: 0 (absent or not clinically significant); 1
(present but of uncertain clinical significance); and 2 (present and clinically
significant). Also there is an 'uncertain' category.

Inter-rater reliability has been shown to be good with kappas of 0.7 or
above for individual PD diagnoses, while test–retest reliability for borderline PD (as shown by testing by another rater prior to discharge from
hospital) gave a kappa of 0.57 (Widiger & Frances, 1987). But this
instrument has been criticized for relying too much on patients' opinions
and self-evaluations, as patients are not encouraged to provide examples to
support their answers. However, it has led to the development of a modified
version, the International Personality Disorder Examination (IPDE),
which has been used in several World Health Organization studies (Loranger *et al.*, 1991).

SIDP-R

The Structured Interview for DSM-III-R Personality Disorders is an
updated version of the SIDP for DSM-III (Pfohl, Stangl & Zimmerman,

1982; Reich, 1989). It provides 160 questions for the subject, which are arranged in 16 sections based on aspects of functioning, such as self-esteem, dependency and social interaction. Questions are open-ended and the interviewer can clarify and probe. Each criterion is scored on a 3-point scale (0,1,2). Although the time required for the interview has been stated to be up to $1\frac{1}{2}$ hours, this has been considered to be an optimistic claim. The interviewer should be an experienced clinician, and a prior assessment of other mental disorders is recommended. If a change in personality has followed the onset of another mental disorder, the predominant features in the last 5 years are accepted (Standage, 1989).

Studies of inter-rater reliability have given kappas above 0.6 for schizotypal, histrionic, dependent, borderline and passive-aggressive PDs (Widiger & Frances, 1987), although in most cases the same interview was assessed by two raters. However, test–retest results after 6 months, involving the same interviewer, gave an acceptable kappa of 0.68 for the presence of 'any PD', and of 0.7 for borderline PD, although there was poor agreement for some other PDs (Reich, 1989).

In a study of 66 patients with depressive disorders (Zimmerman *et al.*, 1988), there was poor agreement between SIDP ratings made on the basis of the interviews with the patient and those involving a close informant; for all individual PD diagnoses, kappas were below 0.35. Informants generally reported more pathology for each individual PD, except for antisocial and schizoid PDs; for example, borderline PD was diagnosed 3 times more often on the basis of the informants' interview.

DIPD

The Diagnostic Interview for Personality Disorders (DIPD) (Zanarini *et al.*, 1987) has 252 questions in 11 sections, based on the DSM-III-R PDs. Each item has 2–3 probes and it has been claimed, again optimistically, that the interview usually takes up to $1\frac{1}{2}$ hours. Additional enquiries based on clinical judgement are encouraged, and prior assessment of other co-occurring non-PD psychiatric disorders is recommended. Each PD criterion is scored as follows: 2 = present and definitely clinically significant; 1 = present and probably clinically significant; 0 = absent and clinically insignificant. Inter-rater reliabilities for a group of inpatients were high (the kappas were above 0.88) for all PDs except paranoid PD, although schizoid PD was never diagnosed. Test–retest kappas after one week were above 0.6 for seven PDs, including antisocial PD (0.84) and borderline PD (0.85).

PIQ-II

The Personality Interview Questionnaire II (PIQ-II, Widiger, 1987) is an interview that has 106 questions divided into eight sections: self-description; self-confidence; work; relationships; emotions; social responsibility; interpersonal sensitivity and aberrant behaviour; and perceptions and beliefs. Each item is scored on a 9-point scale. Although it was originally used by lay interviewers, clinical experience is preferred.

The following structured interviews do not generate DSM-III-R PD diagnoses:

PAS

The Personality Assessment Schedule (PAS) was developed by Tyrer & Alexander (1988) and subsequently revised. It is not based on either the DSM or ICD classifications, but on 24 traits derived from the clinical literature: pessimism, worthlessness, optimism, lability, anxiousness, suspiciousness, introspection, shyness, aloofness, sensitivity, vulnerability, irritability, impulsiveness, aggressiveness, callousness, irresponsibility, childishness, resourcelessness, dependence, submissiveness, conscientiousness, rigidity, eccentricity and hypochondriasis.

Each is assessed on a 9-point severity scale after several specified questions have been presented, although further questions are encouraged. The interview takes up to an hour and can be administered to the subject or an informant. Analysis of the scores can give one of three global categories based on severity: 'personality difficulty', 'personality disorder' and 'severe personality disorder'. Scores can be converted to the ICD PD categories, but while some of the PD categories are similar to those of the DSM-III-R, they are not strictly equivalent.

Good inter-rater reliability and acceptable test–retest reliability have been reported (Ferguson & Tyrer, 1989), but there has been poor correlation between ratings from patients' and informants' interviews (Widiger & Frances, 1987). This instrument has been shown to have predictive validity for improvement of depressive symptoms with drug treatment and for the effects of an alcohol treatment programme (Reich, 1992).

SAP

The Standard Assessment of Personality (SAP) was reported by Mann *et al.* (1981) and is unusual in that it is a short interview (about 20 minutes) with an informant only. A revised version, which was modified in relation to the ICD-10, has been recently published (Pilgrim & Mann, 1990; Pilgrim *et al.*, 1993).

The informant should have known the patient for at least 5 years during which other mental disorders were not apparent. After open-ended questions with prompts, the following ten probes are given:

how does he/she get on with people; does he/she have many friends; does he/she trust other people; what is his/her temper like; how does he/she cope with life; is he/she a calm sort of person; how much does he/she depend on others; how does he/she respond to criticism; does he/she have unusually high standards – at work or home; and what sort of opinion does he/she have of him/herself?

If the informant uses any of a set of key words suggesting PD features, the following eight personality categories are evaluated further: paranoid, schizoid, dissocial, impulsive, histrionic, anankastic, anxious and dependent, with a set of seven questions for each category. The degree of handicap is then assessed by three additional questions, and the informant is also asked about the priority of handicaps if there are more than one PD categories.

Satisfactory inter-rater reliability has been reported, and although test–retest reliability after one year was variable and often poor, the kappa for anankastic (obsessive-compulsive) PD was 0.74 (Widiger & Frances, 1987).

KAPP

The Karolinska Psychodynamic Profile (KAPP, Weinryb *et al.*, 1992) is a structured interview based on psychoanalytic theory in which 18 subscales are evaluated, involving the patient's self-image and relationships with others. But these include items which would appear to present particular problems of reliability, such as 'regression in the service of the ego', while others, such as 'sexual functioning' would be influenced by many variables other than those of PD.

The following structured interviews are directed towards specific features of PD psychopathology (Table 5.2):

DIB

The Diagnostic Interview for Borderlines (DIB, Gunderson *et al.*, 1981) was based on several concepts and meanings of the term 'borderline' in previous literature. Although it reflects a similar concept to the definitions of borderline PD in DSM-III and III-R, substantial 'convergent validity' (i.e. agreement between DSM-III-R and DIB diagnoses) has not been shown (Widiger & Frances, 1987).

The interview takes up to 90 minutes and covers five areas of functioning (sections): social adaptation (e.g. school/work achievement, social activities, appearance/manners); impulse/action patterns (e.g. self-mutilation, manipulative suicide threat or action, drug abuse, antisocial behaviour); affects (e.g. depression, anger); psychosis (e.g. derealization, depersonalization, brief paranoid experiences); and interpersonal relations (e.g. avoids being alone, instability, devaluation of others, and dependency on others). The 165 items involve questions (some related to specified behaviour), together with observations during the interview. Most items are rated as 'absent', 'probable' (some) or 'yes' (much), and scored 0, 1 and 2 respectively. But two items have a maximum score of 4, i.e. 'repeated manipulative suicide attempts' and 'severe dissociative experiences'. Each of the five areas of functioning is then scored separately on a 0, 1, 2 scale, and a threshold score for the sum of the five subscores of at least 7 classifies the patient as 'borderline' (Lewis & Harder, 1991).

The sections that relate mostly to symptoms (affects and psychosis) are generally based on the preceding 3-month period, while the sections involving social adaptation and impulse/action patterns are based on the previous 2 years, and the 'interpersonal relations' section on the preceding 3 years.

Acceptable inter-rater reliability has been reported (Ferguson & Tyrer, 1989), as have examples of convergent validity involving associations with other assessment methods and clinical diagnosis. But although the DIB has not always discriminated between those with borderline PD and those with other PDs (Reich, 1992), this may have been due to high rates of co-occurring PDs. Widiger & Frances (1987) have discussed the various strategies for borderline PD assessment in different settings and populations, involving adjustment of diagnostic thresholds and weighting of the scores of individual sections.

Kernberg's Structured Interview (Kernberg, 1977)

This is based on three areas of 'personality organization': namely, serious distortions in reality testing, a predominant use of splitting defence mechanisms, and serious difficulties in the formation of a cohesive identity. But although this method provides a framework for the evaluation of individual patients, the scores cannot be satisfactorily combined to provide a diagnosis. However, ratings from the three areas have been associated with DSM-III-R borderline PD diagnoses (Lewis & Harder, 1991).

SBP

The Schedule for Borderline Personalities (SBP) is part of a 70-item 'Schedule for Interviewing Borderlines', (Baron, 1981), but has not been widely used. Each item is rated on a 5-point scale.

BPD scale

The Borderline Personality Disorder scale (BPD) (Perry & Klerman, 1980) has 36 items involving questions for nine categories of relevant behaviour. It takes up to 90 minutes to administer and the results can be related to DSM-III criteria.

There is evidence for its reliability and validity but this instrument has not been widely used (Reich, 1992).

SIS

The Structured Interview for Schizotypy (SIS) was designed as a research instrument for assessing schizotypal symptoms and signs (Kendler, Lieberman & Walsh, 1989) and has been applied to 29 pairs of twins (Kendler *et al.*, 1991).

SSP

The Schedule for Schizotypal Personalities (SSP) (Baron, 1981) is part of the 'Schedule for Interviewing Borderlines', together with the SBP as noted above. This assesses ten areas based partly on DSM-III criteria for schizotypal PD: illusions; depersonalization/derealization; ideas of reference; suspiciousness; magical thinking; inadequate support; odd communication; feedback from others; social isolation; social anxiety; and transient delusions/hallucinations. (Abnormal scores in four or more areas identifies DSM-III schizotypal PD.) However, many items rely too heavily on self-evaluation or on previous 'feedback' from others to the patient. But good inter-rater reliability has been shown (Widiger & Frances, 1987).

Symptom Schedule for the Diagnosis of Borderline Schizophrenia

This structured interview was reported by Khouri *et al.* (1980) and covers features such as altered perceptions of body-image/self or of the world around, auditory hallucinations, abnormalities of thought pattern and content, ideas of reference, ideas of persecution, preoccupation with aspects of sex and violence, and episodes of self-harm.

DIN

The Diagnostic Interview for Narcissism (DIN) (Gunderson *et al.*, 1990) takes up to 50 minutes and evaluates 33 aspects of narcissism by 105 questions within the following five sections: grandiosity; interpersonal relations; reactiveness; affects and moods; and social and moral adaptation. The sections cover three time frames: the previous year (affects and mood states); the previous 3 years (grandiosity, interpersonal relations, and reactiveness); and the previous 5 years (social and moral adaptation). The 'grandiosity' section explores whether the person has unrealistic views about special abilities, invulnerability, self-sufficiency and superiority. The section on 'interpersonal relations' focusses on issues such as a tendency to idealize others, lack of empathy, devaluation or exploitation of others, and feeling entitled. 'Reactiveness' is concerned with unusually intense reactions to criticism, defeat or disappointment, within a background of extreme sensitivity. Relevant 'affects and moods' include sustained periods of emptiness, boredom and a feeling of meaninglessness. 'Social and moral adaptation' for the narcissistic individual may be associated with high achievement, but the subject has self-serving values and morals. 'Grandiosity' is assessed first, because it was felt that open responses were more likely to occur early in the interview, as some subjects can become more defensive as the interview progresses. All items are scored as 2 (much), 1 (some), or 0 (none). Good inter-rater reliability has been reported.

SAS

The Suicide and Aggression Survey (SAS) (Korn *et al.*, 1992) is a structured interview that was developed to evaluate various aspects of these complex behaviours and to help the prediction of suicide and violence. The interview provides information about recent and past aggression, as shown by suicidal and violent thoughts, threats and actions. Other aspects covered include predisposing factors, precipitating events, underlying emotions, nature of the action, effects of the action and functions of the act.

The interview consists of five sections: general background; screening for history of self-harm and aggressive behaviours; ratings of such behaviours; the assessment of contextual and cultural factors; and further detailed information related to self-harm and aggressive acts. Aspects that are covered include the use of drugs in relation to an incident, and stressful life events that occurred in the preceding month.

APFA

The Adult Personality Functioning Assessment interview (APFA) (Hill *et al.*, 1989) is based on the concept that most individuals with PD share a 'pervasive and persistent abnormality in social functioning'. This instrument was an attempt to provide a standardized assessment of the subject's functioning over a period, in six different social circumstances (sections): work; love relationships; friendships; non-intimate social contacts; negotiations; and everyday coping. In each section, the interviewer rates level of functioning on a 6-point scale (0 = unusually effective, to 5 = pervasive failure). As social circumstances vary during life, APFA usually rates the period from age 22 to 30, although other age periods can be used, and behaviour is only rated for time periods when opportunities for social interaction have been present. The interviewer is concerned with reported behaviour rather than the subjects' evaluations or attitudes, and high inter-rater reliability has been reported.

Self-report questionnaires (SRQs)

Influential SRQs include the PD scales of the Minnesota Multiphasic Personality Inventory (MMPI), the Millon Clinical Multiaxial Inventory (MCMI), the Tridimensional Personality Questionnaire (TPQ) and versions of the Personality Diagnostic Questionnaire (PDQ). However, the MMPI was not designed in relation to ICD or DSM PD categories, and the TPQ is concerned with Cloninger's three hypothesized PD dimensions.

The following group of SRQs attempt to evaluate a range of PD features (Table 5.3):

MMPI

The Minnesota Multiphasic Personality Inventory has over 500 questions and was developed by Hathaway & McKinley in the 1930s. It also rated other non-PD mental disorders (Widiger & Frances, 1987), but as it was not based on the DSM, relationships between the MMPI scales and DSM-III-R disorders are variable and often uncertain. Therefore, this instrument has not been designed for PD diagnosis using current classifications, although Morey, Waugh & Blashfield (1985) developed 11 scales (the MMPI Personality Disorder Scales) related to the DSM-III PDs.

A currently-available version of the MMPI (from NFER-Nelson, Freepost, Windsor, Berkshire SL4 1BU, UK) takes up to 95 minutes and has 14

Table 5.3 *Self-report questionnaires (SRQs) for assessment of personality disorders (PDs)*

Assessment target	SRQ
A range of PD features:	
PDs (based on various concepts) and other mental disorders	MMPI (Minnesota Multiphasic Personality Inventory)
PD traits that can be related to DSM-III-R diagnoses	MCMI-II (Millon Clinical Multiaxial Inventory – revised)
DSM-III/III-R PD criteria	PDQ and PDQ-R (Personality Diagnostic Questionnaire and the revised version). Also, a modified version: the STCPD (Screening Test for Co-morbid Personality Disorders)
	WISPI (Wisconsin Personality Inventory)
13 proposed PD traits	SNAP (Schedule for Normal and Abnormal Personalities)
Three proposed dimensions of normal and abnormal personality	TPQ (Tridimensional Personality Questionnaire)
'Extraversion/introversion' 'neuroticism/stability' and 'psychoticism' dimensions	EPI and EPQ (Eysenck Personality Inventory and Questionnaire)
Proposed personality dimensions	KSP (Karolinska Scales of Personality)
16 proposed personality dimensions	Cattell's 16 Personality Factor Scales
Specific PD features:	
Borderline PD	BSI (Borderline Syndrome Index)
Schizotypal PD	Claridge's schizotypal and borderline scales and a combined Schizotypal Traits Questionnaire
Narcissistic PD	Narcissistic Personality Inventory; the Narcissistic Trait Scale; O'Brien Multiphasic Narcissism Inventory; scales from the California Psychological Inventory and the MMPI
Antisocial PD	Self-Report Psychopathy Scale; Buss & Durkee's Hostility Inventory

scales: hypochondriasis; depression; hysteria; psychopathic deviate; masculinity/femininity; paranoia; psychasthenia; schizophrenia; hypomania; social introversion and four validity scales.

MCMI-II

The MCMI-II is the updated version of the Millon Clinical Multiaxial Inventory (Millon, 1987) consisting of 175 questions, which are answered as true or false. The original version evaluated eight personality patterns: schizoid, avoidant, dependent, histrionic, narcissistic, antisocial, obsessive-compulsive, and passive-aggressive, together with some features of other mental disorders (Lewis & Harder, 1991). The revised version was designed to bring the scoring more in line with the DSM-III-R PDs and some 8-week test–retest reliability data were described as acceptable (Reich, 1989, 1992).

PDQ

The Personality Diagnostic Questionnaire (PDQ) is a 163-question, true–false questionnaire, which was closely based on the wording of the DSM-III PD criteria. A lie scale and five questions for an 'impairment and distress' scale were also included. The revised version, with 155 questions (PDQ-R) (Hyler *et al.*, 1988) reflected the changes in DSM-III-R and takes about 30 minutes to complete.

It is uncertain whether some items involving socially undesirable behaviour should be evaluated by relatively subtle questions, but it has been generally considered that most patients are compliant and that 'items will perform optimally when their content clearly relates to what they intend to measure' (Wrobel & Lachar, 1982). In the early versions, adequate one-month test–retest reliabilities were found for most scales but were low for narcissistic, histrionic, dependent and passive-aggressive PDs (Hyler *et al.*, 1990). But few data are currently available for the PDQ-R in relation to reliability. The PDQ-R has all questions for a single PD on one page, and around 20% of pathological answers are 'false' in an attempt to reduce a 'true' response-bias. There is a consensus that the PDQ format tends to overdiagnose PDs compared with other methods, especially schizotypal PD (Reich, 1989). But the PDQ-R has been used to identify those questions to be evaluated further at interview, and an informant's version has been developed (Dowson, 1992*b*). It has been claimed that, for many patients, the total score of positive PD criteria is an indication of overall severity, and that a shorter modified version (the STCPD – Screening Test for Co-morbid

PDs) can be used as a screening test for routine clinical evaluation (Hyler *et al.*, 1990; Dowson, 1992*b*). Yeung *et al.* (1993) found that improved concordance with an interview method could be obtained for the PDQ-R by adjusting the threshold for 'case' (i.e. diagnosis) identification.

WISPI

The Wisconsin Personality Inventory (Klein, 1985) has 360 items related to DSM-III PD criteria, interactional styles, social desirability, response bias and global ratings of work and social adjustment. Each item is rated on a 10-point scale. Validation studies are awaited.

SNAP

The Schedule for Normal and Abnormal Personality (SNAP) (Clark, 1989), contains 375 self-report true–false items. It is not based on DSM-III, and has 13 scales with three higher-order dimensions.

TPQ

The Tridimensional Personality Questionnaires (TPQ) (Cloninger, 1987*b*) is based on Cloninger's proposed three dimensions of normal and abnormal personality, i.e. novelty seeking, harm avoidance and reward dependence. It has 100 true–false questions and has been used in a study of patients with alcoholism (Cloninger, 1987*c*). A relationship between the TPQ and DSM-III-R PD features has been demonstrated (Goldman *et al.*, 1994).

EPI and EPQ

The Eysenck Personality Inventory (EPI, Eysenck & Eysenck, 1964) (currently available from NFER-Nelson) takes about 15 minutes to complete, and measures the dimensions of 'extraversion/introversion' and 'neuroticism/stability'.

The Eysenck Personality Questionnaire (EPQ, Eysenck & Eysenck, 1975) (also currently available from NFER-Nelson), in addition to the above dimensions, provides a measure of 'psychoticism'. The questionnaire was standardized on a large normal group and in various groups with psychiatric diagnoses.

KSP

The Karolinska Scales of Personality (KSP) is a questionnaire based on theories of biologically-based personality dimensions (temperaments) (Weinryb *et al.*, 1992).

Cattell's 16 Personality Factor Scale

This system has been used for many years in psychological research but has had little impact on the study of psychiatric populations. Sixteen factors were described in dimensional form, for example, 'outgoing' versus 'reserved' (Frances, 1982).

Various other SRQs relate to specific PD features; for instance, the Borderline Syndrome Index (BSI) (Conte, Plutchik & Karasu, 1980), which has 52 items. This method was not able to distinguish between groups selected on the basis of one of various principal diagnoses, including borderline PD, and was considered to offer a measure of general maladaption with chronic illness (Remington & Book, 1993). Schizotypal and borderline scales were described by Claridge & Broks, (1984); and schizotypal PD can also be assessed by a Combined Schizotypal Traits Questionnaire (CSTQ) (Bentall, Claridge & Slade, 1989). Raine & Allbutt (1989) have described five further scales for related features.

Several SRQs for narcissism have been reported: for example the Narcissistic Personality Inventory (Raskin & Hall, 1979); the Narcissistic Trait Scale (Richman & Flaherty, 1987) with ten items each rated on a 4-point scale; a 41-item O'Brien Multiphasic Narcissism Inventory which has been fully reported (O'Brien, 1988); and narcissism scales from the California Psychological Inventory and the MMPI (Wink & Gough, 1990).

SRQs related to antisocial PD include the Self-Report Psychopathy Scale (Hare, 1985). This has 29 items scored on a 1 to 5 point scale, and varying convergent validity with other assessment methods have been reported (Widiger & Frances, 1987). But there was more agreement between interview-based ratings than between ratings which included a SRQ. (It has been noted that SRQs for antisocial PD have the disadvantage of relying on an antisocial subject's insight and honesty.) Buss & Durkee (1957) fully reported their Hostility Inventory with the following sections: assault; indirect hostility; irritability; negativism; resentment; suspicion; and verbal hostility. Other instruments have been reviewed by Blackburn (1989).

Miscellaneous SRQs include the Lazare–Klerman Trait Scale (Lazare *et al.*, 1970) for histrionic PD; Sandler & Hazari's (1960) questionnaire for obsessional personality; the California Personality Inventory (McCormick *et al.*, 1987); the 54-item socialization scale of Gough's California Psychological inventory, which measures the degree to which a person has internalized social values and considers them binding (Gough, 1969); Quay's behaviour dimensions for delinquents (Quay, 1977); a shortened version of the Michigan Alcoholism Screening Test (Pokorny, Miller & Kaplan, 1972); the South Oaks Gambling Screen (Lesieur & Blume, 1987) which is a 20-item SRQ for the identification of pathological gamblers; and the Interpersonal Dependency Inventory (IDI) fully reported by Hirschfeld *et al.* (1977). The IDI consists of 48 items based on three main aspects: emotional reliance on another person, lack of social self-confidence and assertion of autonomy; and the measurement of dependence was reviewed by Birtchnell (1991). Other SRQs include the Locus of Control of Behaviour (Craig, Franklin & Andrews, 1984); the Interpersonal Sensitivity Measure (Joffe & Regan, 1988) with scales for interpersonal awareness, need for approval, separation anxiety, timidity and fragile inner-self; the Perceptual Aberration Scale, which is a true–false measure of body-image and perceptual abnormalities (Chapman, Chapman & Raulin, 1978), and other scales related to schizotypal PD features (Widiger & Frances, 1987).

Various aspects of validity for SRQs have been studied, in particular convergent validity (i.e. agreement between different methods of assessment), criterion validity (i.e. an association between the assessment and other variables) and predictive validity (i.e. an association between assessment and outcome).

Several studies have compared the convergent validity of the PDQ or PDQ-R with structured interviews, and Hyler *et al.* (1989) compared PDQ diagnoses with clinicians' diagnoses obtained by post. In this study, it was noted that the PDQ diagnosed many more PDs than did the clinicians, for instance, for paranoid PD, 44 versus 8. A similar finding has been noted in a number of studies, and Hunt & Andrews (1992) reported one or more PDs in 67% of their sample as diagnosed by the PDQ-R, while the PDE interview yielded only 7%; also, Reich *et al.* (1987*a*) found a poor convergence between the PDQ and the SIDP interview in 121 patients with panic disorder and depression. In addition, Dubro, Wetzler & Kahn (1988) reported a high rate of 'false positives' (in relation to other methods) with the PDQ, and Hyler *et al.* (1990) described many 'false positives' with the PDQ-R although there were very few 'false negatives'. An exception to this trend was in Zimmerman & Coryell's findings (1990) in 697 non-patients,

17% of whom received at least one PD diagnosis with an interview but only 10% with the PDQ.

However, these reports do not mean there is little or no relationship between some parts of SRQs and other PD assessment methods. Pfohl and colleagues (1989) obtained a kappa of 0.72 for the presence of at least one PD comparing the PDQ and SIDP interview in 45 non-psychiatric patients, and, although concordance between PD diagnoses is not generally good between a SRQ and an interview method, this varies between PD diagnoses. Hyler and colleagues (1990) found kappas of around 0.6 between SRQ and interviews in respect of avoidant and dependent PDs, while Hunt & Andrews (1992) reported correlations of around 0.6 between the dimensional scores from SRQ and interview for antisocial, avoidant and dependent PDs, based on the number of positive criteria for a specific PD. Also, when assessment of individual criteria are compared by SRQ and interview, some provide a good concordance: Clark (1992) has compared a 'true/false' SRQ with the SIDP-R interview, and good convergent validity was found for some criteria for borderline and histrionic PD, involving impulsiveness, recurrent suicidal behaviour, and expressing emotion with inappropriate exaggeration. Conversely, items which showed poor convergent validity included lack of empathy, and unstable and intense interpersonal relationships. Factor analysis of positive scores for PD criteria obtained by both SRQ and interview have shown that factors vary in the degree to which they are influenced by the method of assessment.

Further evidence of examples of good convergent validity between SRQs and other assessment methods has been obtained using a modified version of the PDQ-R, which retained the basic format with wording closely related to DSM-III-R criteria, and provided an informant's version (Dowson, 1992*b*). In a study of 60 psychiatric patients with a provisional diagnosis of PD, and their informants, five PDs gave correlations (between subject and informant) for the number of positive criteria in each PD, which were significant at the 0.05 level, and when individual criteria were considered, for example for narcissistic PD, three of the nine criteria for this PD yielded significant kappas between patients' and informants' ratings, although only one (a sense of entitlement) showed 'fair to good' convergence at a level of 0.62 (Dowson, 1992*a*).

Because of the lack of a clear standard with which to compare the various PD assessment methods, it is important to obtain other forms of validity (or usefulness), namely 'criterion validity' when PD assessment is associated with other types of variable, including theoretical relationships and pre-

Table 5.4 *Clinical ratings for the assessment of personality disorders (PDs)*

Assessment target	Rating method
DSM-III-R PDs	'LEAD' standard (longitudinal expert evaluation that uses all data)
PD related to antisocial behaviour	PCL-R (Hare Psychopathy Checklist)
Criminal behaviour	Criminal Profile Scale
Aggression	MOAS (Modified Overt Aggression Scale)
Risk of aggression	ARP (Aggression Risk Profile)

dicted outcome. For example, the modified PDQ-R was completed by 74 psychiatric patients, and a factor analysis of the scores of positive criteria for each of the PDs yielded three factors which defined three PD clusters (Dowson & Berrios, 1991). These were similar to the three DSM-III-R PD 'clusters' for seven out of the 11 PD categories, as the first cluster included paranoid, schizoid and schizotypal PDs, the second antisocial and borderline PDs, and the third dependent and obsessive-compulsive PDs. A further example of criterion validity of SRQs has been shown in relation to patients with a history of anorexia nervosa who were divided into two groups (Dowson, 1992c), firstly 'vomiters', defined by a history of self-induced vomiting, and, secondly, 'non-vomiters' or 'restrictors' who had maintained low weight mainly or only by diet or exercise. Several previous studies had reported personality differences between such groups and, in this study, vomiters showed significantly higher scores on self-report measures of borderline and antisocial PD criteria. Finally, Pfohl and colleagues (1987) demonstrated predictive validity for the PDQ by relating PD assessment scores with outcome measures, both at discharge and at 6 month follow-up, in a group of inpatients with 'major depression'.

Clinical ratings (Table 5.4)

The 'LEAD' standard
The process of improving the methodology for PD assessment has been handicapped by the lack of an accepted standard with which to compare a particular method. Spitzer (1983) attempted to solve this problem by

proposing that a PD assessment should be compared with a 'longitudinal expert evaluation that uses all data' (LEAD). The three essential ingredients were the opinion of one or more expert clinicians, observations over a period of time, and the use of all available information from past records, informants and other members of a clinical team. Support for this approach has been provided by Skodol and colleagues (1988), who reported evaluations of 20 patients with severe PD, admitted for inpatient treatment. The LEAD procedure involved multidisciplinary conferences at which behaviour in various unit settings was considered. PDs and traits were rated by consensus, on a 4-point scale: 1 = no or very few traits, 2 = some traits, 3 = almost meets DSM-III-R criteria, and 4 = meets DSM-III-R criteria. Although the reliability of this approach is likely to be suspect at times, it is a welcome reminder that an experienced clinician's judgement is also an important assessment method; for instance, when the LEAD procedure was compared with the SCID interview, the interview produced fewer diagnoses of narcissistic PD.

PCL-R

The Hare Psychopathy Checklist (Hare, 1991) is a rating scale for the assessment of antisocial PD. Information is collected from records and an informant (if available) as well as from a structured interview with the subject. This covers school adjustment, work history, career goals, finances, health, family life, sex/relationships, drug use, childhood/adolescent antisocial behaviour, adult antisocial behaviour, and 'general questions' related to aspects relevant to antisocial PD, such as previous guilt. Twenty items are then rated on a 3-point ordinal scale (0,1,2), based on the degree to which the information matches descriptions provided in a scoring manual. The following items are rated: glibness/superficial charm; grandiose sense of self-worth; need for stimulation/proneness to boredom; pathological lying; conning/manipulative; lack of remorse or guilt; shallow affect; callous/lack of empathy; parasitic lifestyle; poor behavioural controls; promiscuous sexual behaviour; early behavioural problems; lack of realistic, long-term goals; impulsivity; irresponsibility; failure to accept responsibility for own actions; many short-term marital relationships; juvenile delinquency; revocation of conditional release; and criminal versatility.

The PCL-R is the result of many years of research on thousands of prison inmates and forensic patients, and there is considerable evidence for its reliability and validity in research settings. The manual recommends that more than one rating for each patient should be made independently and that the scores should be averaged.

Criminal Profile Scale

The Criminal Profile Scale (Gunn & Robertson, 1976) is a rapid and simple 5-point rating (i.e. 0 to 4 based on severity) for each of the following: theft, fraud, sex, violence, motoring, drink, drugs, financial gain and relationship to drinking.

MOAS

The Modified Overt Aggression Scale (Kay, Wolkenfeld & Murrill, 1988*a*) is a revised version of the method of Yudofsky, Silver & Jackson (1986) designed for psychiatric inpatients. The following four categories are rated on a 5-point scale over a specified observation period: verbal aggression, aggression against property, autoaggression, and physical aggression. The rater is asked to rate the most severe point on the scale relating to the most serious aggressive act, and the scores are weighted to reflect the increasing severity of the above categories.

ARP

An Aggression Risk Profile (ARP) for psychiatric inpatients, including those with PD, was reported by Kay, Wolkenfeld & Murrill (1988*b*) and included data on age, sex, previous hospitalization, psychiatric diagnosis, history of aggression and a clinical profile based on information about the previous week.

Routine clinical assessment

Overview

Routine clinical assessment does not generally include a questionnaire, structured interview or formalized rating. However, the clinician needs a procedure and a set of guiding principles.

It can be helpful to keep in mind Walton's (1973) concept of a 'mature' or 'normal' personality, which is an ideal view of good adaptation. A 'mature' person has correct self-perception, can adjust to new situations, can operate with appropriate autonomy, has good reality testing, and has an integrated pattern of attitudes, feelings and behaviour. (A lack of integration would be shown by a policeman who engages in petty theft.) Thus, 'normal' individuals have been able to find ways of expressing their behavioural patterns in adaptive ways. A detailed history of the patient's close and significant relationships is of particular importance in evaluating PD.

Some structure can, however, be appropriate to clinical interviews, for example, the use of screening questions such as those suggested by Leff & Isaacs (1990), i.e. in relation to ICD-10 categories, 'do you find you can trust people?' and 'are you mostly treated fairly?' (for paranoid PD); 'can you mix easily?' and 'do you prefer to be alone or with company?' (for schizoid PD); 'have you been in much trouble with the police?' and 'how do you get on with people in authority?' (for dissocial PD); 'do you frequently lose your temper?' and 'have you ever hurt anyone or caused any serious damage?' (for emotionally unstable PD); 'are you sometimes over-emotional?' and 'do you like to be the centre of attention?' (for histrionic PD); 'do you always try to follow a set routine?' and 'do you prefer things to be very neat and tidy?' (for obsessive-compulsive or anankastic PD); 'do you tend to feel very tense and self-conscious?' and 'do you live cautiously and avoid taking unnecessary risks?' (for anxious or avoidant PD); and 'do you tend to rely on others excessively?' and 'do you prefer others to make decisions for you?' (for dependent PD).

An interview with an informant can often be important, but a judgement has to be made about the accuracy of this account, particularly if the informant's relationship with the patient has significant maladaptive aspects.

It must always be remembered that a 'cross-sectional' evaluation of a patient may not provide a typical example of the patient's behaviour, particularly in the presence of other mental disorders (such as depression or anxiety) or soon after stressful life-events. Under stress, a normally considerate and reasonable individual may become selfish, irritable and demanding, and it is important for the clinician not to allow his/her emotional reaction to the patient to influence the assessment. Also, it is important to remember that there is evidence that clinicians can inappropriately assign PD diagnoses (such as histrionic and antisocial PDs) partly on the basis of the patient's gender (Ford & Widiger, 1989; Adler, Drake & Teague, 1990). As with any patient in psychiatric practice, it is important to understand the relevance of the presenting complaint and why the patient has been referred at that particular time.

The assessment, including family and personal history, should be explored in a systematic way, for example under the following headings: description of patient; the patient's complaints; history of present problems/symptoms; previous contact with medical services; family history; personal history (school record, work record, sexual history, police record, present domestic situation, past and recent social network, recreational habits, and alcohol, tobacco and drug history); aspects of personality (relationships, mood, dependency on others, impulsive aggression, solitariness, inability to cope with routine demands, undue sensitivity to criticism, undue mistrust of others, conscientiousness, a tendency to be excessively methodical and thorough, self-confidence, timidity, worry, level of activity, fantasy, and reaction pattern to stress); and mental state at interview.

Routine assessment of 'cluster A' PDs (paranoid, schizoid, and schizotypal)

Patients with paranoid PD traits may have a variety of presenting complaints, such as tiredness, insomnia, irritability, anxiety and difficulties in coping with work. It may take some time (and several interviews) before the underlying psychopathology is revealed, perhaps by a tendency to blame others, to be easily offended and to feel that others are generally hostile. Initially, such individuals may be more than usually concerned with issues of confidentiality. Accounts of various relationships may indicate a pattern of hostility and varying degrees of conflict. The patient may complain that he/she has been overlooked for promotion or that he/she finds it difficult to assert him/herself.

Those with schizoid and schizotypal PD traits usually appear detached, unemotional, cold, quiet and shy. Persons with schizoid PD traits do not often request medical help and some other 'significant' person may ask for advice. Medical involvement may be precipitated by some event that interferes with the person's long-standing pattern of social isolation, such as a physical illness that makes him/her less independent, or the loss of a job due, perhaps, to the person's maladaptive functioning (Turkat, 1990). At interview, those with schizoid traits often appear unemotional, aloof, uncomplaining and relatively unresponsive to social cues. Schizotypal features may include the patient appearing to be odd, anxious and vague with a bizarre appearance, dress and mannerisms. Some individuals with these features may apparently wish for social relationships but find these difficult, and their talk may have persecutory or grandiose themes.

Routine assessment of 'cluster B' PDs (antisocial, borderline, histrionic and narcissistic)

When individuals with antisocial PD traits present to clinicians, their motivation for seeking advice and help must be evaluated. Sometimes antisocial individuals can have superficial charm, which must not be taken at face value. Turkat (1990) has described three types of presentation: 'clear' sociopaths, when the history of antisocial features is obvious and the person may be requesting help to deal with legal consequences; 'clever' sociopaths, who deliberately present the clinician with a non-existent psychological problem (such as hallucinations or depression) to try and obtain the status of a patient rather than a law-breaker; and the 'hurting' sociopath, who wants relief from genuine symptoms such as anxiety and depression. But of course, these are not mutually exclusive. If the patient appears motivated to change (for instance, in relation to a pattern of domestic violence when his wife has threatened to leave), it is important to explore the patient's expectations and whether these are realistic. Some of the core psychological features of antisocial PD may be indicated by the person continually stating that his/her actions are justified despite the adverse effects on others, and showing a lack of concern for the consequences. If future dangerousness is being assessed, it is important to have a detailed record of previous dangerous behaviour, any precipitating and relevant environmental factors, and the characteristics of any victim (Pollock, McBain & Webster, 1989).

The inconsistency and variety of presenting complaints are often characteristic of individuals with borderline PD, and the complaints may appear unusual. Other pointers to a 'borderline PD' diagnosis include frequent crises, extra demands and phone calls to medical services, apparent misinterpretation of the clinician's remarks or advice, strong reactions to changes in the arrangements (for instance, to a proposal to reduce the frequency of appointments), a low tolerance for direct eye contact or physical contact or close proximity, and ambivalence about a continuing clinical contact (Beck & Freeman, 1990).

Histrionic PD traits may be suspected if the patient draws attention to him/herself in relation to general behaviour, mannerisms, gestures, flamboyant appearance or dress (sometimes with inappropriate sexual seductiveness), and shows some variability of mood in the interview, perhaps becoming suddenly tearful but recovering rapidly. Such individuals often appear generally lively with frequent and exaggerated smiles and gestures. They appear to invite attention, and while some are concerned with eliciting reassurance, approval and praise, others seem to want to control people they come into contact with, by their manipulative, dramatic behaviour (Turkat, 1990). Such persons tend to be self-centred, unaware of the effects of their behaviour on others, and may talk in a vague manner, which may involve exaggerated all-inclusive adjectives but lacks detail. This can be very striking to a clinician trying to take an initial history, who finds the task almost impossible. Patients with histrionic PD often present to medical services when they are unhappy and anxious, perhaps related to 'separation-anxiety' or a crisis in their relationships. This discomfort provides the motivation for seeking help but when these symptoms have improved, the motivation is lost. This explains why many such patients fail to keep subsequent appointments that are made in a time of crisis. An experienced clinician can often predict a high risk of non-attendance at a first appointment by identifying examples of the pattern of behaviour for 'histrionic PD' in a referral letter. Also, presentation of histrionic PD may be associated with substance abuse, conversion disorder and somatization disorder. Useful avenues of exploration are previous close relationships, any complaints that the other individuals in these relationships made to the patient, and activities that are generally enjoyed. Subjects with histrionic PD generally like situations in which they are the centre of attention.

Those with pronounced narcissistic PD traits can appear to be trying hard to impress the clinician by showing 'how good I am' (Turkat, 1990) and can be difficult to interview because of a demanding, arrogant manner with expectations of special consideration. They may question the clinician's qualifications and try to negotiate special arrangements for their appointments. The clinician is either idealized or devalued, and a change can occur rapidly. Attempts to explain the effects of their behaviour on others are considered as criticism and met with anger. They appear to be most comfortable when talking about themselves, often mentioning their abilities, achievements and possessions, while complaining about the shortcomings of others. They tend to pay a lot of attention to their appearance and dress; this concern can be noticeable at interview if the subject frequently smooths his/her hair, adjusts clothes or over-reacts to minor physical problems which affect appearance. They may resent any kind of formal testing, such as completing questionnaires, as this may be taken to imply that their problems can be related to similar problems of others and are not unique. Motivation for clinical consultation can include a depressed mood in the context of relationship difficulties or the patient may wish to show his/her partner that he/she 'is trying' in response to an ultimatum about selfish behaviour.

Routine assessment of 'cluster C' PDs (avoidant, dependent, obsessive-compulsive, and passive-aggressive)

The individual with avoidant PD may complain of anxiety, depressed mood, and associated somatic symptoms, related to a widespread fear of criticism and disapproval, and the clinician must remember that such a patient is particularly sensitive to evaluation.

The person with dependent PD appears submissive and self-effacing, has low self-confidence, is self-critical and, like those with avoidant PD, seeks to please and to receive reassurance. It is particularly important to try and explore the details of the individual's current supportive relationships, how decisions are made and how he/she feels about being alone. At interview, the clinician may observe that the patient avoids conflict where there is disagreement. Presenting complaints often involve anxiety and depressed mood, and the patient's passive helplessness may produce an emotional reaction in the clinician, which can signal the nature of the problem. In this situation some clinicians feel impatient and irritated, while others feel tempted to make special arrangements for extra 'help', because it seems difficult to set a limit to the patient's demands.

Patients with obsessive-compulsive (obsessive) PD show variable combinations of indecision and rigid attention to order and detail. They may be very neatly dressed and initially cooperative, polite and unemotional, giving their history in a very detailed manner, although sometimes there may be hesitancy due to anxiety. But this can cause some problems to the clinician, particularly at the first interview, as it is difficult to interrupt and clarify points of clinical importance. The patient may have a written list of notes and is obstinately determined to tell you what he/she feels is relevant, however long it takes. Such persons try to be unemotionally logical, and find it difficult to describe their feelings and attitudes. Presenting problems include depressed mood associated with failure to achieve unrealistically high standards, or worry about illness. In a clinical situation, obsessive patients are generally unemotional, and are most comfortable when the interaction is organized and when details are considered. In general, cognitive therapy may be better tolerated than unstructured counselling or joint sessions with his/her partner.

Persons with passive-aggressive PD traits may have difficulty in formulating a complaint other than vague dissatisfaction, or that someone else has insisted that he/she takes advice. Because an essential feature of this disorder is poor performance in unwanted tasks, he/she will be a 'poor patient' if not motivated. Even if relief from a depressed mood or anxiety is sought, he/she may blame others for the problems and tend not to cooperate in giving information. Such individuals may give short, incomplete answers and appear irritable. They may feel they should not have to answer some questions and tend to talk about perceived interference from others. But they are less wary than those with marked paranoid PD features (Beck & Freeman, 1990). If they cannot see that they have contributed to the previous problems, a poor response to advice would be expected.

Differential diagnosis and co-occurrence

Reference has been made to the frequent co-occurrence of PDs with other psychiatric disorders. Such associations may involve causal mechanisms or occur by chance but, whatever their nature, co-occurrence and interactions can affect the presentation and outcome of each disorder. Even when there is a clear history of PD, the clinician must be alert to the possibility that there may be additional disorders requiring diagnosis, especially if the history is inconsistent with an apparently understandable interaction between PD and life events. Sometimes PD can mask disorders such as hypomania, an unrelated depressive disorder, or neurological disorder.

The frequent co-occurrence of more than one PD has also been described, and the clinician must be aware that certain PD features are more likely to co-occur than others. For example, histrionic with borderline, histrionic with narcissistic, narcissistic with antisocial, narcissistic with passive-aggressive, avoidant with schizotypal, and avoidant with dependent (Oldham *et al.*, 1992).

Personality disorder assessment: future directions

Despite the aspects of validity that have been demonstrated for self-report questionnaires, those currently available do not appear suitable for the task of assigning specific categorical PD diagnoses in a clinical context, as their diagnostic thresholds are generally lower than those related to interviews or clinical judgement. But despite this and other limitations, a variant of the PDQ self-report questionnaire is currently being used as a screening procedure to identify items for subsequent assessment by the SCID-II interview method. Also, a shorter version of the modified PDQ-R has been used, which assesses those PDs that appear to be most prevalent in routine psychiatric practice, namely borderline, histrionic, avoidant and dependent PDs (Dowson, 1992*b*). This can be used before a routine clinical interview as well as for research purposes. Even this simple approach in routine practice would encourage more clinicians to look for a range of features from several individual PDs. This appears to reflect clinical reality, as discrete PDs are rare.

It is, perhaps, surprising that aspects of validity for such a relatively crude instrument as the PDQ have been demonstrated in several studies. But this is encouraging, and the potential for the increased use of self-report methodology appears to be considerable. Also, an intermediate format between self-report and interview, involving actively supervised self-report ratings, with some explanation and encouragement from the interviewer, deserves further attention.

Self-report questionnaires, structured interviews and clinical ratings will all have a place as part of a range of different methods of assessment, and it has been claimed that 'multiple methods of measurement should be the norm ...'. Also, all methods of PD assessment will need to consider variables such as other co-occurring psychiatric disorders, the time-frame being evaluated, whether questions in structured interviews or question-naires are organized by PD diagnoses or by topics, other personality attributes, the level of impairment and aspects of the environment.

It must be remembered that many patients with PD in psychiatric practice refuse to cooperate with structured assessment methods or even with a detailed unstructured interview; rating procedures by clinicians on the basis of all available information are then required.

Part Two

Clinical management

6

Drugs and other physical treatments

J.H. DOWSON

Overview

For a patient with PD, a drug may act in several ways: by a non-specific beneficial effect on a range of PD features, by a relatively specific effect, or by targeting a co-occurring psychiatric disorder. Also, a placebo effect can be marked.

Drugs are prescribed for many patients with PDs, although their effects are often unpredictable. The most commonly prescribed classes are neuroleptics and antidepressants, while lithium carbonate, anticonvulsants, anxiolytics and psychostimulants have also been used. But an individual patient may benefit from each of several drugs, while an individual drug may have effects on a range of target symptoms and behaviours. Also, there can be a considerable variability of response to a drug regime within a group of patients selected on the basis of PD.

Some of the many factors that account for such variability include an inconsistent placebo response and the heterogeneity of a patient sample in relation to PD features and to co-occurring psychiatric disorders, particularly co-occurring depressive disorders.

Investigations of drug treatments for PD are complicated by methodological problems in the assessment of PDs and by the need to assess a range of outcome measures. Compliance with treatment is often poor and the effects of some drugs may take time to develop, for example several weeks in relation to the effects of neuroleptics on some features of borderline PD. Also, self-reports of change do not always correspond with clinicians' ratings.

However, there is a general consensus that drug treatment can have an important place as part of a range of measures to help some patients with PD (Ellison & Adler, 1990; Stein, 1993).

Most of the empirical evidence in support of the use of drugs relates to borderline PD, in particular to the effects of low doses of neuroleptics, but even for these drugs the results of long-term treatment are unknown. It is generally advised that drug treatment should not be the only intervention for PDs, but be accompanied by psychological treatments, in particular supportive psychotherapy. As some patients with PD show a repeated pattern of self-harm, any drug treatment must take into account the risk of overdose and of paradoxical reactions to drugs, for example, when depressive features can worsen.

Other physical treatments can have a limited role in the management of patients with PDs, and ECT and psychosurgery will be considered.

Neuroleptics

Neuroleptic (i.e. 'antipsychotic') medication has been reported to be associated with a range of beneficial effects in patients with borderline PD, in particular reduced impulsive anger and self-harm, and improved depressive symptoms. Such effects are more evident when the features are severe, and recommended doses are usually considerably less than those used for the treatment of schizophrenia. Also, benefits have been claimed for neuroleptics in relation to schizotypal PD, as well as schizoid and paranoid PDs.

Montgomery & Montgomery (1982), in a non-controlled study, claimed that flupenthixol injections reduced the rate of self-harm episodes in a group with various PDs, and three subsequent placebo-controlled trials found beneficial effects with different neuroleptics on various features of patients selected on the basis of borderline PD. Goldberg *et al.* (1986) compared thiothixene (at a mean daily dose of 8.67 mg) with placebo in 50 outpatients with either borderline or schizotypal PD over 12 weeks. Subjects were recruited by a newspaper advertisement. A beneficial effect, which was positively related to severity of PD, was found for several features including impulsive anger and cognitive abnormalities such as ideas of reference. Soloff, George & Nathan (1986) compared the effects of haloperidol or amitriptyline (at mean daily doses of 7.24 and 147 mg respectively) on 90 inpatients for 5 weeks. Patients were identified by a diagnostic interview before being assigned into borderline, schizotypal and mixed (borderline and schizotypal) PD groups on the basis of DSM-III diagnoses. It was found that haloperidol was superior to amitriptyline or placebo, and clear improvements were noted for several outcomes, including behavioural dyscontrol (i.e. involving impulsive anger/self-harm), depressed mood, hostility, anxiety and features of schizotypal PD. In another placebo-controlled study that used a longitudinal cross-over design, Cowdry & Gardner (1988) investigated 16 outpatients with borderline PD and prominent behavioural dyscontrol, who received the following drugs in varying sequence: trifluoperazine, carbamazepine, tranylcypromine, alprazolam (at mean daily doses of 7.8 mg, 820 mg, 40 mg and 4.7 mg respectively), and placebo. The trial for each drug lasted 6 weeks. There were positive results in relation to carbamazepine and tranylcypromine, and the outcome for those who did not discontinue the trifluoperazine in the first 3 weeks was 'fairly favourable' for anxiety and self-harm as rated by the clinician, and for depression, anxiety and sensitivity to rejection as rated by the patients. However, the most recent placebo-controlled trial of haloperidol for borderline PD, (at a mean daily dose of 4 mg for 5 weeks), did not confirm the efficacy of this drug (Soloff *et al.*, 1993). This study, which also included a group who received phenelzine at a mean daily dose of 60 mg, involved 108 consecutively admitted inpatients, but, in contrast to the report of Soloff *et al.* (1986, described above), patients were encouraged to leave hospital after a minimum of 14 days. Also, all groups received considerable non-specific support. Although phenelzine had a significant beneficial effect on anger and hostility, these effects were not marked, and the findings were largely negative. Soloff and colleagues considered that the failure to confirm their previously reported beneficial effects of haloperidol may have been due to such factors as a high dropout rate in the second study and different sample characteristics, as the former study involved more severe disorders. It was suggested that, in general, neuroleptics may be clinically useful only when relatively severe disorders are treated.

Antidepressants

Most studies of the effects of antidepressants on patients with PD relate to borderline PD, which commonly co-occurs with an additional diagnosis of a depressive disorder. Also, some of the mood states that are an integral part of the borderline PD syndrome consist of depressive symptoms, which have been considered to differ in nature and origin from other types of depressive disorders. Depression with borderline PD is, therefore, heterogeneous (Soloff, 1993), perhaps involving chronic unhappiness related to experiences of boredom and emptiness, a labile depressed mood related to life crises, or a co-occurring syndrome such as 'major depression'. The latter is related to a variable range of causal factors including genetic vulnerability to episodic changes of mood.

Monoamine oxidase inhibitors

Cowdry & Gardner's study (1988, described above), examined the effects of four drugs, including tranylcypromine 40 mg daily, in a placebo-controlled longitudinal crossover study of 16 outpatients with borderline PD and prominent behavioural dyscontrol. Tranylcypromine was found to be better than placebo in relation to a range of effects including decreased depressive symptoms, reduced anxiety, increased capacity for pleasure, and improved impulsivity and self-harm. But it was considered that behavioural benefits were the result of an improved mood rather than reduced impulsivity. Also, Liebowitz & Klein (1981), in a non-controlled trial of phenelzine, found improved mood in patients with 'hysteroid dysphoria', most of whom had DSM-III borderline PD.

Parsons *et al.* (1989) compared the effects of imipramine, phenelzine (90 mg/day) and placebo in over 300 patients with 'atypical depressive disorder' and examined the associations of three to five positive criteria for borderline PD. For those with five or more positive criteria, there appeared to be an association with a good response of depressed mood to phenelzine, compared with imipramine or placebo. But these findings related to depressed mood were not confirmed by Soloff *et al.* (1993, described above), who compared the effects of haloperidol, phenelzine (60 mg/day) and placebo on patients with borderline PD. Although phenelzine was found to be significantly better than placebo on self-report measures of anger and hostility, these effects were small. However, as previously noted, all groups received considerable non-specific support.

Tricyclics

Amitriptyline (at a mean daily dose of 147 mg) was compared with haloperidol and placebo in 90 inpatients with borderline PD for 5 weeks by Soloff *et al.* (1986, described above). As previously noted, haloperidol was superior to amitriptyline on a number of outcome measures, including depression, although a small improvement in depression was found for amitriptyline compared with placebo. But a most important observation was that some patients on amitriptyline became worse, although others appeared to do well. The negative effects included increased paranoid ideas and behavioural dyscontrol, involving impulsive behaviour and threats of self-harm.

Despite generally negative reports of tricyclics, various case reports indicate that these drugs may have a role in the management of some patients with PD. For example, Satel, Southwick & Denton (1988) described a young man with borderline PD and co-occurring attention deficit hyperactivity disorder (ADHD) in whom imipramine produced a marked decrease in anxiety, explosiveness, restlessness and lability of mood.

Bellak (1985) also advocated the use of imipramine in relatively small doses (e.g. 10–30 mg daily) for 'attention deficit disorder psychosis', and noted that improvements in agitation, overactivity, impulsivity and attention span may be found within a few hours of the first dose. Also, Biederman (1988) reported that adolescents with ADHD may respond to tricyclic antidepressants such as desipramine, as well as to various other medications.

Selective serotonin reuptake inhibitors (SSRIs)

There are theoretical reasons why a drug with a relatively selective action on serotonin metabolism may be expected to help to reduce impulsivity in patients with borderline PD, as impulsivity appears to be associated with reduced CNS serotonergic activity, shown by low levels of a serotonin metabolite in the CSF and a reduced serotonin-mediated prolactin response to fenfluramine (Soloff, 1993).

This prediction is supported by several non-controlled studies of fluoxetine in patients with borderline PD. Norden (1989) prescribed fluoxetine for 12 outpatients with borderline PD for up to 26 weeks in doses of up to · 40 mg/day. For most patients, improvements were reported for a number of features such as depressed mood, lability of mood, rejection sensitivity, anger and impulsivity, and such changes usually appeared in the first few days. Markowitz *et al.* (1991) studied eight outpatients with borderline PD, four with schizotypal PD and ten with both disorders, and gave fluoxetine at a dose of 80 mg/day for 12 weeks; clear reductions in self-injury were reported, regardless of diagnosis. Also, Cornelius *et al.* (1991) studied five severely-affected inpatients with DSM-III borderline PD, who had not responded to phenelzine or neuroleptics, who received 20 to 40 mg of fluoxetine daily for 8 weeks. Their findings suggested that this drug improved depressive and impulsive features. Finally, Hull, Clarkin & Alexopoulos (1992) reported the case of a severely-affected young woman with borderline PD who was in hospital for 58 weeks. When fluoxetine was prescribed at week 40 there was a rapid and widespread improvement affecting her symptoms and behaviour.

These preliminary findings are encouraging, and further placebo-controlled trials are needed. However, six reported cases of 'intense suicidal preoccupation' with depressed mood in patients receiving fluoxetine have been described by Teicher, Glod & Cole (1990). Two of these patients had a diagnosis of borderline PD but, in addition, they had co-occurring diagnoses of major depression or temporal lobe epilepsy with episodic alcohol abuse. Also, one patient had an history of attempts at self-harm, and the other had described previous suicidal ideas. In all the six patients there was a tendency for intense, 'obsessive' suicidal ruminations to continue for about 27 days after the drug was discontinued, and these cases suggest the possibility of a rare 'paradoxical' response to fluoxetine.

Lithium carbonate

An effect of lithium on violent behaviour has been claimed in US prison populations. Sheard (1971), in a non-controlled study, reported the effect of the drug on 12 young male prisoners with a history of violence, and it appeared that there was a consequent reduction of serious violent episodes, although most of the improvement occurred in just three subjects. Tupin, Smith & Clanon (1973) studied the effects of lithium on 27 male prisoners, about half of whom had PDs associated with impulsive violence. Their results were encouraging, as 56% showed a clear reduction in aggressive or violent episodes, often associated with a 'reflective delay' when the subject did not appear to respond so impulsively to adverse events. A further study by Sheard et al. (1976) involved 66 subjects with PDs and a history of violent crime who continued to show a pattern of violent behaviour in prison. The placebo-controlled design involved two groups treated in parallel for 3 months, and the lithium-treated group showed a significant and clear reduction in assaults or serious threatening behaviour. Also, this behaviour returned when the lithium was discontinued. It has also been noted that lithium can be of benefit in some patients with mental retardation who show recurrent aggression and self-mutilation. However, there is a possibility that a few patients may become more aggressive.

There is scant information about the value of lithium for subjects identified on the basis of PD, but a placebo-controlled cross-over trial in female adolescents with spontaneous mood swings and 'emotionally un-stable character disorder', found a significant association between treatment with lithium and decreased 'within-day mood fluctuations' (Rifkin, Quitkin & Carrillo, 1972). Other studies have examined subjects selected on the basis of alcoholism, and it was considered that some may benefit, particularly when there is co-occurring episodic affective disorder. Also, Stone (1990) found that some patients with borderline PD and co-occurring episodes of affective disorder, in particular bipolar disorder, benefit from lithium. Although it can be difficult to predict which patients with borderline PD may respond to lithium unless there is a clear history of discrete episodic mood disorder, a trial of this drug may be indicated if there is a family history of episodic affective disorder or alcoholism.

Anticonvulsants

As previously described, Cowdrey & Gardner (1988) included carbamazepine for 6 weeks (at a mean daily dose of 820 mg) as one of the three drug regimes in their placebo-controlled longitudinal cross-over study involving 16 outpatients with borderline PD and prominent behavioural dyscontrol. A significant reduction in the severity of behavioural dyscontrol was found in the carbamazepine group, and this was suggested to involve a 'reflective delay', as with lithium in the studies of prison populations. But one patient became severely depressed and four others developed skin reactions.

It has been claimed that episodes of impulsive behavioural dyscontrol in borderline PD, involving anger and self-harm, may sometimes follow 'an abrupt onset' of intense dysphoria (Monroe, 1982), perhaps triggered by alcohol, drugs or stress. The relationship of these phenomena to epileptic disorders has been a matter of speculation, and some patients have reported prodromal experiences such as anxiety and agitation. Also, after an episode of self-harm or anger, some patients may feel that tension has been relieved. But EEG changes related to temporal lobe epilepsy are not usually found in borderline PD (Stein, 1993). However, in a case report of a patient with the uncommon EEG patterns of rhythmic midtemporal discharges and 6/s spike and wave complexes, carbamazepine produced clear improvement in episodic violent behaviour that was accompanied by anxiety and intrusive self-destructive thoughts (Stone *et al.*, 1986).

Anxiolytics

Although rapidly-acting anxiolytics might be expected to reduce a build-up of tension that can precede an episode of behavioural dyscontrol in borderline PD, anxiolytics are generally contra-indicated for this and other

PDs. This is because of a risk of addiction and of paradoxical reactions, involving disinhibition with an increase in impulsive behaviour. However, a small minority of patients with borderline PD may benefit.

The reported effects have been varied. Faltus (1984) described three male patients with both borderline and schizotypal PDs and noted a favourable response to alprazolam. However, two of these patients were rather atypical as examples of PDs as they had hallucinations. Also, Reus & Markrow (1984) studied the effect of alprazolam in 18 inpatients with borderline PD in a cross-over design, and claimed a favourable response in over half the subjects. In contrast, Cowdrey & Gardner (1988) used alprazolam, at an average daily dose of 4.7 mg, in their placebo-controlled cross-over study of 16 outpatients with borderline PD. Those receiving alprazolam showed a clear increase in the severity of impulsive behaviour involving self-harm and aggression, compared with placebo, although two patients showed improvement. It was considered that this drug often has an adverse disinhibiting effect.

However, there have been case reports in favour of clonazepam for borderline PD, and preliminary results for buspirone in borderline PD indicate that beneficial effects may occur (Soloff, 1993).

Psychostimulants

Various psychostimulants, including methylphenidate, pemoline, amphetamine and levodopa have been reported to produce beneficial effects in some patients with borderline PD, or with PD co-occurring with present or past ADHD (attention deficit hyperactivity disorder).

For example, in a case report, methylphenidate benefitted a patient with borderline PD and co-occurring ADHD, and this drug has also been claimed to be of value for the impulsivity of adult minimal brain dysfunction (Wood et al., 1976), for residual ADHD (Wender et al., 1985), and for ADHD in children (Pelham et al., 1985). In addition, it has been noted that a history of ADHD in borderline PD predicted a favourable response to tranylcypromine, which has a stimulant action in addition to its effect on monoamine oxidase (Cowdry & Gardner, 1988). Also, Stringer & Josef (1983) described two inpatients with seriously disturbed behaviour in the context of antisocial PD and repeated aggression, who improved considerably while on methylphenidate, 20 mg twice daily.

Pemoline was reported to be better than placebo for improving concentration and reducing impulsivity in adults with a history of severe ADHD (Wender, Wood & Reimherr, 1984), and levodopa was claimed to benefit patients with borderline PD and histories of drug abuse (Bonnet & Redford, 1982). The use of dexamphetamine for borderline PD has also been the subject of favourable case reports, although this drug is generally contra-indicated because of its addictive and abuse potential. But a 30-year-old man with repeated aggressive and violent behaviour apparently responded dramatically to 20 mg dexamphetamine twice daily. It has been claimed that childhood hyperactivity and an history of drug abuse are predictors of response to both psychostimulants and monoamine oxidase inhibitors (Stein, 1993).

Other drugs

Propranolol has been reported to benefit brain-damaged patients who show unprovoked rage attacks (Ratey, Morrill & Oxenkrug, 1983), as well as some patients with behavioural dyscontrol (Mattes, 1988). Also, clozapine may be useful for borderline PD associated with severe or prolonged 'psychotic' features (Frankenburg & Zanarini, 1993).

It has been suggested that abnormal functioning of the endogenous opioid peptide system is associated with repeated self-harm and feelings of boredom and emptiness in borderline PD, which may predispose some individuals to self-medication by substance abuse (Soloff, 1993). Increased levels of plasma β-endorphin were found in five subjects with borderline PD who were bored, unhappy and drug abusers (Bonnet & Redford, 1982), and as dopamine inhibits the release of pituitary β-endorphin, these authors prescribed levodopa and carbidopa, with apparently beneficial effects. Further evidence for the involvement of endogenous opioids in borderline PD was provided by Coid, Allolio & Rees (1983), who found high levels of plasma metenkephalin in ten borderline PD patients with a history of self-mutilation. These observations and associated hypotheses have led to an interest in the effects of opioid antagonists such as naltrexone, in particular for self-mutilation and narcotic drug abuse. A case report with apparent benefit of naltrexone was described by Soloff (1993).

Drugs that influence hormones related to sexual drive can be prescribed for subjects who show sexual violence or distressing sexual preoccupations, and PDs may often co-occur with these phonemena in groups who repeatedly commit criminal offences with a sexual motive (Bowden, 1991). Cyproterone acetate competes with testosterone at receptor sites, and also inhibits hormonal release by the hypothalamus and pituitary, leading to a reduced production of testosterone. However, side-effects are often problematic and, while sexual drive is reduced, sexual aggression is not necessarily affected. Other agents that produce reduced levels of plasma testosterone include medroxyprogesterone acetate, which is given by regular intramuscular injections, and goserelin acetate, which is administered by subcutaneous injection. The practical and ethical problems of using these agents have been discussed by Bowden (1991). Despite such difficulties, such interventions do appear to enable some individuals to interrupt a pattern of criminal activity, although these drugs should be used in the context of counselling and practical support.

Drug treatment: borderline and related personality disorders

As has been described, borderline PD often co-occurs with other features of PDs, and with other psychiatric disorders that may merit treatment in their own right. Within the range of borderline PD features, targets for drug treatment include affective instability, chronic dysphoria and behavioural dyscontrol involving anger and self-harm. It is important to recognize that, in general, the prescription of a drug should not be the only intervention and that the patient's expectations should not be raised too high. While there are anecdotal accounts of apparently dramatic responses to drugs, a more modest effect is generally anticipated.

The best evidence in favour of drug treatment for borderline PD relates to neuroleptics in low doses, monoamine oxidase inhibitors (MAOIs) and carbamazepine. But MAOIs are dangerous in overdose and require dietary compliance, while carbamazepine has been associated with a worsening of depressed mood in some subjects. Selective serotonin-reuptake inhibitors (SSRIs) such as fluoxetine require further studies of their use for PDs, but early reports are promising, and these agents are relatively safe if taken in overdose. The effects of tricyclic antidepressants and anxiolytics appear to be much less predictable, as a worsening of symptoms and behaviour have often been reported, although a minority of subjects may benefit. Other drugs that have been associated with favourable case-reports include lithium, psychostimulants and β-blockers.

Some guidelines for prescribing for patients with borderline PD have been suggested: if there is a possibility of a co-occurring episodic depressive, manic or bipolar disorder, then lithium may be indicated, unless the risk of overdose or dangerous noncompliance appears significant. If behavioural dyscontrol is associated with EEG abnormalities, then carbamazepine should be considered, while if chronic depressive features are prominent, an MAOI may be prescribed if the patient is compliant and not at risk of self-harm. When behavioural dyscontrol predominates, a low dose of neuroleptic (perhaps given by depot injection), or carbamazepine, may be of benefit.

It should be noted that the evidence in favour of these agents relates to short-term use of up to several months, and the effects of longer periods of drug treatments are unknown. A therapeutic trial of a sequence of several drugs may be appropriate.

Drug treatment: schizotypal and related personality disorders

Low doses of neuroleptics have been reported to produce improvement in features of schizotypal PD, such as ideas of reference, anxiety, derealization and depersonalization (Goldberg *et al.*, 1986; Ellison & Adler, 1990). Also, patients with paranoid PD may respond to low doses of neuroleptics, although compliance is usually poor and empirical evidence is lacking (Tyrer & Seivewright, 1988*a*).

Drug treatment: other personality disorders

Several case reports suggest that some patients with avoidant PD may respond to a MAOI or fluoxetine. Delito & Stam (1989) recommend a 2–3 month trial of these drugs in this context.

Drug treatment: target features

Ellison & Adler (1990) have considered drug treatment of PDs in relation to various target symptoms, namely transient psychosis (related to borderline PD, schizotypal PD, or co-occurring substance abuse), cognitive abnormalities (related to schizotypal, paranoid and borderline PDs), impulsivity (related to borderline, narcissistic and antisocial PDs), mood instability (related to borderline and histrionic PDs), dysphoria (with chronic low energy and depressed mood related to borderline, antisocial and some other PDs), and anxiety (related to many PDs). Such an approach can provide an additional framework to guide drug treatment for patients with PD.

It appears that transient psychosis, and some cognitive abnormalities, respond to relatively low doses of neuroleptics, which act more quickly than when these drugs are used for the treatment of schizophrenia. Suggested regimes have included trifluoperazine 2–4 mg/day.

Impulsivity may respond to neuroleptics, MAOIs or carbamazepine, and preliminary reports of fluoxetine, which is relatively safe in overdose, are encouraging in this respect. Also, trazodone, which has some serotonergic reuptake inhibiting activity, has been reported to reduce aggression in patients with structural brain disorders (Simpson & Foster, 1986). Lithium may also improve impulsivity in some subjects.

Mood instability, with vulnerability to environmental stress including relationship difficulties (i.e. 'rejection sensitivity'), may respond to a MAOI, or to other agents, such as neuroleptics or fluoxetine. For those patients with a co-occurring pattern of episodic mood disorder, lithium may be indicated.

Chronic dysphoria may also respond to a MAOI, and a MAOI has been reported to be beneficial for avoidant PD. In addition, Reich, Noyes & Yates (1989) found that alprazolam helped features of avoidant PD. Ellison & Adler (1990) suggested that if anxiety is present with PD, a beta-blocking agent should be considered if somatic symptoms are pronounced, but while alprazolam is a treatment option, it should be avoided if there is a perceived risk of impulsivity or the development of addiction. The use of an MAOI requires compliance and a low risk of overdose.

Drug combinations

As has been described, indications for the prescription of drugs are often unclear in patients with PD, and it is not surprising that the role of drug combinations is obscure. However, anecdotal case reports have involved drug combinations, and it is likely that some patients could benefit. For example, Ellison & Adler (1990) reported a patient with impulsive behaviour who appeared to respond to fluoxetine and lithium.

Other physical treatments

Electro-convulsive therapy (ECT)

ECT is mainly indicated for certain types of severe depression, treatment-resistant mania, and certain features of schizophrenia, such as excitement, stupor or drug-resistant distressing hallucinations. ECT may act in different ways in relation to these syndromes; for instance, while it appears to have a relatively specific effect on certain mood disorders, such as bipolar manic-depressive disorder and its variants, it may also have a non-specific and short-lived effect on other types of depression. In relation to this latter effect, ECT can be considered to have a place in the management of any type of severe depressive disorder, if the patient's life is at severe risk.

Zimmerman *et al.* (1986) reported 25 patients with 'major depression' who received ECT; ten had various PDs, while the remaining 15 had depression only. The short-term effect of ECT was considered to be good in both groups but, at follow-up after 6 months, five of the patients with PD had been readmitted in contrast to only one of the remaining 15. While Black, Bell & Hulbert (1988) also found an apparently good response rate to ECT in patients with major depression alone, and with depression and PD, Pfohl, Stangl & Zimmerman (1984) reported that the absence of PD was associated with a better response.

In conclusion, ECT does have a place in the management of depression in patients with PD, in particular borderline PD. This treatment is particularly indicated for those patients who have PD and a co-occurring affective disorder of the type that shows a relatively specific response to ECT. In such patients, a pattern of episodes of severe depression may be superimposed upon a more chronic dysphoria. But for any patient with borderline PD who develops a severe episode involving repeated impulsive self-harm, ECT may produce a rapid response. Such an effect is usually short-term, but, nevertheless, it may interrupt a vicious circle of escalating risk.

Psychosurgery

In a recent review, Dolan & Coid (1993) concluded that there is 'no clear justification' for the use of psychosurgical procedure for PD. However, there are many uncontrolled reports of favourable outcomes, for example, in relation to impulsive aggression, following a variety of procedures.

Andy (1975) described six patients with antisocial behaviour, four of whom showed marked improvements after thalamotomy, and Laitinen (1988) concluded that posteromedial hypothalamotomy could be indicated for 'restless, aggressive and destructive behaviour'. Dieckmann, Schneider-Jonietz & Schneider (1988) reported a follow-up of 14 subjects with 'aggressive sexual delinquency' who received unilateral ventromedial hypothalamotomy. In general, improvements in several aspects of functioning were claimed. van Manen & van Veelen (1988) described 54 patients who had received psychosurgery for various psychiatric disorders including self-mutilation, aggressive behaviour with temporal lobe epilepsy, and aggression in the setting of mental retardation. Operative procedures involved lesions in the fronto-basal region, cingulum, para-cingular white matter, anterior corpus callosum, amygdala and thalamus. In Japan, Sano & Mayangi (1988) reported 'good results' from stereotactic posteromedial hypothalamotomy for 'violent, aggressive behaviour'.

Physical treatments: psychological aspects

A decision to prescribe medication for a patient with PD may produce a range of reactions apart from compliance with realistic expectations. Some patients may perceive this as the clinician 'giving up', or, in the case of an individual with narcissistic PD features, as a severe blow to self-esteem (Ellison & Adler, 1990). Others perceive this as a welcome message that they can be dependent patients and wait for their problems to be resolved.

Several studies have noted that there is often a powerful placebo effect of drugs in patients with PDs, and the patient's psychological reactions can depend to some extent on the characteristics of the underlying PD. Borderline PD may be associated with the drug having a 'soothing' effect due to its association with the clinician, patients with paranoid PD may become defensive and suspicious as they feel some control has been lost, and histrionic PD may be associated with exaggerated complaints of side-effects. Patients who are prone to manipulative behaviour may use their medication in such interactions, for example by threatening an overdose, while others may develop marked psychological dependence, or physical addiction due to non-compliance.

One model of service delivery separates the psychological and pharmacological management of patients (particularly those with borderline PD), so that two clinicians are involved. But although such an arrangement may be necessary if the psychological management is provided by a non-medical clinician, the two roles can be successfully combined.

It is important to stress to the patient that a course of medication is being advised on a trial basis. The patient should be told that individuals respond differently to a particular drug and that it is uncertain whether benefits will be obtained. It may also be appropriate at the outset to outline the possibility of future trials with other drugs. Patients should usually be encouraged to take an active part in the evaluation of the effects of a drug regime by noting improvements and side-effects, and, if appropriate, reducing the dose accordingly. It is most important to assess the risk of overdose, in particular in the context of impulsive self-harm, and if a significant risk is identified the prescription of drugs which are relatively toxic must be avoided.

Physical treatments: a summary

Drug treatments have a role in the management of PDs, in particular borderline and schizotypal PDs. Most of the literature has been concerned with borderline PD, and it must be noted that patients with this diagnosis have a high rate of co-occurrence of other psychiatric disorders. Also, compliance is often poor and there is a danger of overdose. As favourable results of drug treatment are generally modest, the patient's expectations must not be raised too high, and drug treatment should take place in the context of other interventions, in particular supportive psychological management.

In relation to borderline PD, low doses of neuroleptics can be of benefit for a range of features, but Soloff (1987) has recommended that treatment duration should be generally brief, i.e. up to 12 weeks. Although clinical experience suggests that longer periods of 'continuation' treatment may help in some cases, a placebo-controlled trial of haloperidol or phenelzine for 16 weeks in patients with borderline PD did not provide clear evidence in favour of continuation treatment, even though modest improvements were reported (Cornelius *et al.*, 1993). Some antidepressants and carbamazepine can also benefit some patients, as can benzodiazepines, lithium and psychostimulants, but the effects of several of these drugs are unpredictable and may worsen symptoms and behaviour. In particular, behavioural dyscontrol may be worsened by anxiolytics or tricyclics, while carbamazapine may be associated with an increasing depression.

It may be appropriate to arrange a therapeutic trial of a sequence of drug treatments for an individual patient and, as anecdotal evidence suggests that drug combinations may be of benefit, combinations can be evaluated in certain patients with severe chronic disorders.

ECT can be indicated for management of some patients with severe life-threatening depression in the context of PD, as outlined above.

Finally, it is important to recognize that some patients with severe PD have co-occurring affective disorders of the type that responds well to medication or ECT. But episodic mood changes due to such co-occurring disorders are often obscured by a chronic pattern of maladaptive behaviour. If such co-occurence is suspected, the patient should receive a trial of appropriate medication such as lithium or an antidepressant.

Future directions

Future research may enable a range of psychotropic drugs and drug combinations to be targeted more specifically in patients with PDs. The evidence of cerebral serotonin abnormalities associated with impulsivity is partly based on abnormal neuroendocrine responses to drug 'challenges' that affect serotonergic function, such as the administration of *m*-chlorophenylpiperazine and fenfluramine (Coccaro *et al.*, 1989), and future studies are needed to investigate the associations between such challenges and subsequent treatment response. This strategy may also prove useful in relation to short-term changes in mood as a result of an 'amphetamine challenge', in which 30 mg dexamphetamine is given daily, for example for 2–3 days, and ratings of mood are compared with those associated with placebo (Fawcett & Siomopouloo, 1971). A significant improvement of mood in relation to amphetamines has been associated with a history of childhood attention deficit hyperactivity disorder and may predict a favourable response to other stimulants or antidepressants, in particular MAOIs (Stein, 1993).

7

Psychological management

J.H. DOWSON

Definitions and overview

'Psychological management' is a broad term encompassing a range of theoretical frameworks and techniques, such as psychoanalysis, various forms of psychotherapy, behaviour therapy, supportive psychotherapy and counselling.

Some methods focus on an evolving interpersonal interaction between therapist and patient (i.e. a 'psychodynamic' psychotherapy approach), while others are mainly concerned with a patient's thoughts (i.e. a 'cognitive therapy' approach) or behaviour (i.e. a 'behaviour therapy' approach).

Psychological management can be defined as the alleviation of problems by behavioural interventions designed to influence the patient's higher mental activity. Such behavioural interventions include what the therapist (or other relevant individuals, e.g. in group psychotherapy) says and does (or does not say or do), together with any modifications that the therapist may encourage in the patient's social environment, such as admitting a patient to hospital or a day centre. Higher mental activity can be considered as those mental processes that are experienced in conscious awareness, or have this potential, and includes thoughts, memories and emotions. Higher mental activity also involves so-called 'unconscious' mental processes, an example of which would be an instruction given in an 'hypnotic state' that is subsequently carried out without the individual being consciously aware of the reasons for his/her actions.

The term 'psychotherapy' has usually implied an emphasis on interpersonal interactions between therapist and patient, and the American Psychiatric Association's Committee on the Practice of Psychotherapy has defined psychotherapy as

a method of treating mental disorders, the cornerstone of which is the development of experiential understanding of the meaning of symptoms and/or ... those

249

characteristic patterns that cause the patient to suffer limitations and pain. In contrast to somatic or pharmacological intervention, psychotherapy relies on verbal means and techniques to modify characteristic ways of thinking, feeling, and behaving that interfere with the patient's capacity for maximal functioning.

In similar vein, the British Association of Psychotherapists (1993) note that the 'method employed is verbal communication' for

> those who are experiencing difficulties within themselves or in their relationships with others . . . Psychotherapy is a process of exploration undertaken by two people, therapist and patient, in the context of a personal relationship between the two. In this exploration, the patient takes the lead by relating thoughts, associations, feelings, memories and dreams. The therapist follows, clarifying what is happening by drawing the patient's attention to habitual modes of behaving and by making links between conscious and unconscious, present and past experience. All this has the aim of promoting the patient's self-understanding and capacity to view the world objectively and less coloured by personal wishes, fear and prejudices.

Such descriptions refer to a process that is generally time-consuming (i.e. 1–3 hours per week for up to several years), that is not readily available to patients in psychiatric services, and is relatively inaccessible to evaluation because of the degree of variability of this type of intervention.

PDs are characterized by long-term disorders of social functioning together with associated features, and it has been claimed that 'the personality disorders constitute one of the most important sources of long-term impairment in both treated and untreated populations' (Merikangas & Weissman, 1986). However, the provision of psychological management for those with PDs must recognize that apparent short-term improvement in symptoms or behaviour can be misleading and may reflect an environmental change, as, by definition, these disorders consist of deeply ingrained patterns of behaviour. Nevertheless, psychological management can often help to relieve a patient's symptoms (e.g. a depressive disorder) that are secondary to problems engendered by PD; this may then lead to a temporary respite in a pattern of maladaptive behaviour such as substance abuse or self-harm episodes. But although overt patterns of PD-related behaviour may show apparently rapid changes, the patterns of cognitive processes associated with PD, if they do respond to psychological management, do so at a relatively slow rate. If a clear change takes place this is usually over a time-scale of many months or years, and realistic goals of treatment of PDs usually involve only modest cognitive changes. However, this need not discourage the therapist, as even a modest change (e.g. teaching a patient to act in a different way when he loses his temper) can have major beneficial effects on social functioning.

Shea (1993) has reviewed the claims for several approaches to psychological management of PDs, including various types of psychodynamic psychotherapy, in particular for patients with borderline PD; one approach involved a focus on the use of interpretations by the therapist, another advocated more supportive interventions, while some treatment programmes have been time-limited, in contrast to most 'psychodynamic' psychotherapy. Another approach for those with borderline PD has been to focus on interpersonal interactions in a series of 30 sessions of group psychotherapy, while 'cognitive' interventions have provided very different strategies for the treatment of PDs, as they have been directed towards the maladaptive patterns of thoughts and feelings (also known as 'schemas' or 'cognitive structures'), which are claimed to produce biased judgements and interpretations in selected situations. Cognitive approaches usually incorporate a behavioural dimension, as the process of developing new schemas, and the modifications of old schemas, includes planning changes in the patient's behaviour. Cognitive therapy has been applied to the treatment of some depressive disorders, with attention to the thoughts and behaviours related to a depressed mood, and for PDs a wide range of schemas need to be addressed. Although 'behavioural' treatments theoretically involve a specific focus, most specified psychological interventions are invariably supplemented by other potentially therapeutic aspects, such as the nonspecific ingredients of a therapist–patient relationship, involving empathy, advice, and personal warmth. The 'behavioural' approach of Linehan *et al.* (1991) for patients with borderline PD is of particular interest, as its efficacy has been supported by experimental data; this treatment programme involved training the patient in interpersonal skills, in emotional regulation and expression, and in distress tolerance. Other behavioural approaches such as desensitization with gradual exposure to feared situations have been used to treat patients with avoidant PD.

For patients with borderline PD, uncontrolled studies of various forms of psychological management, in particular psychodynamic psychotherapy, have indicated a tendency for a high drop-out rate in the first months of outpatient treatment sessions. However, ten controlled studies of a defined psychological management for patients with various PDs have evaluated a range of behavioural treatments and other forms of psychotherapy (Shea, 1993). For avoidant PD, three studies reported a significant beneficial effect of behavioural treatments, which included graduated exposure, social skills training and systematic desensitization (Marzillier, Lambert & Kellett, 1976; Cappe & Alden, 1986; Alden, 1989). Also for avoidant PD, Argyle, Bryant & Trower (1974) found beneficial effects of either social skills training or psychodynamic psychotherapy, while improvements following social skills training have been found in other studies (Trower *et al.*, 1978; Stravynski, Marks & Yule, 1982; Cappe & Alden, 1986). But, while these reports indicated improvement on such measures as frequency and range of social contacts, avoidance, and pleasure in social activities, such benefits were often modest, and the effects of social skills training were generally limited to superficial relationships. Control groups were often waiting-list patients or patients undergoing a different type of treatment, and none of these studies controlled for non-specific factors of a treatment situation, such as the placebo effect and the therapist's interest and concern.

Linehan *et al.* (1991) have provided impressive empirical evidence in favour of a form of psychological management in relation to patients with borderline PD who had a history of repeated self-harm episodes. A regime of group and individual psychological management sessions for one year (Dialectical Behaviour Therapy, DBT) was compared with the effects of 'treatment as usual'. The clear benefits of DBT (which will be described subsequently) included a reduction in frequency and severity of self-harm behaviour, so that these results have important implications for the appropriate provision of psychiatric services for a group of patients who present considerable management problems. Another study of borderline PD investigated the effects of intensive, brief psychological management (4 hours/day for 8 days, using either behavioural methods or a psychodynamic psychotherapeutic approach) and found that both treatments had some effect, while the group treated with behaviour therapy had less frequent suicidal thoughts on follow-up (Liberman & Eckman, 1981).

Winston and colleagues (1991) investigated the effects of two forms of brief psychodynamic psychotherapy on patients with various PDs, but excluded those with schizoid, schizotypal, narcissistic or borderline PDs. Patients were involved with weekly sessions for 40 weeks, and patients on a waiting-list formed the control group. Both forms of psychotherapy were associated with significant improvements.

Investigating the effects of treatments for patients with PDs presents two main methodological problems. Firstly, a patient sample based on the diagnosis of a named PD will show considerable heterogeneity, as another psychiatric disorder (such as a depressive disorder or anxiety state) may be present, more than one PD may co-occur, PDs defined by polythetic criteria are heterogeneous, and a specified PD exhibits a range of severity. Secondly, a co-occurring psychiatric disorder can not only influence the assessment of PD but can also affect the evaluation of change in response to treatment. Other problems include a high drop-out rate from a treatment programme in relation to some PDs, variability in the skills of therapists for psychological management techniques, the effects of various aspects of the patient's life situation (or other uncontrolled variables) on PD behaviour, and the difficulty in obtaining suitable control or comparison groups. As it is unethical to form a 'no-treatment' control group (such as a waiting-list group) over a period in excess of that which would normally be the waiting time, alternative research strategies are needed, such as comparing the effects of a standard treatment on groups of patients with different PDs, or comparing the results of a standard treatment 'package' with those of a similar regime that omits certain specific interventions. However, the findings using the latter approach can be influenced by interactions between the various ingredients of a treatment programme.

The evaluation of treatments for PD may be assisted by the identification of 'core' PD features that could provide the focus for outcome measures. This would be a change from the approach derived from current polythetic criteria sets in DSM-III-R and ICD-10, in which equal weight is given to all the criteria listed. The selection of patients partly on the basis of core features might also increase the homogeneity of the sample. Outcome of treatment programmes for patients with PD can sometimes be expressed in monetary terms in a cost–benefit analysis, perhaps by taking into account the cost of medical resources and the costs to society of antisocial behaviour, but, in the organization of clinical services, such analyses have to involve additional clinical and social judgements. In clinical practice, the evaluation of monetary benefits have to be considered together with effects that are measured in different units, such as symptom scores and levels of social functioning (Krupnick & Pincus, 1992).

There have been many reports that a patient's personality and PD can influence the outcome of various forms of psychological management in psychiatric practice (Conte *et al.*, 1991). Not surprisingly, poor outcome has been associated with mistrust, hostility and problems with intimacy, while good outcome has been related to a good 'therapeutic alliance', non-aggressive problems, assertiveness and sociability. An approach that has identified the importance of PD for the outcome related to various psychiatric treatments, including psychological management, has been to study the results of treatment of non-PD psychiatric disorders in patients with and without co-occurring PDs. Tyrer *et al.* (1990) reported 210 patients with anxiety or depressive disorders, of which 30% also had a PD.

The latter subgroup had more severe symptoms, and those with a depressive disorder and PD responded less well to treatment than those without PD.

An overview of psychological management for patients with PDs must consider some implications of the use of the PD diagnostic categories, in particular the attitudes of professionals in psychiatric services to patients whose symptoms and behaviour have attracted these diagnostic labels. Clinicians' attitudes often relate to their concepts of a patient's personal reponsibility for his/her actions and whether he/she is 'in control'. In this context, patients with PDs are often considered as distinct from those with other forms of psychiatric disorder, in that they have 'control' and 'responsibility' for their actions. But such an analysis is simplistic, inaccurate and inappropriate, as shown by the evidence that genetic and other biological factors are associated with personality and PD. Although the behaviour of many patients with PD can be aggravating and unpleasant, clinicians must not allow themselves to reject such individuals inappropriately.

Psychodynamic psychotherapy

Overview

Psychodynamic techniques focus on the interpersonal interactions between the therapist and patient and, in relation to PDs, have been mainly investigated for those patients with borderline PD.

Certain hypotheses related to the development of borderline PD have been influential in providing a rationale of treatment, in particular that a person has developed borderline PD as a result of bad parenting and other traumatic experiences such as physical and sexual abuse (Masterson, 1981). But although many patients with borderline PD (and other PDs) do give such histories, there is no good evidence that such experiences are essential. However, despite the uncertainties surrounding the hypothesis that borderline (and other) PDs are mainly the result of faults in the previous behaviour of 'significant' others, which would always give the patient victim status, a major role of psychodynamic psychotherapy has been conceived of as allowing the patient to re-experience past adverse relationships and to build new ways of thinking, feeling and reacting, in the context of an extended relationship with the therapist. Sessions may be regularly provided for up to several years and the patient's feelings towards the therapist (the 'transference') are usually a major focus of discussion. Although this format is subject to certain techniques and theories, it is relatively unstructured, compared with cognitive and behavioural regimes.

As there are considerable methodological problems in evaluating the processes of psychological management, and of changes in PD, a lack of evidence in favour of a treatment regime for PD does not exclude the possibility that there are some benefits. But reviews of published studies have not concluded that psychodynamic psychotherapy is superior to placebo. Andrews (1991) considered that 'dynamic psychotherapy . . . has not been demonstrated to be superior to placebo in the neuroses or personality disorders. The case reports of improvement during long-term dynamic therapy for personality disorders may be due to the combined effects of normal maturation and the non-specific effects of continued clinical care'. In a review of 19 studies, it appeared that short-term psychodynamic psychotherapy was associated with beneficial effects at the end of treatment but not at follow-up after 6 or 12 months (Svartberg & Styles, 1991). But even these improvements were not as beneficial as those associated with other forms of psychological management, mainly involving cognitive-behavioural regimes.

Such studies have generally evaluated relatively short periods of treatment, and it can be argued that they are not relevant to the considerably longer periods of psychodynamic psychotherapy which are often undertaken. But it has been pointed out that at least 50% of patients with borderline PD will no longer meet criteria for this diagnosis after 10 years, and that specific effects of treatment must be distinguished from natural remission and placebo responses. These latter variables could account for the modest improvements that were found in patients with borderline PD who received 100 hours of psychodynamic psychotherapy over 2 years (Stevenson & Meares, 1992).

Andrews (1993) has considered that apart from lack of evidence for efficacy, additional arguments against the provision of long-term psychodynamic psychotherapy (other than in private practice) are the high cost (in an Australian survey each patient received an average of 330 hours of treatment) and possible side-effects such as inhibiting normal remission, encouraging undue dependency, encouraging emotional arousal which cannot be satisfactorily dealt with by the patient, and sexual abuse of the patient by the therapist.

'Psychodynamic psychotherapy' includes a range of techniques, and one important variable is duration of treatment, which can vary from up to several sessions a week for several years to once a week for a few months. Another variable is the degree of the therapist's 'neutrality', which is defined as how much he/she shows his/her thoughts, feelings and opinions, and how much active encouragement and support is given. There is also variation in the focus of strategy; some therapists mainly try to uncover and explain hidden aspects of mental functioning with an emphasis on past experiences, while others concentrate more on the 'here-and-now' pattern of feelings and interpersonal reactions.

Intensive psychoanalytic psychotherapy

This strategy of psychological management has been advocated by a minority of psychiatrists for patients with features of borderline and/or narcissistic PD. At the most intensive end of the spectrum of such intervention is 'psychoanalysis', which involves sessions of up to 1 hour, four or five times a week, with the patient lying on a couch (i.e. not in face-to-face contact with the therapist) in a setting that encourages the patient to experience strong emotions (Higgitt & Fonagy, 1992). However, this format is considered by many psychiatrists to be generally contra-indicated for individuals with borderline PD, as the emotional experience in relation to the therapist can often become excessively hostile and destructive, with a degree of anger that can lead to aggressive or self-destructive behaviour that is the opposite of therapeutic (Gunderson & Sabo, 1993a).

At a modest distance from this end of the spectrum, 'intensive psycho-analytic psychotherapy' involves two or three hourly sessions per week, involving face-to-face contact between therapist and patient, and can continue for between 2 to 7 years. Such a regime is believed by some therapists (but probably not by most psychiatrists) to be the treatment of choice for patients with severe borderline PD. Within this format, the focus is on the interpretation of the transference, which can be defined as aspects of the patient's emotions, attitudes, motivations and behaviour that are directed to the therapist and are derived in part from past experience. Transference phenomena may be present at the beginning of treatment as well as developing subsequently. The process of interpretation involves providing the patient with links or associations between aspects of the transference and hidden mental processes that relate to past experiences. The psychological means by which the patient keeps such mental processes hidden are known as 'defence mechanisms'; examples are 'denial' and 'avoidance', which will be described subsequently.

Transference reactions in patients with borderline PD can involve sudden intense emotion, which often leads to anger, and Kohut (1977) has described three common patterns, mainly in relation to features of co-occurring narcissistic PD. In a 'merger' transference, a grandiose patient may see the therapist as part of his/her omnipotent influence, and expect the therapist to be owned by the patient and exclusively committed to his/her treatment. This is similar to a 'mirror' transference, in which the therapist is expected to focus on and admire the patient's special qualities, while an 'idealized' transference involves the therapist being perceived as the provider of unlimited safety and support. Another pattern that is often seen with borderline PD patients is a tendency to see the therapist as 'all good' or 'all bad', and to change from one perception to the other (perhaps alternating) in the course of treatment.

For borderline PD patients, some therapists have believed that the main ingredient of treatment is for the therapist to identify and point out (interpret) negative feelings in the transference (i.e. anger and mistrust), as well as the patient's hidden motivations of sadism, destructiveness, aggression and the wish to control others (Higgitt & Fonagy, 1992; Gunderson & Sabo, 1993a). However, there have been disagreements whether all these 'hidden' aspects are invariably present, about the timing of such interpretations, and about their relative importance.

In routine psychiatric practice, several strategic guidelines have emerged for psychological management, some of which contrast with the approach of intensive psychoanalytic psychotherapy. Many psychiatrists believe that, compared with some other patients, those with borderline PD require a relatively active therapist, as excessive silence is not well tolerated. Also, in general, a limit-setting approach with few interpretations appears to be needed, in which the therapist repeatedly draws the patient's attention to the adverse consequences of his/her behaviour. The therapist has to be able to tolerate considerable anger and child-like or regressive behaviour, involving tantrums and demands for instant gratification. Common mistakes include not challenging the patient's view of the therapist as 'heroic' or 'good' when the patient is in a phase of idealization, or being excessively rejecting in response to provocation.

Kernberg's expressive psychotherapy

Kernberg's treatment model is a type of intensive psychoanalytic psychotherapy and was developed from ideas based on the Psychotherapy Research Project of the Menninger Foundation (Kernberg *et al.*, 1972). It was considered that this study indicated that patients with borderline PD did best with intensive psychotherapy aimed at hypothesized core psycho-pathology, rather than with a supportive approach aimed at improving social adaptation.

Kernberg advocated the importance of transference interpretations, in particular in relation to the patient's mistrust, anger and aggression, which were considered to form the core of borderline PD psychopathology. Indeed, he considered that a supportive approach, which avoids or damps down anger by positive and caring responses, may cause an increase in hidden anger as it cannot readily be expressed.

The format involves sessions at least twice weekly, in which the patient faces the therapist and there is a fixed timetable of appointments. This precludes responding to phone calls or approaches at other times. Limits are set in relation to destructive behaviour such as missing appointments, physical aggression, substance abuse and self-harm. A written contract at the start of treatment can be signed, and the therapist's options are to stop or postpone treatment, or to refer to another clinician if the contract is broken. Sometimes any attempt at this form of treatment may produce an increase in destructive behaviour and if a decision is made to proceed, this may have to be within the setting of a long-term inpatient admission. At times, regular contact between the therapist and significant persons in the patient's life may be indicated.

The therapist should be neutral in that he/she should not be directive or display much of his/her own feelings and attitudes. But this is not a 'blank screen' approach, as a caring attitude, personal warmth, showing respect and being active in treatment sessions is necessary. Interventions include clarification, confrontation and interpretations, and are aimed mainly at current situations and relationships. Clarification includes inquiring, in a non-challenging way, about incomplete, vague or contradictory aspects of the patient's statements, while a confronting therapist may tell the patient how such statements appear to others. Interpretations involve suggestions about possible underlying (hidden) motives and feelings associated with the patient's behaviour; at first these can be limited to 'here and now' situations, but later may be linked with past experiences, particularly when interpretations about the transference are involved. For instance, a comment may be made about the patient's negative reactions to the therapist that appear disproportionate to the reality of the situation, or about inappropriately positive feelings. But appropriate positive feelings can be accepted without interpretation, and the patient must not be made to feel that their every feeling and reaction is invalid and unreal. Often it may be useful to point out a similarity between the transference relationship and other current relationships with 'significant others'. If the patient distorts the nature and meaning of the therapist's interventions, this may form the basis for further interpretation, as can contradictory or maladaptive views of self and others that can be expressed at different times. For example, a patient may variously consider him/herself as a child, a victim, as all-powerful, or as a person with a need to control others (Goldstein, 1990). Patients often have difficulty in integrating different views of themselves and others, and need to learn that an individual has different facets and modes of behaviour, so that 'all-or-none' concepts are inaccurate.

While countertransference can be viewed as 'the therapist's emotional reactions to the patient that are based on the therapist's own unresolved unconscious conflicts' (Goldstein, 1990), Kernberg had a broader concept that incorporated both conscious and unconscious reactions to the patient, including those based on reality as a result of the patient's behaviour; the latter component has been called the 'objective countertransference' (Winnicott, 1949). It is important that the therapist monitors his/her reactions and uses this information objectively to try to understand the patient. If objectivity is lost, countertransference can be antitherapeutic in many ways; limits may fail to be set because of the therapist's inability to tolerate anxiety, or the therapist's anger may lead to a harmful rejection or an inappropriate encouragement for the patient to experience a destructive anger. This could increase the risk of suicide.

Masterson's confrontative psychotherapy

Masterson (1976) has described another variant of psychodynamic psychotherapy for borderline PD patients (Goldstein, 1990). This involves the therapist being ready to express a wider range of personal views and attitudes than in Kernberg's approach, with a focus on the depressed mood such patients have when they feel alone and abandoned. It was considered particularly important to help the patient to cope with the ending of treatment, so that any efforts to develop autonomy are encouraged and supported. Various countertransference problems were identified which apply to psychological management in a range of settings. These include inappropriate anger if a patient shows destructive behaviour (this may precipitate further self-harm), an inability to set limits that are necessary for treatment to continue, an excessive need to have the patient's approval, and an excessive need to be in control and directive, thus preventing autonomous behaviour.

Conclusion

The role of psychodynamic psychotherapy for PD, in particular for borderline PD, is controversial. Gunderson & Sabo (1993*a*) have noted that there is increasing evidence (Wallerstein, 1986; Kolb & Gunderson, 1990) that less intensive and more supportive strategies appear to be associated with changes that have been believed by some to result only from more intensive transference-based regimes; 'Such observations cast doubt on accounts of psychoanalytic psychotherapy that propose that change relies on insight without recognizing the corrective role of such unspecific "supportive" interventions'. Although it is possible that, for certain patients, their unique experiences of intensive psychodynamic psychotherapy are of benefit, it seems that there is insufficient evidence to recommend such expensive and time-consuming procedures.

However, many of the strategies derived from these approaches may be of benefit in relatively brief, more supportive forms of psychological management, which will now be described.

Brief (psychodynamic) psychotherapy

There have been several attempts to develop brief programmes of psychological management for use in routine psychiatric settings that incorporate some theories and strategies derived from psychodynamic psychotherapy (Weissman, Klerman & Prusoff, 1981; Luborsky, 1984; Horowitz, Marmar & Weiss, 1986). Such interventions have been provided for patients with a range of psychiatric disorders, including depressive disorders and PDs.

Brief (short-term or time-limited) psychotherapy involving 10–20 sessions over 6–12 months was at one time considered inappropriate for those with borderline PD (Mann, 1973), but some clinicians consider that such regimes can be useful if sessions are focussed on specific situations or interpersonal problems, and the patient is not encouraged to develop strong transference feelings. This is achieved by avoiding explanations of transference phenomena, and providing direction and structure to the content of the sessions.

Gunderson & Sabo (1993*a*) have considered that this strategy may be appropriate for those patients with borderline PD who would drop out of more intensive treatments and who would find it very difficult to cope with becoming dependent on a therapist. Also, brief psychotherapy can be given intermittently on a long-term basis (Silver, 1985).

Winston and colleagues (1991) have examined the efficacy of two forms of brief psychotherapy for patients with PDs, but excluded borderline, narcissistic, paranoid, and schizoid/schizotypal psychopathology. Patients were seen once a week for a maximum of 40 sessions. One treatment format was called 'short-term dynamic psychotherapy' (STDP) and the other 'brief adaptational psychotherapy' (BAP). Both therapies involved clarification, confrontation and interpretation, and attempts were made to link present patterns of thinking, feeling and behaving to past events and relationships. In general, STDP was the more active method involving the confrontation of psychological defences and the encouragement of emotional arousal, while BAP was a more cognitive therapy which focussed on the origins and determinants of maladaptive patterns of distorted thoughts and on the patient–therapist relationship, with less pressure on the patient to remove psychological defences. The findings suggested that STDP, with the emphasis on confrontation and eliciting emotions, can be antitherapeutic if inappropriately used, although if the patient has the resiliance to tolerate the stress involved without dropping-out, or engaging in destructive behaviour, higher levels of improvement may follow. Also, STDP seems more effective than BAP in improving mood in some types of co-occurring depressive disorder. This is consistent with the hypothesis that, for depression which is causally associated with certain experiences, the expression (release) of any anger can be therapeutic. But there is a great danger of assuming that all depressed patients can be improved by the therapist eliciting (or even provoking) anger; such a strategy can have disastrous consequences.

The results of this study in relation to those PDs involved (which excluded borderline PD), indicated that these treatment strategies were associated with significant improvement in target complaints and social adjustment, compared with a waiting-list control group. A subsequent report from Winston *et al.* (1994), with a larger patient group, which also excluded 'cluster A' and borderline PDs, concluded that BAP and STDP were effective for patients with certain types of PD, but that the two approaches did not differ in overall outcome.

Supportive and related psychotherapies

Overview

'Supportive psychotherapy' encompasses many theoretical perspectives and techniques, including some derived from psychodynamic psychotherapy. But in contrast to the latter, the main aim is to restore, maintain or improve adaptive functioning, at the expense of self-destructive behaviour. The focus is on the current reality of the problems of daily life, and psychological defences are generally strengthened unless they are seriously maladaptive. Exploration of unconscious processes by interpretation is generally avoided. The patient is not encouraged to develop the type of relationship with the therapist that involves considerable emotional expression, excessive dependence or the experience of strong anger. But a patient can be encouraged to realize that it is possible to deal with anger in a way that is not always destructive.

The techniques used in supportive psychotherapy include allowing patients to express their thoughts and emotions, appropriate reassurance, rational discussion, education, advice, encouragement, promotion of problem-solving behaviour, suggestion, and environmental manipulation. However, some non-confrontational interpretations may also be useful. There may be flexibility about timing of sessions or unscheduled contracts, (for example, by phone), and a high degree of availability of the therapist (or colleague) can be a successful strategy in responding to a crisis, without allowing excessive dependency to develop.

For borderline PD patients, supportive psychotherapy may take place once a week or less frequently, and continue for up to several years in patients with severe disorders. For such patients a variety of schedules may be appropriate, so that frequency of sessions may range from once a week to once every 1–2 months, depending on the current level of social adaptation. A 'holding environment' is often important for borderline PD patients, which requires the therapist to offer a degree of personal warmth, consistency, and flexible availability, within stated limits. 'What these patients need is an experience, not an explanation' (Fromm-Reichmann, quoted in Higgitt & Fonagy, 1992). Higgitt & Fonagy (1992) consider that, on available evidence, techniques derived from both psychodynamic and supportive psychotherapy may be useful for some patients with borderline and narcissistic PD. Although Kernberg believed that supportive techniques for some borderline PD patients were harmful, because dependence on a therapist would be added to the problems without significant benefit, he subsequently described a variant of supportive psychotherapy for patients with borderline PD (Kernberg, 1984). In this approach, the aim is to improve the patient's adaptation and to increase his/her control over destructive behaviour. The therapist is less neutral than in psychodynamic psychotherapy and the frequency of sessions can vary in response to a crisis. The therapist's role is 'a teacher about the nature of reality and appropriate behaviour' (Goldstein, 1990), which involves the identification of negative feelings in the transference and maladaptive psychological defences, and the process of relating these to the problems they have caused. But further interpretations are avoided which would link them with past events and relationships. For example, if the process of 'splitting' is identified (i.e. a type of psychological defence, perhaps involving an attitude that a person is either 'all good' or 'all bad'), such a distortion is challenged; i.e. 'is she really as bad as you think she is?'. But even in this treatment format, Kernberg believes that attention must also be given to the negative transference involving feelings of mistrust and anger towards the therapist, and that some insight into this tendency, with the encouragement of some adaptive strategies for coping, is necessary if the patient is to be able to form and maintain more positive attachments. Thus, the therapist tries to get the patient to recognize such negative feelings, even if they may not be apparent; for example, a patient may be reminded that although he/she feels positive today, a few weeks ago he/she was full of complaints.

Kohut's psychotherapy

Kohut (1977) stressed the importance of focussing on the patient's inner world in an attempt to understand and empathize with his/her thoughts and feelings. However, it was suggested that this approach should be based on theories that are controversial, namely that anger in individuals with borderline PD is due to 'severe and repeated assaults they experienced in early childhood', and that such a patient 'should have had a lot more attention and encouragement ...' (Goldstein, 1990). It is important to remember that an indiscriminate use of such unproven statements may not only be inaccurate but could set up additional family conflicts. Some interpretation of psychological defences, such as lateness, is advocated by Kohut, although this should not usually be attempted in the early stages of treatment, while empathy should not extend to approving dysfunctional behaviour. Indeed patients should be confronted with the effects of their behaviour.

Adler and Buie's model of psychotherapy (Adler & Buie, 1979; Adler, 1985)

This approach, for patients with borderline PD, is closer to psychodynamic than supportive psychotherapy, but is more flexible than the former, as it draws on a wider variety of techniques. The main aim is to help patients develop their impaired capacity to evoke and experience positive attitudes to others in their absence or when frustrated by them. The therapist tries to be empathic and supportive, in the hope that the patient will develop a positive image and attitude to the therapist, which is then 'internalized'. Such a strategy is based on an assumption that a patient with borderline PD does not have sufficient positive memories and attitudes to previously significant persons, and that an 'internalized' positive role model of the therapist will allow more positive feelings to develop in future relationships. This is in contrast to Kernberg's view that good and bad feelings are 'split', in that they cannot be experienced together about another person; in Adler and Buie's model, the capacity for 'good' feelings is missing.

This strategy, emphasizing the provision of safety, security and trust, involves two to five sessions per week but the arrangements can be flexible with a defined provision for unscheduled phone calls and extra sessions. Additional security can be offered by such techniques as offering to return any phone call, the provision of the therapist's holiday address so that the patient can write, and sending the patient postcards when on leave. But although the therapist is relatively flexible, limits still have to be set for the continuation of treatment, for example in relation to physical violence. Other techniques used include clarification, confrontation and interpretation.

Problems related to the therapist's feelings and attitudes (countertransference) are similar, whatever form of psychological management is used. The therapist can feel helpless, hopeless about the outcome, and guilt that more has not been achieved. Such feelings can lead to inappropriate withdrawal, excessive dedication with the setting of unrealistic goals, or the denial of the patient's hostility.

The Blancks' psychotherapy

Another approach for patients with borderline PD, advocated by Gertrude and Rubin Blanck (Goldstein, 1990), aims to build up the positive and adaptive aspects of the individual's functioning.

The patient's achievements and abilities are identified and commented upon, which can include pointing out the positive aspects of otherwise problematic behaviour. For example, the frequent expression of inappropriate anger may be maladaptive but the patient is told that it is better to express anger directly than drop out of treatment. Adaptational strategies can be encouraged or developed, and patients can be helped to identify triggers for maladaptive anxiety or anger, together with alternative ways of coping. Care is taken not to encourage patients to express anger to the therapist early in treatment if it is not balanced by more positive feelings, which are identified and reinforced. Patients are encouraged to tell the therapist about the details of their thoughts, although many patients find this difficult and have an unrealistic wish to be understood without the effort of verbal explanation. Attention is also given to helping the patient to recognize and describe their various mood states and to understand how these may be part of their patterns of maladaptive behaviour. Patients can be regularly asked for their suggestions, rather than allowing an implicit expectation that all the wisdom and effort resides in the therapist. Also, some psychological defences can be adaptive and should be recognized as such; for example, it may be appropriate for a patient to want a break from treatment sessions to prevent the development of excessive dependency. The development of the patient's autonomy is encouraged, perhaps involving less dependency within the therapeutic relationship and the development of new social and recreational activities. The therapist needs to recognize that some patients become more demanding during the time that improvement in symptoms or functioning is taking place, because of their concern that their treatment and support will be lost if it is no longer needed.

This approach may involve one to three sessions per week or less often for longer-term maintenance. The therapist takes an active interest in the patient, is flexible within defined limits, and positive feelings for the therapist are encouraged. In addition, some explanation and interpretation aimed at distortions of the here-and-now relationship with the therapist can be appropriate.

Psychotherapy of borderline personality disorder: methods compared

Much of the literature on psychotherapy for PD has been concerned with borderline PD, and the clinician is faced with a confusing array of theoretical frameworks, techniques and formats for the provision of services.

While individuals with borderline PD form an heterogeneous group that requires a range of psychotherapeutic approaches, there is uncertainty about aspects of the theoretical frameworks on which some types of psychological management are based. For instance, Kernberg has argued that the patient's anger needs to be addressed before more positive, adaptive, feelings can develop. But excessive early confrontation and encouragement of the expression of anger can be harmful, and this approach may allow a therapist to ignore that some of the patient's anger to the therapist may be justified and is not necessarily a distorted reaction. Also, the hypothesis that the encouragement of positive feelings should be delayed can be used to justify the therapist's relative non-involvement with the patient, although an active approach is generally considered to be helpful for most patients. According to Kernberg, an early focus on anger is the most effective means of significant change for the most destructive patients and, while this is possible, it is unproven. Such a strategy must take into account the risks of excessive anger leading to violence to others or to self, and drop-out from treatment. Other authors have noted the importance of several ingredients in the therapist–patient relationships for the management of borderline PD; namely, initial acceptance of childlike, dependent behaviour, rather than confrontation (Masterson); encouragement of the development of positive, adaptive, examples of the patient's behaviour (the Blancks); a human empathic approach (Kohut); and availability and flexibility (Adler & Buie).

In routine psychiatric practice, it would seem appropriate to adopt a flexible integrated approach, which draws on many of these styles and formats, for the majority of patients with borderline PD (Goldstein, 1990). A positive, empathic relationship with the patient is attempted and, in general, the emphasis is not on confrontation or on interpretations that attempt to link hidden feelings to past experiences. However, a limited number of interpretations that help the patient to recognize and manage hidden emotions, attitudes and fears can be useful, particularly if insight can be gained into current behaviour; for example, the patient may recognize that unexpressed anger, or fear of being alone and abandoned, can be a problem in close relationships. Some limits need to be set for therapist availability, while so-called 'transitional objects' or situations can be provided; for example the patient phoning the therapist (or a colleague) under certain circumstances and times, the provision of vacation addresses so the patient can write when appointments are not available, and a diary in which the patient is encouraged to note thoughts and feelings to be shown to the therapist at the next meeting. The degree to which the clinician should gratify excessive dependency needs of the patient is subject to theoretical disagreements, and the appropriate decision is likely to vary. For some patients, acceptance of requests for frequent appointments and toleration of destructive behaviour without initial confrontation may be necessary for engagement in treatment, but there are limits to what the therapist can tolerate both emotionally and practically. There has to be a limit to the availability of the therapist's time, while physical destruction or violence to others must trigger containment measures or discharge from treatment, above a certain threshold. It may be important to pay attention to the patient's family and social environment, by involving significant others in psychotherapeutic sessions.

Cognitive psychotherapy

Overview

Cognitive therapy (CT) is a form of psychological management in which the therapist talks with the patient, focussing on how recurrent maladaptive conscious thoughts are used to assign meaning to events, how these may contribute to the patient's current behaviour and problems, and how the patient can develop skills to change such patterns of thinking and behaviour. Such an approach requires a good therapist–patient relationship with shared goals. Maladaptive patterns of thoughts can give rise to emotional changes, and CT has been shown to be useful in the management of some types of depression and anxiety, but has also been applied to PDs. It is a relatively short, time-limited treatment, perhaps involving from between 10 and 30 sessions, and patients are told in advance that the aim is for them to develop problem-solving skills that will be available to them after treatment ends.

Beck & Freeman (1990) have termed stable, ingrained patterns of conscious thought as 'schemas', which select and synthesize information and assign meanings to events. Schemas can be considered to consist of a set of related cognitions, or smaller units each involving a relatively narrow belief, and can be evaluated in relation to their breadth, flexibility, prominence and threshold for activation. Schemas can be considered as one type of basic unit of personality and most PDs; for example, 'I am helpless' would relate to dependent PD. Most PDs have characteristic schemas, although Beck & Freeman (1990) have noted that borderline and schizotypal PDs appear not to have specific beliefs. Schemas have been called 'rules for living', and maladaptive examples associated with achievement, acceptance by others and personal control are often found in individuals with PDs.

Maladaptive schemas, involving a patient's dysfunctional thoughts, attitudes and beliefs, are explored in CT, and the associations between the schemas and the patient's problems are identified. Three types of cognition are relevant: core assumptions (e.g. 'I am a helpless person'); conditional assumptions (e.g. 'If a person does not show me a lot of concern, he/she does not care about me at all'); and goals that are the result of core assumptions (e.g. 'I want people in my life who can give me the help I need') (Beck & Freeman, 1990).

The process of modification of such schemas involves a variety of procedures: the patient prepares a written record and evaluation of his/her cognitions and behaviour; irrational beliefs are discussed, disputed and tested; and new skills and strategies are devised and practised in 'homework assignments'. Evaluation of schemas may include examining the antecedents and consequences of behaviour, as well as the mediating thoughts, beliefs and feelings. The goals of CT include not only a change in overt behaviour, but also a modification in irrational or unproductive thoughts, beliefs and emotional responses to various stimuli.

Despite its structured theoretical framework, CT is not a fully automated treatment, and the relationship between therapist and patient is of crucial importance, requiring an atmosphere of collaboration and trust. A positive, non-judgemental approach by the therapist is needed and, at times, the transference relationship should be discussed if the patient's distortions of the reality are interfering with the progress. Also, the therapist may serve as a model for new patterns of behaviour.

Another dimension to this form of treatment, which is relevant to all forms of psychological management, is the degree of emotion (anxiety, happiness, depression or anger) experienced and displayed. As with other clinical settings, it is believed that the degree of change in conscious thought processes often depends on the patient experiencing a certain level of the appropriate emotional accompaniments.

The patient's written notes of problems and associated mental activity are usually a central focus of CT treatment sessions. For each problem the 'ABC method' can be used for the patient's record: in column A the activating event which triggers a problem is noted; in column B, the beliefs, feelings and behaviour in relation to the situation are recorded; while C, the third column, records the consequences. A final column D, for the later stages of treatment, notes the patient's plans to 'dispute' and modify the sequence (Beck & Freeman, 1990).

Practical strategies

The first stage of CT, the exploration of schemas of maladaptive thoughts and feelings, occurs in regular sessions supplemented by the patient keeping a written record of relevant beliefs, feelings and behaviour (together with triggers and consequences).

Relevant incidents that have an association with the patient's PD are identified, and the patient is invited to talk about his/her associated cognitive processes, perhaps helped by trying to relive an incident in the imagination. The patient has to try and recognize 'automatic thoughts', in certain situations and any core assumptions, conditional assumptions and associated goals. A series of questions (cognitive probes) may be needed to help the patient to arrive at a 'core assumption' which underlies other types of automatic thought. Beck & Freeman (1990) have given the following example:

> 'Linda is ignoring me'
> Q: 'What did that mean?'
> 'I can't get along with people'
> Q: 'What does that mean?'
> 'I will never have any friends'
> Q: 'What does it mean "not to have friends"?'
> 'I am all alone'
> Q: 'What does it mean to be all alone?'
> 'That I will always be unhappy'.

It is necessary to identify which automatic thoughts are 'core assumptions', as these need to be the target of methods designed to modify cognitive processes. These can be explored by repeatedly asking 'What does that mean for you?'.

The second stage involves attempts to restructure (i.e. replace or modify) irrational thoughts, beliefs, emotional responses and behaviour, although a more modest aim may be to help the patient alter behaviour and its consequences, without a significant change at the cognitive level. Identified schemas that are inaccurate, distorted or wrong, can be repeatedly challenged in an organized process. This can involve writing down and discussing alternative rational approaches. The patient can be encouraged to ask the following: 'What evidence is there?'; 'what alternative views are there?'; 'what are the advantages and disadvantages of this way of thinking?'; and 'if my interpretation is correct, are things as catastrophic as they seem?' (Moorey, 1991). Often there is a tendency towards all-or-none thinking, so patients can be asked to rate certain variables on a 5-point scale; for instance, whether a person is 'worthless'. It can also be useful to explore with the patient various aspects of maladaptive cognitions and behaviour, such as certain advantages (e.g. avoiding the risk of a close relationship), as well as disadvantages (e.g. loneliness). Other procedures include planning for the patient to test whether some of his/her attitudes are correct (e.g. 'I can't cope with certain situations and something will go wrong'); encouraging the patient to imagine the worst possible outcome (deliberate exaggeration) before identifying any discrepancy between this and what is likely to happen; asking the patient to list other possible outcomes of a situation if a negative outcome is always anticipated; and discussing various explanations for other people's behaviour. A diary related to ongoing maladaptive thoughts and feelings, with their associations, can be supplemented by 'predictive diaries' in which the patient anticipates the outcome of certain situations on the basis of their maladaptive automatic thoughts. Subsequently, the patient notes what actually happened. Another diary method involves the patient analysing events in terms of alternative schemas.

Cognitive therapy is often called cognitive-behavioural therapy as it can be used with other techniques that focus on behaviour. These include planning behaviour to minimize anxiety (anxiety management), and assisting decision-making by setting priorities amd listing pros and cons, perhaps weighting individual items. Other relevant behavioural techniques are assertiveness training, role playing (including roles as the patient in various situations or as other people), relaxation training, distraction techniques, '*in vivo*' exposure to feared situations, encouragement to be involved in activities that give pleasure or a feeling of achievement, the realistic anticipation of future problems, and time management planning. The use of imagination has also been claimed to be useful for patients with PD, and can involve reliving certain childhood experiences and traumatic events. This can be associated with some 'restructuring' of the experience, when other methods of coping are rehearsed, perhaps with associated role playing. For example, unfair criticism which had been previously accepted without comment can be recalled but this time the patient argues in his/her defence.

As with all forms of psychological management, non-collaboration may be a problem due to factors such as lack of patient's capacity to develop new skills, lack of experience and skill in the therapist, advantages to the patient in maintaining the PD features, lack of motivation to change, the setting of unrealistic or vague goals by patient or therapist, and frustration at the slow rate of progress.

Andrews (1993) has reviewed the evidence from controlled trials that cognitive and cognitive-behavioural treatments can benefit some depressive disorders, generalized anxiety disorders, obsessive-compulsive disorders, bulimia nervosa and social phobias. In relation to depressive disorders, Robinson, Berman & Neimeyer (1990) found that cognitive-behavioural treatments were better than other verbal psychotherapies, which did not differ from placebo, while in a multicentre trial of treatment for depressive disorders, cognitive-behavioural techniques were associated with modest benefit in excess of improvement on 'routine clinical management', which was the placebo condition (Elkin, Shea & Watkins, 1989). These results are likely to have some relevance to PDs, which may present with symptoms of depression and anxiety, and may lower the threshold for the emergence of other disorders (such as eating disorders) in vulnerable individuals. There is less clear evidence for the efficacy of CT or cognitive-behaviour therapy for features of PD, but claims have been made in relation to avoidant PD and recurrent self-harm behaviour (Linehan, 1987; Alden, 1989). Also, in a study of opiate addicts in a methadone maintenance programme, Woody *et al.* (1985) found that those with both antisocial PD and a depressive disorder responded to CT, showing improvements in psychiatric symptoms, drug use, employment status and illegal acts. But those with antisocial PD and no depression showed little response. It is likely that CT is less prone to harmful effects such as a transference with excessive violence or dependence, and, compared with psychodynamic psychotherapy, it is less expensive. Also, staff training to an acceptable standard is more readily achieved.

Despite these encouraging reports and the belief among many clinicians that some patients with PD can benefit from cognitive and behavioural techniques, these treatments require further controlled evaluation. It is important to remember that depressive disorders are heterogeneous from both the clinical and aetiological perspectives.

Cognitive analytic therapy (CAT)

Ryle (1989) has described an approach to psychotherapy that draws upon concepts derived from psychoanalytic, cognitive and behavioural treatments, with an emphasis upon the cognitive elements. Although various techniques are used, the focus is on helping the patient to identify and understand 'procedures', i.e. 'linked sequences of mental and behavioural processes', which overlap with the concept of 'schemas'. An example of such a sequence would be: dislike of self, avoidance of others, being seen as hostile by others, being rejected or ignored by others, a feeling by the patient that he/she has deserved this, and reinforcement of dislike of self.

The patient is encouraged to identify 'procedures' associated with problems, and to work out ways of changing the usual sequence. The first three or four sessions involve the identification of relevant problem-related 'procedures', and the patient is asked to keep a daily self-monitoring diary. Once a list of relevant procedures has been completed, written copies are provided for both therapist and patient. A contract is then made, usually for 12 sessions, with the aim of their modification. Although subsequent sessions are relatively unstructured, the 'procedures' form a framework for other techniques such as discussing current relationships or the transference. During treatment, the patient is asked to continue daily diary self-monitoring, based on the identified procedures. Ending of treatment should be anticipated and discussed during the final three or four sessions, when attention is paid to the transference in this respect. The patient should be reminded of his/her new strategies and ways of thinking, and the aim of increasing self-control. A follow-up appointment after 2 months may be appropriate.

Behaviour therapy

In the consideration of cognitive therapy, it has been shown that techniques of psychological management that focus on thoughts, feelings and beliefs, are also usually concerned with some aspects of the patient's behaviour. But although the separation between cognitive and behaviour therapy is somewhat arbitrary, techniques that are aimed primarily at the patient's behaviour can be termed 'behaviour therapy'.

A particular regime for patients with borderline PD who show repeated self-harm episodes has been developed and evaluated by Linehan and colleagues (1991) and is known as 'Dialectical Behaviour Therapy' (DBT). This treatment, for a clinically important and problematic patient group, was compared with 'treatment as usual' at completion of treatment and at 1-year follow-up, and it was found that those who received DBT for 1 year had a significantly lower drop-out rate and less self-injury, despite both groups showing only slight improvement in depression. The superiority of DBT over 'treatment as usual' was still evident at a 1-year follow-up (Linehan, Heard & Armstrong, 1993).

Details of this treatment have been described by Shearin & Linehan (1993) and involve an individual session and a group meeting each week. Individual sessions last at least 1 hour, while the group meeting, with two co-therapists, lasts for at least 2 hours. The initial emphasis in the group is on the teaching of behavioural coping skills, but subsequently it can also function as a general support group. In addition, phone contacts in a crisis (mainly with the individual therapist), are encouraged on an as-required basis.

In the individual sessions, patients are encouraged to acquire new behavioural skills, and particular behaviours are targeted for discussion; for instance, self-harm behaviour, behaviour that interferes with treatment or with quality of life, behaviour related to past stress, and behaviour related to the patient's level of self-respect. It is particularly important to identify self-harm behaviour (and thoughts), and patients are asked to complete a daily diary card noting any self-harm items. At all times self-harm behaviour is given the highest priority, while behaviour that interferes with treatment must be targeted before focussing on other topics, as the process of treatment requires the patient's collaboration.

In relation to self-harm behaviour, the therapist needs to obtain information about preceding and subsequent events, so that a more adaptive strategy to similar situations in the future can be discussed. At all times the therapist emphasizes that self-harm behaviour is taken seriously and that such behaviour reduces the opportunity to discuss other issues. The aim is for the patient to feel that self-harm behaviour, in particular suicidal behaviour, will not be ignored and that it should be thought of as a signal to try out active coping strategies, such as phoning the therapist. The next priority is to address behaviours that interfere with treatment, such as not completing diary cards or avoiding other 'homework' tasks, and it has been noted that reinforcement (e.g. by praise) of partial task completion (shaping) can be effective. It is also important for the therapist to be aware of the counter-transference, and to resist inappropriate acceptance that the patient should discontinue treatment. Priorities will need to be set when targeting behaviours that interfere with the patient's quality of life, and may involve focussing on substance abuse, maladaptive sexual behaviour, criminal behaviour and the selection of abusive partners. Further goals of individual or group sessions in DBT are to help the patient acquire new behavioural skills such as carefully observing the environment; learning to put up with distress using methods of distraction and comfort; regulating the expression of emotion; setting realistic goals; avoiding or controlling stimuli that trigger maladaptive behaviour; and increasing the patient's interpersonal skills, such as assertion, communication, or assessing the motives of others. The latter may involve pointing out that the patient must not habitually judge people or situations as either 'all good' or 'all bad', which is commonly found in relation to borderline PD. Certain behaviours related to past stress may be modified by discussing their antecedants, for example, childhood abuse, which may have contributed to a patient's self-blame and low self-esteem. Again, the tendency to have a judgemental 'all-or-none' thinking needs to be challenged. Finally, behaviours are encouraged that increase the patient's self-respect; for instance, maintaining opinions even when opposed, attempting problem-solving behaviour, and improving self-care.

While the focus of DBT is the patient's behaviour, aspects of cognitive therapy can be incorporated; for example, dysfunctional beliefs can be challenged. Also, the therapist–patient relationship is of major importance, as it is with all forms of psychological management. A degree of self-disclosure and responsiveness on the part of the therapist is considered appropriate and can include telling the patient about the negative effects of the patient's behaviour on the therapist's motivation to continue. Flexible availability of the therapist (or colleague) by phone is an important part of the regime, and the patient is expected to call if he/she feels suicidal. The therapist requires a high tolerance of criticism and hostility, and an ability to experience a patient's distress without feeling forced to 'do something' as a response to his/her own reaction, rather than to the reality of the situation. Appropriate goals need to be set, and care must be taken to help the patients prepare to end their contact with the treatment programme. An inpatient regime for patients with borderline PD, based on DBT, has been described by Barley *et al.* (1993).

Good clinical care

Overview

Andrews (1993), on the basis of Australian data, has estimated that, at any time, 1600 persons from a catchment area of 100 000 would be receiving some kind of intervention from medical services for non-psychotic psychiatric disorders, including PDs. While some of these patients may respond well to medication, such as those with some types of depression and anxiety disorders, psychological management would probably be appropriate for the majority. But the provision of psychodynamic psychotherapy or even shorter courses of cognitive behaviour therapy would only be available for a minority.

Andrews has pointed out that before the era of a range of effective treatments in medicine, doctors had a major role in explaining, reassuring and providing regular contact with people to help them cope with chronic disorders. Such a process can be called 'good clinical care' and involves establishing a good professional relationship with 'therapist genuineness, empathy and non-possessive warmth'. This 'holding' process involves non-specific support, as well as the recommendation of any appropriate specific treatment, and there is considerable overlap with various forms of supportive psychotherapy. As gradual improvement can occur in many PDs, an explanation of what kind of problem the patient has can help him/her to accept what cannot be significantly altered in the short-term, and to make the best of adaptive aspects of personality. This can be combined with advice given within a relatively simple problem-solving approach, which initially involves the identification of any problems that trouble the patient, the clinician or significant others. Some of these may be amenable to improvement by certain actions on the part of the patient, which can be specified. The clinician needs to be able to tolerate 'not doing anything' (despite pressure from patients or relatives), if there is nothing to be done other than to maintain concern about the patient with a chronic disorder and to be prepared to see the patient again, for instance, 'to see how you are getting on'. Faced with this task, clinicians who find it difficult not to be in control of the patient's disorder or not to be offering specific treatment, may inappropriately discharge the patient, providing themselves with the excuse 'there is no further treatment I can offer'.

It is probable that the psychological management of most patients with PD who are seen within clinical services consists of 'good clinical care', which, in broad terms, has been considered to be 'more effective, cheaper and less harmful than dynamic psychotherapy, and less efficacious but more broadly applicable and comparable in safety and cost to cognitive behavior therapy' (Andrews, 1993). Despite the limitations of such a generalization, these claims concentrate the minds of those who have the task of planning services and allocating limited resources. But although 'good clinical care' can appear to be deceptively simple, it requires considerable skill and experience and deserves more attention in training and research.

Practical strategies

Within the general heading of 'good clinical care', psychological management in a routine medical setting can draw upon psychoanalytic, cognitive and behavioural techniques, with considerable flexibility. Sessions with partners and family, together with the patient or separately, may also be appropriate. Although this might seem to be a recipe for everlasting chaos, certain principles can be identified, which are then applied to the management of each individual patient.

The main format for intervention involves one-to-one sessions, each lasting from a few minutes to an hour. The frequency also varies considerably, from several times a week to once every 3–6 months. Even an infrequent appointment may provide an important 'holding' function for a patient with a chronic disorder. Some of the goals may be that symptoms do not increase, self-harm does not occur, and a series of unproductive referrals and investigations is avoided. Sessions are generally unstructured, although cognitive and behavioural elements can be included. The therapist should not demand early extensive self-disclosure.

For psychological management in the common setting of 'good clinical care', the main framework is usually 'supportive' psychotherapy, which implies that the clinician provides a consistently active input. The therapeutic ingredients include advice, explanation, instruction, suggestion, a caring attitude with active listening, reassurance, encouragement, persuasion, permission for the display of emotion (in particular depression related to loss), and environmental manipulation if this is possible and desirable. The focus is usually on the present and future, rather than on the past. However, more 'explorative' techniques can be incorporated, directed towards the past and an awareness or understanding of hidden (unconscious) mental activity; this may involve an examination of transference, countertransference, psychological defence mechanisms, and resistance. The latter is defined as obstacles to the aims and procedures of treatment that arise from within the patient. Techniques of asking the patient to 'free-associate' (i.e. to talk about what comes into his/her mind) or to discuss dreams, may occasionally be appropriate in this setting but are generally reserved for more time-intensive psychodynamic psychotherapy.

Several studies have claimed that certain characteristics of a therapist are associated with beneficial effects, such as an ability to empathize with the patient and to be personally concerned about his/her welfare, together with emotional warmth and genuineness (Malan *et al.*, 1976). The 'treatment alliance' (Sandler *et al.*, 1970*a*), refers to the common aims of therapist and patient, and its development can also be beneficial, as can the provision of new learning situations; for instance the patient may learn that it is possible to be assertive without loss of temper.

Cognitive and emotional components of a learning process can usefully be distinguished, although, in practice, these are never completely separated. Cognitive learning may involve conscious mental activity, which includes the registration of new experiences, or, by the process of insight, the development of an awareness of attitudes, feelings or conflicts that had not been fully available to consciousness. Insight can be induced or assisted by suggestions (interpretations) from the therapist, which are directed towards the defence mechanisms responsible for the patient's transference or resistance. However, even though a patient may develop some insight, perhaps by becoming aware of the maladaptive nature of a behaviour pattern or attitude, this may have little impact if the learning process did not involve an emotional dimension, which was concerned with motivation and mood. If emotional arousal occurs during a series of learning experiences, the effects are more likely to include an emotional as well as a cognitive change, so that emotional arousal has been termed the 'motive power of psychotherapy'. Psychological events that are associated with the experience and expression of emotion are usually necessary for significant personality adjustment in a psychotherapeutic context. Although insight accompanied by little or no emotion can be of benefit, some patients' behaviour does not change even though they appear to understand why they are behaving maladaptively and the consequences of their actions.

Psychological defences include denial (a special type of denial is known as 'isolation', when different components of a reaction are separated, for example, when an emotional reaction to bereavement is not consciously experienced); avoidance; projection (when unconscious mental events in the patient are attributed to others, for example, 'my sister distrusts doctors'); sublimation (when unconscious mental events produce conscious experiences that are similar but more acceptable, for example, anger can be harnessed to produce success in aggressive contact sports); intellectualization (when mental events are disguised by complex argument and discussion); rationalization (when mental events are hidden by apparent explanations that are wrong, for example, 'I became manic again just because I was upset, not because I stopped taking my lithium carbonate'); reaction formation (when the opposite of unconscious mental events appear in conscious awareness, for example, an angry patient may appear excessively deferential); displacement (when mental events remain hidden because the patient concentrates on other aspects of life); and regression (when a person may return to a childlike pattern of thinking and behaving, for example, becoming excessively dependent with frequent temper tantrums). But not all psychological defence mechanisms are maladaptive, and psychological management is often directed towards a strengthening of these unconscious manoeuvres to hide or distort reality, if they provide the best method of coping with an insoluble situation or a severely maladaptive personality structure. This might involve encouraging the patient to continue to avoid certain situations, even though this avoidance may cause some problems.

Patients can often be helped to recognize what they can achieve by their own efforts, while identification with the therapist, involving the patient modelling him/herself on the therapist's attitude and behaviour, may also be of benefit. Another therapeutic ingredient is the instillation of hope, but this must not involve making wild promises and predictions which, if unrealized, will produce despair and loss of confidence. A patient's hope is often a reflection of a positive approach by the therapist and, even when severe and intractable problems exist, it may be possible to comment on the patient's fortitude, transient symptomatic relief or the hope of a natural remission. Also, the therapist's continued concern and interest encourages a positive attitude in the patient. Another important therapeutic ingredient can be catharsis, involving the patient's expression of anger, depression, anxiety or, more rarely, positive feelings. Catharsis can be therapeutic in itself, as was shown by a young man with a severe depressive disorder and anxiety following, and causally related to, the death of his alcoholic father. Although he clearly recognized his feelings of intense anger towards his father for ruining the life of his family, these conflicted with positive feelings, and it was not until he had repeatedly expressed his anger that his symptoms were relieved. Self-disclosure, particularly if this involves confessions, may also provide relief of some forms of depression and anxiety in association with PD, even if this does not generate specific advice or other interventions.

For patients with chronic disorders who receive 'holding' and 'support' on an indefinite basis, the clinician needs to remember the aims of such a strategy. These may include the prevention of deterioration in functioning, even when there is little or no 'treatment alliance', so that the patient may have a different view of what is happening; for example, he/she may be hoping for and expecting a new treatment. Sometimes this can be acknowledged, by telling the patient that while his/her disorder is being monitored at the regular visits and that no change in treatment is likely to help at present, the possibility of a change in management will be regularly reviewed. In relation to PDs, the patient's presenting complaint may be of a mood disorder, perhaps resulting from social difficulties. After listening to and sharing the patient's account of the various problems and symptoms, it may not be possible to give any specific advice or treatment and the clinician needs to be able to 'do nothing', while still taking an interest in the patient and arranging a further appointment. For example: 'I am very sorry that you have had such a bad time in recent weeks and I know how difficult it has been for you to keep at work. But I am glad you were able to share this with me. I am afraid we have run out of time this session; let me give you another appointment'. This approach can be difficult with those patients who engender feelings of guilt in their therapists and demand action or specific advice. If challenged directly, the clinician can only state the reality, namely that he/she is not able to make any other specific suggestions but that a further appointment is recommended.

Couple, family and group treatment

'Significant others', mainly those living with the patient, may be incorporated in programmes of psychological management, in particular for those with borderline PD. There is a range of formats for such involvement, including sessions with the patient and partner/family (conjoint sessions) as the only input, and sessions with significant others in parallel with, or in sequence with, individual sessions with the patient. One therapist may be involved throughout, but a second therapist may be a co-therapist or sole therapist for partner/family or conjoint sessions.

For borderline PD, couple/family sessions may be useful when the relationships seem to be aggravating or perpetuating problems, or where the significant others are participants in dysfunctional beliefs, attitudes and behaviour (Goldstein, 1990). Such sessions are often appropriately offered to younger patients who are emotionally or financially dependent on their family, who may seem overinvolved. In such cases the patient may not have been given an appropriate degree of independence.

The patient may display transference feelings to a partner/family member, which can be the focus of discussion and attempts at modification. The variety of techniques available for individual sessions can be considered for conjoint treatment but, in general, experienced clinicians have recommended that the focus should be on the 'here-and-now', and that the therapist should be active in setting a clear structure with limit setting, the facilitation of communication and trust, and the containment of anger. The participants in conjoint sessions can be encouraged to identify maladaptive interactions and sequences of behaviour within their relationships, to be less defensive and to be more aware of underlying feelings and motives. This may involve some interpretation of psychological defences, such as questioning whether there is just one good or bad member of the partnership/family. Participants can be encouraged to understand the feelings of others, and positive behaviour can be reinforced with the aim of increasing self-esteem and cohesion. Sometimes it can be useful for the participants to understand how their present behaviour is linked to past experiences.

If the patient has been the victim of childhood sexual or violent abuse, or neglect, family therapy presents particular difficulties and risks. Strategy has to be determined by an evaluation of the individual family by an experienced clinician, and care must be taken not to produce an emotional experience of an intensity that cannot be satisfactorily handled and resolved. But patients are often ambivalent about their feelings to their abusers and may direct their anger and dislike onto themselves; in such a situation, some exploration of the abuse may be appropriate, although most of this work may need to be done in individual (one-to-one) sessions.

The partner/family may be angry with the patient for being 'in treatment' if this requires their participation, and be worried that they will be blamed for the patient's problems. It may be necessary to see parents (or relevant others) alone at least once to give as much reassurance on this aspect as is possible.

Whatever the therapist's views about the distribution of blame and the causes and effects within a family, an acrimonious and angry content of sessions is generally counter-productive. A positive, educational, supportive atmosphere should usually be fostered.

Various forms of group psychotherapy may also be part of a treatment regime for patients with PD. For those with borderline PD, a group focussing on behavioural skills was part of the regime of 'Dialectical Behaviour Therapy', and it has been suggested that parallel group sessions can be used with sessions of individual psychodynamic psychotherapy for some patients with borderline and narcissistic PD (Higgitt & Fonagy, 1992). Most clinicians with special experience have believed that, for borderline PD, group treatment should not completely replace individual sessions, but can be a useful adjunct (Gunderson & Sabo, 1993a). Sometimes a patient's peers in a group session are better able than the therapist to effectively confront maladaptive behaviour, as other group members are not subject to such strong transferences as is a single therapist. Also, various self-help groups, such as Alcoholics Anonymous, may be helpful to some patients with PD.

Treatment settings

Any psychiatric service must provide a range of interventions with in-patient, daypatient, outpatient and non-hospital-based facilities.

Borderline PD is the most common PD diagnosis in psychiatric inpatient units, and such patients are usually admitted for relatively short periods (i.e. from a few days to less than 4 weeks) in response to a crisis involving self-destructive or antisocial behaviour. A low threshold has been advocated for the admission of apparently suicidal borderline patients, with the aim of defusing the crisis and organizing outpatient or other alternative input (Gunderson & Sabo, 1993*a*). The length of inpatient stay will be related to the level of social support and to the degree of problems in the social environment. Long-term hospital treatment for those with PD, in particular with borderline and antisocial features, is rarely available but, for a small minority, a long-term residential treatment programme may seem appropriate. Alternatives to a residential hospital place include hostel accommodation combined with day or evening treatment programmes, and such arrangements may be better for those individuals who tend to get excessively dependent on long hospital admissions. Such dependency may cause 'regression' to a childlike overdependence, self-preoccupation and intense anger at the inevitable limits and controls of a hospital regime, with demands for instant gratification. For those borderline PDs in hospital, a structured timetable is advisable with psychotherapeutic sessions and other occupational, social or recreational activities. Group meetings can be a useful adjunct with, for example, discussion of abuse experiences, family problems and work plans.

Management of specific problem-behaviours related to personality disorders

Self-harm and suicide

Self-harm involving 'recurrent suicidal threats, gestures, or behaviour, or self-mutilating behaviour' is part of the syndrome of borderline PD (American Psychiatric Association, 1987). Although there are associations between self-harm with other PDs, such as antisocial PD, the focus in the literature of PD in relation to self-harm and suicide has been on patients with predominant features of borderline PD. Self-harm is a broader category than suicidal behaviour, as it includes self-mutilation, such as inflicting multiple superficial cuts on the wrists and arms, or more severe examples such as hitting limbs with a hammer. But there may be various motives, or combinations of motives, for self-harm behaviour, including the expression of anger, the relief of tension or a wish to influence the behaviour of others. Self-harm must invariably be taken seriously, as several studies have shown that the history of frequency of self-harm episodes is significantly related to completed suicide (Paris, 1993).

Several long-term studies of suicide in groups of borderline PD patients have indicated a significant risk, in the order of 1 in 10, for those who have a history of repeated self-harm and have become known to hospital services (McGlashan, 1986; Paris *et al.*, 1987; Stone, 1990). Also, Stone (1990) found the co-occurrence of substance abuse with borderline PD was significantly associated with suicide, and Rich, Fowler & Fogarty (1988) have reported that the large ($\times$ 3) increase in youth (mainly male) suicide in North America from 1960 to 1980 was associated with substance abuse. Other data (Runeson & Beskow, 1991; Paris, 1993), from retrospective studies of suicides, suggested that about 30% of male youth suicides merited a diagnosis of borderline PD. Another factor that may be associated with suicide is relatively high educational achievement, and it has been suggested that this reflects higher expectations that have been thwarted (Paris, 1993).

The outcome of severe borderline PD gives some hope as well as confirming the serious risk of suicide, as about 75% of those who survive are considerably improved after 15 years (Paris *et al.*, 1987) and suicide after the age of 30 is relatively uncommon. There is, as yet, no evidence that interventions or treatment make any difference to the incidence of suicide in borderline PD or to the process of natural remission, but our present understanding suggests that interventions can prevent completed suicides and that if the patient can be kept alive, in particular by help in a crisis, the outcome of patients with even very severely maladaptive behaviour can be surprisingly good.

The management of self-harm, particularly in those with borderline PD, presents common practical problems and different theoretical approaches. Controversial aspects are the role of extended inpatient or other residential treatment for those who are chronically suicidal, and the emphasis on suicidal thoughts and actions during treatment sessions.

Although the approach in Dialectical Behaviour Therapy (Linehan *et al.*, 1991), which has been shown to produce short-term improvements in self-harm behaviour, gives priority to the consideration of self-harm thoughts and behaviour, this is within the context of a structured programme. But in routine psychological management some limits have to be set with regard to how the therapist responds to talk of suicidal intent.

For some patients, displaying the power to commit suicide may seem the only way to obtain some control over themselves and their environment; in this sense it is a coping strategy that needs to be replaced before it can be discarded. This might be achieved if the patient can develop successful relationships or a career but this takes time, and the practical problem remains: how should the clinician respond to threats of suicide? There is a general consensus that relatively brief hospital admissions can be appropriate for exacerbations in the severity of suicidal or self-harm ideation and intent, usually associated with a life crisis, but for those who are chronically suicidal, 'extended inpatient treatment is unlikely to be of benefit and may perpetuate the behaviour by leading to regression and excessive dependence on hospitalization' (Ennis, Barnes & Spenser, 1985). Such generalizations are deceptively simple as, in practice, the boundary between a crisis and fluctuating chronicity is often unclear. What is certain is that there is no strategy that eliminates a risk of completed suicide, and that the clinician has only a limited ability to prevent suicide. It is often appropriate to make this clear to the patient and the patient's family, who may encourage such patients to recognize their own responsibility and independence (Ennis *et al.*, 1985). When in doubt about the severity of a particular crisis, it is probably best to give the patient the benefit of such doubt by arranging a period of inpatient management, but making it clear that the aim is for a short stay (a few days or up to 2–3 weeks) in the context of planning subsequent outpatient or other support. Sometimes a clinician may decline to admit a patient to hospital, or may discharge a patient, despite the persistence of threats of self-harm or suicide, if it is considered that the further inpatient care would increase the risk of such behaviour still further.

Aggression and violence

Aggression has been defined as coercive action, involving the use of threats or punishments to influence social interaction (Blackburn, 1989). Violence denotes the use of physical force and is an extreme form of aggression. Anger is often associated with aggression, but not invariably so, and this definition of aggression could include self-defence.

Although any example of aggression can be viewed as a specific interaction between the persons involved, a tendency to repeat aggression in different situations over time can be identified as a characteristic of some individuals. But such a concept distinguishes between the personality trait involving a capacity for aggression and the aggression itself, which is shown only in certain situations. This means that the identification of the trait of aggression predicts a series of aggressive acts rather than specific examples of such behaviour. Various studies have found that a tendency towards aggression can be a stable trait, and Olweus (1979) stated that 'there is substantial stability in aggression which cannot be attributed to situational constancy'. This has been shown in various samples including schoolchildren (Feshbach & Price, 1984), a community sample (Huesmann *et al.*, 1984), and those with a history of criminal violence (Farrington, 1978;

Robins, 1978). For example, Robins (1978) found that fighting in child-hood predicted violence in later life.

But even when an aggressive trait has been identified in an individual, the contexts in which aggressive acts occur are important as additional determinants of the person's behaviour. Analysis of the interaction of various causal factors for aggression has been based on hypotheses that implicate a range of variables, including genetic factors (Rushton *et al.*, 1986), witnessing and experiencing aggression in childhood (the more someone has been exposed to aggression, the lower the threshold may be for the perception of aggression in others), inadequate parenting with lack of appropriate punishments and rewards, and any social learning that pro-motes aggression. Even if genetic influences are of major importance in an individual, these are mediated by cognitive processes that interact with the environment. Therefore, examination of the cognitive processes preceding aggression is necessary to understand the relative importance of the various causal factors in any example of such behaviour.

Whether aggression and violence occur in a given situation may depend on such factors as the behaviour and status of the other person or persons involved, anticipation of rewards and punishments, the capacity of the person to show alternative coping behaviour, the degree of control in relation to the expression of anger, personality attributes that oppose aggression (such as a tendency to social anxiety and withdrawal, Black-burn, 1989), and general intellectual ability (IQ). Heilbrun (1982) found that, in prisoners with antisocial PD, low IQ was associated with a history of relatively violent crime, while a degree of social withdrawal has been found to be negatively correlated with violence in a prison environment (Heilbrun & Heilbrun, 1985).

The potential aggressor's cognitive appraisal of a situation is an import-ant variable in determining the subsequent behaviour. If a provoking event occurs, such as an insult, threat or violence, this is usually judged in relation to the person's own standards of what 'ought' to happen, whether the other person's behaviour is intentional, and the degree of maliciousness in any such intent. (If someone is insulting only when under the influence of alcohol, this may be considered as less provoking.) Certain appraisals may be related to a low self-esteem, and involve an emphasis on the need for 'respect' and 'rights', or on the importance of what is considered to be a masculine self-image. If repeatedly aggressive individuals have some co-occurring obsessive-compulsive personality traits such as perfectionism, they may be particularly liable to bear a grudge for a perceived unfairness; for example, in relation to the way the rules have been applied in a prison regime. Other examples of relevant aspects of such cognitive appraisals can include frustration due to delayed gratification if the delay is judged to be unnecessary, and whether certain incentives such as status or money will be achieved by not showing aggression.

A tendency to repeated aggression has been a feature of various definitions of antisocial PD or psychopathy, but while there is a definite association between antisocial PD and violent crime, and between aggression, hostility and impulsivity, a group of individuals selected on the basis of violent crime does not have an homogeneous personality structure. Of course, a single act of violence may not reflect an aggressive tendency.

Violent offenders have been divided into two broad types: 'undercontrolled' and 'overcontrolled' (Megargee, 1966). The undercontrolled offenders have weak inhibitions and engage in more regular violence, while the stronger inhibitions of overcontrolled offenders lead to rarer but more intense episodes of violence. Lane & Kling (1979) found evidence that overcontrolled offenders were more rigid in attitudes, and more reluctant to admit to psychiatric symptoms, and Blackburn (1968) reported that offenders with relatively severe examples of violence were more controlled, inhibited and defensive, and were less likely to have a criminal record or a diagnosis of antisocial PD.

Two subgroups of each of these categories have been identified, so that four main types of violent offender can be described (Blackburn, 1971, 1975, 1986; McGurk, 1978; Henderson, 1982). Undercontrolled offenders can be divided into 'primary' or 'secondary' psychopaths, while the two types of overcontrolled offenders are those who are 'inhibited' (with social withdrawal and anxiety) or 'conforming' (with sociability and lack of anxiety). This classification is supported by Blackburn's finding (1984) that 52% of primary psychopaths (as described below) had a history of repeated violence, in contrast to only 8% of the inhibited overcontrolled offenders.

Primary psychopaths are impulsive, aggressive, hostile and extraverted, and while secondary psychopaths share the first three of these characteristics, social anxiety and withdrawal is found instead of extraversion. Both groups have antisocial PD traits, and it has been claimed that primary psychopaths have more narcissistic and histrionic PD features, while secondary psychopaths are associated with more features of borderline and paranoid PDs.

The inhibited group of overcontrolled offenders appear introverted, unaggressive and withdrawn, and these features have been associated with low self-esteem, social anxiety, offences involving sexual coercion and features of avoidant, schizoid and passive-aggressive PDs. The conforming group of overcontrolled offenders seem defensive, unaggressive and sociable. Such individuals do not appear anxious, deny anger and are often dependent on approval. Associated PD features are from the dependent and obsessive-compulsive PD syndromes, and their offences may be triggered by perceived loss of status.

Management of aggression and violence in psychiatric inpatient units involves a range of perspectives including how to respond to a particular incident, the design and layout of offices and institutions, and specific programmes of psychological management. In relation to aggression in society, wider issues are also relevant, such as social supports and institutions, the availability of illegal drugs and alcohol, the socio-economic structure of society, and social alienation of groups such as the young or members of ethnic or cultural minorities.

The immediate response to a patient's aggression requires a judgement of the characteristics of the particular situation, but certain principles can be used as guidelines. The first priority is to try to calm the aggression, which often involves anger and agitation, using both verbal and non-verbal techniques (Davies, 1989). The clinician should try to empathize with what the aggressor is trying to communicate, perhaps by summarizing the content of what has been said. The initial emphasis is listening, asking questions and identifying the reason for the anger without arguing, although some clarification of fact may be appropriate. Sometimes it may be helpful to 'depersonalize' an accusation, by pointing out that a member of staff has to act according to hospital policy or the limited availability of services. Alternatively, if the anger is directed to the institution or to clinicians in general, the clinician may try the opposite tactic by pointing out that he/she is not just doing a job, but is also a person in his/her own right. This can be reinforced by sharing some personal details with the aggressor. Another technique that has been advocated in certain situations is to repeatedly ask for the required behaviour ('Please stop shouting at me') with increasing force and authority, but maintaining emotional control and courtesy. Other strategies include disengagement, when the patient is told that the clinician is leaving and the reasons; offering to get a senior colleague; promising to try and help; and giving the patient a choice, for example to wait or be seen again later.

Although it is generally considered sound advice to 'keep calm', Davies (1989) has pointed out that if this is perceived as unconcern and inaction, the aggressor's anger may be further fuelled. The motivation of some aggressors is to continue until a required response, such as fear, is obtained;

therefore it may be appropriate to contain aggression by a statement such as: 'What you are doing is really worrying me'. Also, it may help for the degree of arousal in the clinician to approach that of the aggressor to demonstrate empathy and concern. If a very agitated and angry aggressor is met with an apparently unconcerned and 'laid-back' approach, this may provoke further anger, and it may be appropriate for the clinician to show an increased activity and arousal level by non-verbal gestures (nodding, eye contact) and frequent verbal statements.

The nature of bodily confrontation also requires consideration. The clinician should, if possible, not be closer to the aggressor than would be normal in social interaction, and it is best not to face the aggressor directly. But if violence is still a possibility, or if the aggressor moves to a direct face-to-face position, it can be helpful for the clinician to move to a non-threatening stance, for example, moving the body's weight to one leg and placing one hand on the chin (Davies, 1989). A normal pattern of eye contact should be attempted, involving a variable repetition of holding gaze for a few seconds and then changing gaze, even if the aggressor is engaged in a fixed, hostile stare.

After the immediate threat of violence has subsided, the next step is to explore the background to the aggression and to apply a problem-solving approach. However, if violence does occur, an organization requires procedures to manage the after-effects on those who have been assaulted. Such individuals may need support from colleagues and management and, in general, should be encouraged to return to work as soon as possible to prevent the build-up of fear and loss of confidence.

Various steps can be taken to reduce the risk of violence in clinical settings. With regard to office design, chairs should not directly face each other, as a confrontational bodily stance may enhance aggression, and the clinician's access to the door should not be obstructed by the patient. There should be an absence of heavy ornaments or other potential weapons, and it should not be possible to lock the door from the inside. Ideally, the door should open outwards so that it cannot be barricaded, and contain a non-breakable glass panel to enable colleagues to see what is happening if a situation develops when a good deal of noise can be heard by others in the building.

More general organizational policies may include keeping the addresses of staff secret, wearing safe clothing and jewelry (i.e. not earrings in pierced ears), and letting colleagues know your schedule if home visits are planned to potentially dangerous individuals. It may be appropriate to arrange to phone a colleague at a prearranged time after a visit to confirm that all went well. Of course, when a serious risk is perceived, home visits should not be made alone.

Within a psychiatric unit, aggression and violence is reduced by a well-functioning unit, with good communications, good handover between different shifts, sufficient experienced staff on each shift, and clear contingency plans for violent incidents involving a consistent but flexible approach. Staff must try to allocate sufficient time for individual sessions with each patient and manage each session with clear explanation and courtesy. It is often advisable to tell patients how long you have got to see them, so that resentment may be limited if a longer session is expected.

While various studies have examined the effects of variables such as time of day, architectural blind spots, overcrowding and staffing levels on violence in psychiatric inpatient units, no clear patterns have been demonstrated. However, such factors appear to be of major importance in some incidents. Other important variables related to ward violence are the personalities and behaviour of staff and the nature of the social environment. Several studies have found that, in many short-stay adult psychiatric units, patients are unoccupied for long periods, in which there is minimal interaction with staff or with fellow patients, and there is some evidence to support the view that there can be a link between levels of violence and lack of planned activities.

Staff should be trained in techniques for physical restraint, and, if a person is subject to compulsory treatment, have policies for the use of sedation and seclusion. The latter may involve putting the person alone in a 'seclusion room' for periods from a few minutes to several hours. However, the degree of seclusion may vary; the patient may be alone with the door closed (but under regular observation through a glass panel), the door may be ajar with a nurse just outside, or a nurse may be with the patient continually or intermittently. Such arrangements provide some practical and psychological containment in an environment that has reduced stimuli, and can assist in the resolution of an aggressive episode. When physical restraint is required, it is important that the aggressor is faced with considerably superior force, as a more equal balance of force will lead to a higher risk of injury to both staff and patient.

Various treatment programmes have been tried in the management of aggressive individuals in both clinical and non-clinical populations, such as inpatient 'therapeutic community' regimes, individual psychological management sessions including behavioural approaches, and drug treatments (Suedfeld & Landon, 1978). But methodological difficulties allow only broad conclusions to emerge from published studies: psychological management needs to be in a framework of clear rules and support; medication can be a useful adjunct; therapeutic communities may be helpful for some individuals; and improvement tends to occur with the passage of time. Several studies have reported the effects of inpatient management in specialized units (with emphasis on control, confrontation and peer group support), outpatient group psychotherapy and a therapeutic community (Vaillant, 1975; Carney, 1977). Although McCord (1983) reported an association between reduced re-offending in young individuals and exposure to a therapeutic community, empirical evidence of benefit for a therapeutic prison regime was not found in another study (Gunn *et al.*, 1978). There is evidence that various forms of psychological management for aggression are more likely to be associated with improvement if the individual is also depressed or has reasonable social skills (Copas & Whiteley, 1976; Woody *et al.*, 1985). Behavioural approaches to aggression have included 'token economy' regimes (i.e. inpatient or custodial settings in which certain behaviours are rewarded), social skills training, cognitive therapy, and self-control procedures (Cavior & Schmidt, 1978; Templeman & Wollersheim, 1979; Frederiksen & Rainwater, 1981; Moyes, Tennent & Bedford, 1985).

Several studies have reported the effects of social skills training on self-referred individuals with problems due to aggression. This approach is an example of 'indirect' control measures, which aim to teach non-aggressive alternative behaviour, and contrast with 'direct' methods, which try to change the pattern of reinforcement of aggression. The procedures of social skills training include identifying target behaviour and associated circumstances, teaching alternative responses and arranging practice. Desired behaviour can be modelled by the therapist, new behaviour can be rehearsed using role play, video recording and corrective feedback, and subsequent encouragement can provide reinforcement. Such an approach has been applied to various non-clinical and clinical populations, and Henderson (1989) has concluded that some positive effects and generalization have been reported, but that such results have been limited to verbal aggression. Henderson (1989) has also described a social skills training programme for male prisoners in a UK prison that involved group meetings. Twelve prisoners with convictions for violence completed the programme, which was aimed at increasing skills in the following three areas: assertion (the ability to express negative feelings without aggression); self-control (the ability to identify and control anger, and to prevent irritability or loss of temper); and reduction of social anxiety, which may provoke aggression when the person feels threatened or anxious. Six to eight trainees met with two co-trainers for sessions that involved instruction, modelling, videotaped behavioural rehearsal and group discussion. The results were assessed by ratings and self-report questionnaires, and, at follow-up, improvements were found in assertion, social anxiety, self-confidence and global measures of social skills. Although there was little change in aggression for the group as a whole, individual prisoners appeared to respond and it was considered that this programme may be 'an effective intervention method for violent offenders'. Blackburn (1989) considered that there are 'still insufficient empirical data to justify any single approach to the treatment of aggressive individuals who are deviant in personality. Examples can be found of successful outcomes for most forms of psychological treatment, but the evidence suggests that none is consistently successful'.

Chronic somatization

'Somatization' is a process in which 'there is an inappropriate focus on physical symptoms and psychosocial problems are denied' (Bass & Benjamin, 1993). Often this is associated with 'primary gain', when the patient is relieved of responsibilities as he/she is 'ill', or 'secondary gain', such as a gratifying response of caring and concern from others.

PD is often implicated as a causal factor. For instance, obsessive-compulsive PD is associated with a tendency to worry (involving a reduced threshold for somatic preoccupation), while those with dependent or histrionic PDs obtain secondary gain from reassurance. Also, those with narcissistic PD receive reinforcing gratification from medical attention.

Bass & Benjamin (1993) have outlined general management strategies for somatization including the avoidance of a 'dualistic approach', which sees patients as having physical or mental disorders but never both. Creed & Guthrie (1993) have stressed the need for the clinician to develop a good rapport with 'somatizing' patients, involving questions, empathic response and comments that link somatic symptoms and psychological experiences. Often patients can be persuaded to collaborate with psychological management that has the stated aim of helping the patient to cope with the symptoms. This may prevent an endless pursuit of a somatic cause by repeated investigations. Sometimes a cognitive or cognitive-behavioural approach is needed to help patients address dysfunctional beliefs, such as the need to avoid all exercise. It is important to acknowledge that the patient's experience of symptoms is 'real', and to state that a physical illness can never be completely ruled out even if tests are negative, and that this will be kept under review. Patients can then be told that people with chronic symptoms can often be helped to feel better and cope with their disability more effectively.

Substance abuse

A variety of programmes for alcohol abuse and other substance abuse disorders can involve various formats: inpatient units, therapeutic communities, outpatient clinics and self-help groups. Many such individuals have PD, in particular with antisocial and borderline features, and this needs to be considered when the aims and outcomes of a service are being evaluated.

In a study of 20 social and personality variables in the treatment of heroin addiction, the counsellor–patient relationship was related to final outcome, and those who had a single counsellor did significantly better than their peers who were transferred from one counsellor to another (Cohen *et al.*, 1980). Individual counselling was ranked the most important of several treatment components by alcoholic individuals who accepted a 2-year outpatient programme (Ojehagen & Berglund, 1986*b*).

Sexual offenders

Sexual violence involves a victim who is unwilling or unable to consent. Various studies of treatment interventions have been mainly concerned with rape, offences involving children, and genital exhibitionism to adult females (Marshall & Barbaree, 1989). Rapists have been subdivided in relation to different forms of sexual gratification, displaced aggression, the degree of sadism, and impulsive or opportunistic acts. The latter characteristic is often associated with a history of other offences, and features of antisocial PD (Perkins, 1991).

The first stage of management is a detailed assessment including the individual's sexual preferences. The penile plethysmograph (PPG) can indicate male arousal to a variety of stimuli, perhaps presented as projection slides, and can indicate inappropriate denial of specific sexual interests or fantasy. Various behavioural techniques have been used in attempts to modify sexual motivation, aimed at reducing deviant sexual interest, increasing social skills and addressing relevant cognitive processes.

Deviant sexual interests can be the target of an aversive stimulus such as an electric shock to the leg or an unpleasant smell (e.g. strong-smelling salts), which are paired with deviant fantasies or stimuli. Related techniques include masturbatory reconditioning, where masturbation is encouraged when paired with non-deviant stimuli or fantasies, and sensitization, when the patient is encouraged to fantasize a sequence of images of offending behaviour with unpleasant consequences. These techniques can sometimes be extended from the consulting room to real life; if a sequence of triggering stimuli and offending behaviour is identified, the patient can be encouraged to interrupt this, for example, by the use of strong-smelling salts (Perkins, 1991).

Social skills training can be provided in a group format, as for individuals with aggressive behaviour. A problem-solving approach is indicated, which may examine triggering situations and alternative behaviours, and involve modelling, role play, rehearsal and feedback.

Many patients require basic education about sexual behaviour and further understanding of their motivations for offending (together with behavioural antecedents and the consequences), if a logical strategy for the patient to avoid further offences is to be devised. Many subjects deny aspects of their offences and four main types of offender have been identified: 'rationalizers', who admit offences but deny harm is caused to their victims (in particular involving homosexual offences against boys); 'externalizers', who blame others including their victims, who are typically young women; 'internalizers', who admit the offence and the effects but claim a temporary aberration of behaviour; and 'deniers', who present with absolute denial (Kennedy & Grubin, 1992). It is helpful to encourage subjects to reduce the level of denial so that behavioural approaches can be more readily applied. Also, personal skills can be encouraged, involving obtaining a job, reducing alcohol intake and organizing leisure activities.

Various evaluations of behavioural treatment for sex offenders have demonstrated some positive effects within institutions (Burchard & Wood, 1982; Rutter & Giller, 1983) but there is little evidence of specific effects on the reduction in subsequent offending. However, Davidson (1984), in a 2–5 year follow-up of individuals who had experienced a prison-based treatment programme of psychotherapy and behavioural techniques, found evidence that the programme was of benefit for those whose offences involved children, although the recidivism rates for men who had sexually attacked adults were not different from an untreated group. But recidivism rates are unreliable data due to a high level of under-reporting (Furby, Weinrott & Blackshaw, 1989), and the long-term outcome of institutional programmes requires further research. While some subjects have been shown to benefit within institutions, such treatment programmes may be a necessary but not sufficient intervention to reduce further offending. The provision of further outpatient and non-hospital-based individual and group support may be an important development for the long-term management of this group of offenders, as continuing intervention may be able to build upon the gains in a prison or hospital-based programme.

8

Group psychotherapies

J.H. DOWSON

Overview

Historical development

Since Moreno introduced the term 'group psychotherapy' in 1931, many theoretical frameworks and techniques have emerged for use in a wide variety of settings. These include the short-stay psychiatric unit, the outpatient clinic, the medium- and long-stay units of psychiatric hospitals, specialist psychiatric units for alcoholism or forensic problems, and self-help organizations (Ryle, 1976). Regular group meetings may also involve non-patients, such as trainees in those professions where increased self-awareness and an ability to communciate are particularly important.

Research in this field has been limited and, in general, theoretical considerations have determined clinical practice (Malan, 1973). Three approaches have been derived from psychoanalytic theory; the first examines the relationship of each individual patient to the group or therapist, the second is concerned with the relationship of the group as a whole to the therapist, while the third approach emphasizes treatment by the group itself, focussing on general aspects of the group such as themes, communication patterns, values and cohesiveness. In this last approach, the therapist ignores, as far as possible, his/her own relationship with individual group members or with the group as a whole. The first two strategies have been termed psychoanalysis 'in' groups and 'of' groups (Wolf & Schwartz, 1962), while the latter, the so-called group-analytic method (Foulkes & Anthony, 1965), encourages the therapeutic ingredients to be provided 'by' the group (de Maré & Kreeger, 1974).

Despite the differences between these various approaches derived from psychoanalysis, they share the underlying assumption that therapy largely consists of exploring unconscious mental processes by means of interpretations directed towards resistance and transferences. However, although these approaches may be useful with carefully selected groups of out-patients, other strategies are more commonly found in most types of group psychotherapy that are routinely practised within a psychiatric service. These involve the provision of more focus and instruction than is found in groups that mainly aim to explore mental processes.

A major difficulty that is encountered by investigators of group psychotherapy is that, like individual psychotherapy, the procedure is very variable even if the same approach is used. In addition, the treatment goals and criteria for the definition of improvement are varied. Beneficial effects may be judged on the basis of changes observed in the group, disappearance of symptoms, improved subjective well-being, the views of the conductor, the opinions of friends or relatives of the patients, increased self-knowl-edge, increased competence at work, or changes in social behaviour (Yalom *et al.*, 1977). However, there is often a low correlation between various outcome measures. Apart from the methodological problems in measuring outcome, the results are often affected by spontaneous recovery and many non-treatment variables. Also, if a particular psychotherapeutic method is being investigated, many non-technique variables are relevant, such as the 'helping relationship' with the therapist, although this may be of less importance in groups compared with individual psychotherapy (Gurman & Gustafson, 1976). As each group is unique, control data must be interpreted with caution.

Group psychotherapy and PD

Various forms of group psychotherapy have been advocated for individuals with borderline PD, antisocial PD and for certain offender groups, as well as for some other individuals with a PD diagnosis, who present with secondary symptoms such as anxiety.

The literature contains a general consensus among clinicians that individuals with borderline PD can benefit from a treatment regime that includes relatively structured group methods (Blum & Marziali, 1988), involving a format in which tasks of the group are defined, rather than just telling each patient that his/her task involves self-disclosure, listening and interacting with others.

Group treatment for patients who have all received the diagnosis of borderline PD is often combined with individual psychotherapeutic ses-sions and, with such a regime, there has been debate as to whether the therapist for individual sessions should also be involved in the group treatment. Not surprisingly, there is not a clear consensus on this issue, as individuals with borderline PD (and therapists) are heterogeneous. Also, management decisions have to take into account many other aspects apart from patient variables, such as the availability of resources and the level of experience of staff in group treatment methods.

With regard to other PDs, a group of patients with avoidant PD were reported to be helped by just five sessions involving either social skills training or group sessions (Stravynski *et al.*, 1989), and an intensive 4-day group treatment for avoidant PD was associated with clinically-significant improvements that were evident at 1-year follow-up (Renneberg *et al.*, 1990). Also, various programmes have been devised for offender groups that can be assumed to contain many individuals with antisocial PD. For instance, a London prison provided a regime for rapists, which involved 50 group sessions with a structured educational content, focussing on such issues as attitudes to victims, effects on victims, how to avoid situations in which offences may occur, adaptive relationships with women, and control of alcohol abuse. Also, an 18-month therapeutic community experience has been attempted for rapists within a prison system, although such an approach does not appear to be indicated for those who refuse to take any responsibility for their actions. Dolan & Coid (1993) concluded that the literature on therapeutic community approaches to antisocial behaviour have shown 'the most promising results', although there is a lack of controlled studies.

Finally, patients who completed their treatment in a day hospital substance abuse programme and continued to attend self-help groups, had relatively low rates of substance abuse during follow-up (McKay *et al.*, 1994).

Despite the variety of selection criteria, formats, goals and strategies, certain principles for group psychotherapy can be identified in relation to therapeutic ingredients, group-specific phenomena, the organization of groups and the therapist's (i.e. conductor's) role. These will be considered in relation to groups that are relatively unstructured, but are also relevant to groups that have defined procedures and tasks.

Definition and therapeutic ingredients

Group psychotherapy encompasses a variety of forms and goals, which include relief of psychological symptoms, modification of social or family relationships, and a permanent change in attitudes or other aspects of the relatively stable organization of an individual's mental activity and behaviour, which comprise personality.

A group of individuals, who are appropriately called patients within the setting of a psychiatric service, meet regularly with one or more trained professionals to interact by verbal interchange and other communicative behaviour (Frank, 1979).

All the phenomena that are found in individual psychotherapy may also be present in group psychotherapy although some, such as the importance of the relationship between patient and therapist, are attenuated, while others, such as the provision of new interpersonal situations from which the patient may learn, receive an extra dimension in groups.

As with individual psychotherapy there are two main approaches, which can coexist. The 'supportive' approach implies that the therapist accepts a degree of dependency from the patients and provides an active input to their relationships, while the approach derived from psychoanalytic theory is directed towards an increasing awareness and understanding of unconscious mental activity, with a focus on the past.

Group psychotherapy can provide new learning situations that are derived from a much wider range of interpersonal interactions than is possible in individual psychotherapy. Insight may be obtained by observing 'unconsciously' motivated behaviour in other group members, while increased self-awareness is produced by the patient finding out, by 'feedback', how he/she is perceived by others. Each patient is usually encouraged to display his/her own psychopathology by ensuring that he/she feels 'safe' enough to do so, and he/she may have the opportunity to develop and test new patterns of social interaction. Insight can be variable in relation to a beneficial instance of new learning, and may be minimal or non-existent. Thus, a patient with limited capacity for insight or abstract thought may increase his/her self-confidence by being able to advise or comfort other patients, without being aware that a poor opinion of his/her value to others was one of the main problems.

Group psychotherapy can also provide therapeutic events that are specific to this form of treatment. An atmosphere of trust, openness, concern, tolerance, and support, with controlled negative feedback, has been termed 'group cohesiveness', and may be therapeutic in itself. It is also well known that any group of individuals can exert powerful pressure to conform to the attitudes of the majority, and this force may be harnessed to the correction of maladaptive behaviour. The experience of universality, in which the patient realizes that other people have problems, sometimes similar to his/her own, has often been cited by patients to be therapeutic, and the process of sharing problems encourages group members to become less self-absorbed. The opportunity to be altruistic may also reduce self-absorption and increase self-esteem. In some groups, re-enactment of family relationships may take place if other group members resemble various members of the patient's family, and this process may assist the development of insight. For some patients, such as those with social phobias, groups provide the feared situation and a setting in which coping strategies can be developed, while a collective approach to problem solving can sometimes lead to the optimum solution for certain problems.

Group psychotherapy usually provides various additional indirect benefits, the importance of which should not be underestimated. If the group meetings take place in a psychiatric unit, the interest and morale of the staff may be increased, and the assessment and monitoring of the patient is improved. For inpatients, the relief of boredom associated with this or any other activity may also be of considerable, if non-specific, value.

Group-specific phenomena

Psychotherapy in groups incorporates various communication patterns involving both verbal and non-verbal behaviour.

The possible benefits of so-called group pressures have already been considered; groups have the capacity to define, by consensus, acceptable attitudes or behaviour and then to exert pressure to conform to these standards. Behaviour that is generally acceptable may be rewarded by positive regard, while deviance can be punished by criticism, hostility or by being ignored. But at times, the overt consensus attitude may be more extreme than the most widely-held viewpoint. Another property of groups is their ability to define what appears to be reality to the majority; for example, the staff may be considered to be uncaring, or it may be assumed that all patients have similar problems. Such assumptions may be far from accurate. Resistance may involve the collaboration of group members to prevent the consideration of reality, perhaps by means of silence or changing the subject by directing attention to another group member. Although at such times the patients may not be fully aware of what is happening, on one occasion every member of a group made a deliberate decision before the meeting that no one would utter a word! A common example of an unconscious collaborative defence is that of scapegoating, when one individual receives hostile feelings that have been displaced by several group members from their appropriate target; this often occurs when a new member enters a group.

When emotion is expressed in a group there is a tendency for it to precipitate the experience of a similar feeling in several other group members. Thus, a sharing of expressed emotion often occurs; one angry complaint about the staff may initiate a chorus, while a weeping patient may elicit several complaints of depressed mood.

Another group process has been called the 'chain phenomenon' when several members contribute to a group theme, while an examination of the pattern of interaction in a series of meetings invariably demonstrates a tendency for the form and content of the meetings to undergo constant change. Irregular cycles are often seen in which, for example, a meeting (or series of meetings) characterized by the patients being constructive, caring and active will be followed by withdrawal, hostility and hopelessness, before the original form eventually returns.

Finally, a consideration of group-specific phenomena would not be complete without mention of interactions that take place at times other than the group meetings, but which would not have occurred if the patients had not been members of the same group.

Organization

Groups may be 'closed' (and time limited) when the same individuals meet for a set number of occasions, or 'open', when individuals join and leave the group at different times.

The goals of group psychotherapy vary considerably and, although many patients in a psychiatric service may be included in a group at some stage, some are not suitable for this form of treatment and certain principles of selection should be observed. Severely psychotic patients and those with marked paranoid or schizoid PD traits should generally be excluded; the paranoid patient often evokes hostility, which reinforces his/her pathological ideas, while the severely schizoid person will usually find a group too threatening. Also, excessively narcissistic individuals with a minimal capacity to take note of others should not usually be selected. Sociopathic individuals, addicts of both drugs and alcohol and those whose problems centre on sexual deviation must be included only after careful consideration in a group of individuals with a range of psychiatric problems, and, in general, there should not be more than one patient with any of these problems in each group unless a group is selected on the basis of a diagnostic category such as substance abuse, borderline PD or antisocial PD (Bloch, 1979).

Certain characteristics of a patient imply suitability for relatively unstructured group psychotherapy irrespective of the presenting psychiatric syndrome, and such a patient should be judged to have sufficient psychological reserves to tolerate the anxiety-provoking situations that invariably arise in such groups. The patient who is likely to derive significant benefit from an unstructured group will usually have had at least one 'meaningful' relationship, have the capacity to participate in discussion and to use abstract concepts, be committed to active cooperation, be able to experience and express emotion, and have a clearly defined area of conflict (Marmor, 1979); however, these qualities are not essential for a patient to be included in some types of group therapy. The group conductor should avoid selecting a patient who would be conspicuously different from the other group members on such dimensions as age, social class, intelligence or verbal ability, and the inclusion of too many patients who are likely to say very little must be avoided. Patients whose major difficulty is that they become emotionally dependent on others to an excessive extent often do better in groups than in individual psychotherapy, as a pathological and disabling dependency upon one individual is usually avoided in a group setting. The group conductor should interview each prospective member and consider the current state of the group, the nature of the patient's problems and personality, and the conductor's attitudes towards the patient; if the conductor feels considerable hostility towards an individual, this may preclude selection. The patient can be asked to provide a written account of his/her history and present problems, which can indicate motivation as well as providing information (Bloch, 1979). If a patient is selected, the conductor must then consider the best time for entry to an open group, as joining when patients are particularly hostile or apathetic may not be appropriate.

After a patient has been selected, he/she can be seen individually by the conductor or other staff member for a preparatory session (Yalom *et al.*, 1967). Certain rules are usually made: patients should not meet socially outside the hospital or clinic, any significant change in life situation must be reported to the group, notice must be given if attendance is not possible, and confidentiality must be maintained. If necessary it should be made clear that repeated disruptive behaviour other than verbal interchange may lead to exclusion. For unstructured groups, the patient is told that the meetings have no set agenda and that the tasks will be to talk about his/her problems, feelings and thoughts, and to interact with other group members. It may be appropriate to ask that the patient makes a commitment to attend a minimum number of meetings.

The optimum number of patients is generally agreed to be about eight, with a range of three to 12 (de Maré & Kreeger, 1974). Each meeting usually lasts for 1 hour and takes place one to three times weekly, although Linehan's regime for patients with severe borderline PD includes a weekly group of $2\frac{1}{2}$ hours (Linehan, 1987). Sessions should be as evenly spaced as possible. Group members sit in a circle so that non-verbal communication is apparent.

The group conductor should have some experience and must be assisted by at least one other staff member. During each meeting one individual can be clearly designated as the conductor, but two, or even three co-conductors may alternate this responsibility. Not more than three staff members should accompany a group of about eight patients. One, preferably two, staff should be regular group members, while the third may be a student or trainee who can attend for a limited number of meetings. Although two or three staff members may be sufficiently experienced to share the task of conducting the group, one therapist may wish to retain continual responsibility as the conductor; in this situation other staff members can act as 'participant observers' who are relatively inactive. The staff can meet for about 15 minutes after each session when the conductor can compare his/her impressions with those of colleagues. A written summary or report may then be prepared, which may be given to the patients at the next meeting (Yalom, Brown & Bloch, 1975). For many group members, group psychotherapy is part of a varied treatment programme and the conductor must ensure that good communications exist between staff in the group and other staff members in the various professional disciplines.

For an unstructured group, each patient is told that his/her task in the group involves self-disclosure, listening and interacting with others. However, for the many groups that have more structure, group members are provided with defined tasks. For unstructured groups, the emphasis is on verbal communication by which each patient reveals various aspects of psychological functioning, such as attitudes, patterns of social interaction and psychological defences. Transferences to several group members may develop, involving unrealistic feelings and attitudes, which indicate unconscious mental activity.

Awareness of non-verbal behaviour is important. When a patient is speaking, the other group members will be engaged in various forms of silent participation: emotions may be shared, self-examination may be taking place, and the silent patient may be learning from events that involve others. Overt non-verbal activity such as facial expressions, fidgeting, moving restlessly in the chair, tapping the foot, or playing with an ashtray or cigarette, should be noted and may be informative. More rarely, unacceptable and dramatic behaviour may occur: objects are thrown, physical violence or attempts at self-harm take place, or a patient rushes out of the meeting.

Goals of group psychotherapy

Although the patient and therapist may not be able to agree the aims of treatment, the conductor should formulate realistic goals for each group member during the selection process, bearing in mind the likely capacity for change and the time that will be needed to achieve the desired effects. It is a common mistake to underestimate the time required to produce clinically important changes in a patient's personality structure. A minimum of 6–12 months is usually necessary to encourage even modest changes in the personality traits that comprise the major syndromes of PD.

Sometimes the treatment goal does not involve change but an attempt to support the patient who cannot manage his/her life without some help. Support may be provided for a limited time during a resolving crisis, but group attendance may also play its part in the management of more chronic problems. In a crisis, attention must be paid to the precipitating events, which may have involved loss, change, interpersonal difficulties or a conflict between alternatives.

Group treatment may involve discussion of the cause or effects of psychological disorder; thus, attention may be directed towards a lack of trust in others that has led to anxiety and unhappiness, while a patient who has suffered repeated episodes of psychosis may be helped to adjust to residual deficits and vulnerability to stress.

Treatment goals can involve the relief of symptoms that include what Frank (1974) has called 'demoralization'. This involves a feeling of isolation, shame, and a loss of long-term goals. Group psychotherapy may be used to enhance a patient's capacity to relate to others, so that he/she may be more able to achieve close personal relationships, perhaps by being less assertive or histrionic, less uncomfortable in company, less mistrustful of others or more independent. Another goal may be to modify various aspects of personality, such as low self-esteem, lack of purpose and self-confidence, an inability to express emotion, or a tendency to behave impulsively with poor control of emotional expression.

At times, psychological defence mechanisms should be strengthened, perhaps by encouraging avoidance of certain problems but, if defences are maladaptive, another goal may be to assist the patient to discard these or to substitute less harmful manoeuvres. The dismantling of defences usually involves the development of insight; for example a patient may be encouraged to accept that a particular problem is insoluble, or that a decision has been avoided.

Another important aim of group psychotherapy can be the regular monitoring and assessment of the psychological state and life situation of each group member. Group psychotherapy provides an opportunity for this to be achieved in a way that is particularly valuable if the availability of staff for individual interviews is limited. Group psychotherapy can also encourage staff interaction with patients, improve staff morale and foster cooperation across professional boundaries.

The group conductor's role

The conductor bears ultimate responsibility for the group and undertakes the various administrative tasks that have been described. The conductor must also open and close each meeting, monitor the proceedings, and intervene appropriately. The relationship of each individual patient to the group must be borne in mind and group processes should be identified. Both verbal and non-verbal behaviour is noted and patterns are sought. The conductor should also be aware of his/her own emotional reactions.

To achieve the treatment goals for the individual members, and to foster the therapeutic activity of the group, the conductor can use a wide range of interventions. The first priority must always be to do no harm, and a vulnerable patient who cannot cope with certain stressful situations has to be actively protected and, if necessary, withdrawn from the group. The conductor must set a standard of behaviour involving tolerance, concern, perseverance and, above all, calm in difficult situations. He/she should encourage an atmosphere of openness, trust and hope that is 'safe' for self-disclosure and will, by a variety of methods, further the specific treatment goals that have been formulated.

The conductor's contributions are both verbal and non-verbal. Various comments and questions can facilitate a climate of communication, concern, mutual support and the sharing of experience or emotion. Interventions may be relatively non-directive, or be aimed specifically at one group member or a particular topic. At times the conductor should encourage the sharing and expression of emotions, perhaps by drawing attention to depression or anger in the meeting, and by inviting others to share their own feelings or experiences. However, it is not a good policy constantly to encourage the expression of anger or depression. The opinions of the conductor and other staff are often an important class of intervention, as these may help to counteract pathological opinions and behaviour patterns that are shared by most of the group members. Other types of intervention include clarification, the promotion of problem-solving behaviour, confrontation, directives and interpretations. Clarification of a situation may be the first step in solving a problem; Goldfried & Goldfried (1975) have described subsequent stages in this process: the identification of methods for the solution with an examination of their consequences, the choice of one of these possible methods, and the planning of the various steps for its performance. Confrontation refers to the technique of repeatedly bringing the group face to face with a situation, while directives, although usually kept to a minimum, can be essential. Interpretations are the final major category of verbal input and refer to comments designed to produce insight.

Non-verbal activity includes silent participation involving attentive listening. Gestures, facial expression and movements will convey varying degrees of information about the conductor's underlying thoughts, while another type of non-verbal intervention is that of physical activity. Although the need for this should be rare, the conductor and other staff may occasionally have to stop a fight, or prevent an attempt at self-injury.

A flexible approach to the conductor's role is essential in this type of group as changes of strategy are often required. Although the conductor may have no alternative but to encourage a leader-centred communication pattern, in which he/she interacts with several group members in turn, there should be periods when most interactions are between group members. Group communication is encouraged by such techniques as asking a question of the group rather than of an individual, inviting the expression of views from previously silent members and focussing on themes that are of general relevance. In a series of meetings, there should be a balance regarding the content of topics discussed; although events in the remote past and a quest for explanations may be important, the 'here and now' should predominate in most routine practice settings, both inside and outside the group. Also, the future should be considered.

At any moment, the conductor has a choice from a range of overall strategies for the conduct of the group. At one extreme the conductor is authoritative, active, and freely gives his/her opinions and reactions; his/

her main aim is to provide a setting in which patients feel minimal anxiety, where conflicts are diffused or avoided, and where sharing of problems, mutual support and group cohesion are encouraged. The focus is on the problems and symptoms of the here and now. At the other end of the spectrum, the conductor is minimally active and non-directive; no attempt is made to avoid anxiety and hostility, even though this adversely affects group cohesion. With this approach, emotional expression is encouraged, and the focus is on relationships, the awareness of the effects of behaviour on others, defences, and group or individual transferences.

Most unstructured group meetings in a psychiatric service involve an amalgam of strategies, and during each meeting the conductor's tactics may undergo several changes in response to events in the group. However, in general, strategy is weighted towards the former end of the spectrum in routine practice settings, so that group psychotherapy should provide a situation in which patients can usually feel safe and do not often experience a high level of anxiety. The members should generally feel able to join in, and have trust in the staff. Unfortunately, some staff members are not suited to be group conductors in this setting by virtue of their personality or theoretical bias; Yalom (1975) has described the aggressive, confronting, excessively self-revealing, controlling and charismatic group conductor, and it is likely that this type of conducting can often be harmful unless the group is carefully selected. In general, the conductor must strive to ensure that group meetings are usually characterized by attentive concern, so that the members feel relaxed and able to contribute. Of course, emotions are expressed and tensions appear, but these can be tolerated if the background atmosphere is one of trust. The conductor must act naturally and should generally be prepared to voice his/her own opinions or to demonstrate personal concern when this is appropriate. A conductor who displays nothing of his/her views or reactions encourages the development of marked hostility which may not be adequately resolved unless the group members are highly selected. However, the conductor must limit the degree to which his/her own personality becomes apparent and some formality is required, in keeping with the professional nature of the conductor's role. The conductor must constantly review the degree of his/her activity, whatever the overall strategy. This must be considered every few minutes, and the staff should not be so active throughout a meeting that the patient members of the group are seldom given a chance to interact. Often it is appropriate for the conductor to say very little during the first part of the meeting, but if interactions do not develop, or break down, a more active and directive approach is usually necessary; in these circumstances a subsequent attempt should be made to provide a period when the staff is minimally active.

Resistance has been defined as all the obstacles to the aims and procedures of treatment that arise from within the patient, and may include both conscious and unconscious mental activity (Sandler, Holder & Dare, 1970*b*). The latter may involve the various defence mechanisms and a 'negative therapeutic reaction' in which improvement, or the expression by the therapist of an opinion that the patient has improved, is followed by a worsening of the patient's condition. Resistance can involve a varying proportion of group members; examples include persistently coming late, refusing to discuss a particular topic, ignoring staff comments, meeting socially, the formation of subgroups whose interactions persistently exclude other group members, scapegoating, showing hostility to new members, and (in unstructured groups) taking turns to speak or preselecting topics for discussion. Although psychological defence mechanisms may fulfil a useful function, and should not always be considered as resistance, they can lead to the avoidance or distortion of reality and impede the treatment process. Another phenomenon that can result from the use of defences is that of 'splitting', when the ambivalence of feelings to a person or situation is not recognized and the opposing emotions or attitudes are separated; one or more parts may be masked or distorted by defence mechanisms, for example, people are considered to be 'all-good' or 'all-bad'. Transference and counter-transference also involve unconscious mental activity which, if unresolved, can interfere with treatment; for example, one or several group members may develop unrealistic expectations of treatment, or excessive emotional dependence on the conductor (Sandler, Dare & Holder, 1970).

Several techniques are available for overcoming resistance either in the group as a whole or in individual members. The conductor may ignore it, encourage a safe, supportive group atmosphere, mobilize the group members to share their experiences in relation to the topic under discussion, and wait. But if aspects of a particular situation are persistently avoided or distorted, the resistance can be side-stepped by asking a direct question about the topic that is being avoided, if this is known. If this procedure is not effective, the conductor may draw the attention of the group to the resistance itself; for example, if a long silence is considered to be a resistance, the group may be encouraged to consider their feelings about the silence and the possible reasons why this situation has occurred. A fourth technique for overcoming resistance is to provide an interpretation, if unconscious mechanisms are involved. For example, a suggestion was made to a husband who had been deserted by his wife, and who was depressed and excessively protective to his children, that he may have mixed feelings towards his children, as many people in his situation resent such responsibility. This helped the patient to recognize that he felt intensely resentful towards his children as well as towards his wife. But sometimes, all the conductor's efforts to overcome resistance will be in vain, and if the resistance is in the form of a long silence, this will continue. At this stage the conductor has no option but to accept that, for the moment, he/she has done all that is possible. The conductor does not bear all the responsibility for the efficacy of the group, as this is shared to some extent between all its members. Thus, in the case of a prolonged silence, the ball can be repeatedly put back into the group's court by the conductor pointing out that he/she can only do so much. Sometimes the anxiety provoked by an extended silence is a useful catalyst to increased effort and self-reliance by the group members, but, in general, the conductor should try and help the group to avoid this situation.

The conductor may open each group meeting formally, and introduce any new member. He/she may then state the reasons for any absences and, if these are unknown, should encourage the group to consider if any action is appropriate; in a hospital setting a patient may volunteer to look for a missing individual. At this point in an unstructured group, the conductor can wait for a patient to start the proceedings, as part of the overall policy for the staff to be minimally active for at least part of the meeting. This allows the group to assume some responsibility for selecting the topics to be considered. However, if an initial silence continues for a minute or more, interactions may be encouraged by non-directive interventions which prompt the group as a whole.

During the final 15 minutes, the conductor should be aware that the end of the meeting is near. He/she may then decide to prompt previously silent members by directly asking them for their comments and, in the final few minutes, the patients can be invited in turn to give their reactions to the meeting or to each other. The conductor should try and ensure that the scheduled time for ending the meeting does not arrive during an unresolved period of emotionality but, if this occurs, the meeting may have to be extended. This should be avoided if possible, and an alternative technique for dealing with a patient who is very distressed or angry at the end of the meeting is to say that, although it is time to finish, a staff member will remain with the patient. This should also be a rare event, and patients should not be encouraged to expect individual attention immediately after a meeting.

The inexperienced conductor often finds it difficult to decide on concluding remarks. At times, it may be appropriate to summarize the events of the meeting or end on a hopeful and encouraging note. But the conductor must not feel that it is his/her duty to do either, and when the mood is one of hopelessness or resentment, or when the meeting ends in the middle of the consideration of a problem, a statement can be made which merely clarifies the situation; for example 'one of the main problems seems to be that everyone has given up hope of any improvement', or 'although we have to finish now, we must come back to this problem next time'. On other occasions the conductor need not say anything other than to formally close the meeting by a comment such as: 'I am sorry to interrupt you but we have come to the end of our time'. This may be quite difficult, as he/she may come under pressure to say something 'clever' or reassuring, or to prolong the meeting. If group members ignore a concluding remark, the conductor may need to repeat the closing statement. If necessary he/she should interrupt the group by standing up with other staff members.

Emotionality

Although mental events have both a cognitive and emotional component, it can be useful to isolate the emotional content of each group meeting for consideration. Anger, depression and anxiety are of particular relevance, but disgust, positive attraction, happiness and elation should also be noted. If personality change is a goal of treatment for some group members, a degree of emotional arousal may be facilitative and, at times, essential, while varying degrees of emotionality are an inevitable part of all types of group psychotherapy.

Anger may occur in many disguises, such as a show of boredom, sarcasm, or the excessive politeness resulting from the use of the defence mechanism of 'reaction formation', in which the opposite of an underlying feeling appears in consciousness. The conductor should not necessarily draw the group's attention to signs of anger, which can often be ignored, but if these are persistent, exploration may be indicated. Underlying attitudes can be considered, and group members may be helped to handle the experience or expression of anger more appropriately. When anger is overt, the conductor or other group members may face considerable hostility. If the conductor is on the receiving end he/she must remain outwardly calm, and wait for the feelings to have been expressed before making any comments. Even after a delay he/she must not be in too much of a hurry to defend; the views of other group members should be invited, and he/she may decide not to give a specific reply. However, if the anger is directed to another group member, the conductor may need to be actively protective. If the staff are being accused of having various shortcomings, it is usually better not to argue, and an angry response on the part of the conductor is invariably inappropriate, especially if it involves a lack of the self-control that is an essential tribute of the role. It is often helpful to try and identify a pattern of inappropriate emotional arousal or expression, as the group experience may be representative of behaviour that repeatedly occurs in other situations.

A patient who is depressed and tearful is often ashamed at exhibiting emotion and if there are clear signs that a group member is upset it is often reassuring if the conductor indicates that this has been noticed. This implies that it is 'all right' to be upset and the conductor may then try and encourage sharing of similar feeling, either past or present, and mobilize the group's support. However, the tearful patient may find it very uncomfortable to remain at the centre of the group's attention, and the conductor should consider shifting the focus without necessarily changing the subject; for example, a patient who had been upset the previous week could be asked how he/she has been feeling. Talk of suicidal ideas may reduce the likelihood of subsequently putting these thoughts into action, but it may be necessary to arrange to see the patient individually after the meeting, if, at the end, he/she appears to be actively suicidal. However, the motivation behind some patients' talk of possible self-injury is the expression of anger or an attempt to manipulate the attitudes and behaviour of the group. In such cases it may be necessary to state clearly that the group or staff cannot always accept responsibility for a person's actions. At the same time it is important to maintain a sympathetic approach, which can be difficult, as the behaviour of some patients in such situations often arouses hostility.

Emotions can be 'acted-out' by disruptive non-verbal behaviour which, if it is not modified or contained by group pressures, may require a patient's exclusion from the group by the conductor. Physical intervention by the staff may very occasionally be necessary to stop aggression or self-injury, and, if a patient leaves the meeting, it may be appropriate for a member of the group to try and persuade him/her to return.

The conductor's own emotions must not be forgotten, and a capacity for self-control with regard to their expression is an essential skill, which may require experience for its development. If the conductor expresses strong emotions, this should only occur after a decision that this feedback would be helpful to the group. If, occasionally, this ideal is not realized, and the conductor's involuntary expression of strong feeling is apparent, it is probably best to acknowledge to the group that he/she is feeling angry, depressed or anxious. This tactic may defuse tension or embarrassment.

Positive emotions should not be discouraged, but laughter or jokes are often defensive and inappropriate. They should be accepted at their face value only with caution.

Patterns of group interaction

Various developmental stages have been described in 'closed' unstructured groups (which rarely admit new members), and these can also be seen, albeit less predictably, in 'open' groups (Schutz, 1958). In a closed group, an initial 'forming' stage has been identified in which members are often anxious, defensive and ambivalent. The group is dependent on the therapist for guidance and takes few risks. Members are on their best socially acceptable behaviour as they attempt to find out what is permitted and the nature of their task (Bloch, 1979). The middle stage has been termed the 'working' group and involves several patterns of group activity: 'storming', in which conflicts are expressed (often accompanied by criticism of the conductor for not being sufficiently directive), 'norming', in which cohesion develops, and 'performing', in which self-disclosure occurs and solutions to problems may emerge. In addition there may be periods when defence mechanisms are predominant (Bion, 1961). The final stage of a closed group is that of 'termination', which is analogous to the discharge of individual members from an open group. Termination should occur if no further significant benefits are possible, and leaving the group may be, in itself, a therapeutic process, during which further steps are taken towards an appropriate degree of emotional independence.

Although the above stages are not delineated so clearly in an open group, phases of group interaction, e.g. involving dependency, cohesion or emotionality, are often experienced. Thus, if a group is constructively discussing problems in a relaxed and supportive atmosphere, this does not usually last for more than, at most, a few meetings; conversely, the conductor can predict that meetings characterized by despondency, hostility and apathy are likely to become more positive.

Although patterns of communication that involve several group members should be encouraged, lengthy dialogues may also be appropriate, if these do not lead to undue exclusion of other group members. Overt or covert structuring of communications, such as turn taking or assuming that certain questions must never be asked, should be generally avoided in an unstructured group but, as previously described, patients may be asked in turn for their comments near the end of the meeting. The conductor should remember that the communication pattern of a group has a life of its own, which is not entirely dependent on the staff activity, and that members interact to a considerable extent outside groups if they are inpatients.

The degree of staff activity is a common topic for discussion in staff meetings. As part of the flexible approach that is required, the conductor must be prepared to vary the pattern of staff activity; constant intervention by the conductor stifles the group processes, but a directive and active approach by the staff may be needed when the group members lack the capacity to provide a positive input.

Certain themes are commonly encountered in unstructured groups in psychiatric practice, such as previous treatment, symptoms, problems of being a patient, and the relevance, function and difficulties of the group itself. Dependency, trust, self-confidence, loss of hope, future plans, coping with emotions, loneliness, difficulties with authority, childhood experiences, recent life events and marital problems are also often discussed. Responsibility for one's actions is another recurrent theme and group members may share unrealistic expectations of some kind of magical treatment that will involve little effort on their part. Although many psychiatric syndromes respond well to physical treatments, the kind of problems that are considered in groups invariably require some effort and motivation from the patients.

If membership has been beneficial, leaving the group can be a significant event, even in patients who have not participated actively. The setting of a target discharge date is necessary for those patients who have developed a significant degree of dependency on the group, and the discussion of reactions to discharge may be an important part of treatment. The conductor should mention when it is a patient's last meeting and, if appropriate, emphasize that follow-up arrangements have been made. Psychological defences are often intensified before discharge, so that emotionality and exploration of unconscious processes should be minimized during a patient's final meetings. Timing of discharge is vital, as if it is too late a damaging over-dependence may have resulted. The optimum time for each patient will be determined, to a large extent, on the goals that have been formulated.

The conductor's problems

Personality, knowledge and experience determine the efficacy of a group conductor, and it must be recognized that certain traits, such as excessive emotional coldness or obsessionality, can disqualify an individual for this task. Conducting a group can be a stressful experience, and the relatively inexperienced conductor should always have the assistance of at least one other staff member, together with regular supervision. Various maladaptive behaviour patterns have been described in trainee psychiatrists who, together with other professionals, often find that working in groups is one of the most demanding of all their duties. The conductor is also involved in the group processes and may be caught up in contagious emotion. He/she may be the focus of hostility and be subjected to unreasonable demands, which require a firm stand against pressures to conform. Faced with stressful situations, the conductor's defence mechanisms may distort judgement and he/she may take refuge behind a professional mask, by showing his/her 'wares' in the form of long summaries, involved interpretations or the use of jargon (Yalom, 1966).

The main attributes of an effective group psychotherapist are a degree of self-awareness and self-control, together with a confidence to doubt and question his/her own actions. The potentially harmful effects of countertransference or the conductor's defences can be minimized by supervision, feedback from other staff members in the group, and the conductor's increasing recognition of certain characteristics of his/her own personality. Self-control involves an ability to endure difficult interpersonal situations by 'sitting it out' and keeping relatively calm. This does not imply that the conductor is not experiencing strong emotions, but their expression is being controlled. Reacting with anger and getting caught up with a prevailing feeling of despair are two of the most common pitfalls.

Various situations are commonly found in relatively unstructured group psychotherapy, for instance, group members may sit expectantly, awaiting direction from the conductor in the hope that someone else can sort out their problems without any effort on their part. This attitude may need to be discussed and the conductor should repeatedly clarify what can and cannot be done without the members' active participation. This may reduce the hostility that usually accompanies unrealistic and unfulfilled demands.

There are many kinds of silence that reflect apathy, active consideration, a brooding hopelessness, perplexity, anger, tension, stubbornness, or, especially with new members, uncertainty as to what they should be discussing in unstructured meetings. In general, long silences are not beneficial, but their resolution will depend on the underlying cause. Of course, it should be remembered that although the predominant mood or attitude of the group in a silence (or in any other situation) can often be identified, it may not be shared by all the members. Some of those who do not share the prevailing attitude or emotion understandably find repeated references to the opinions of 'the group' rather irritating, and the conductor should always bear in mind that a group is composed of individuals.

If the conductor does not know what to do in any situation, the answer is often 'nothing', apart from putting up with the situation while continuing to try and help the group to function. The burden of responsibility for the proceedings of the group is shared by all its members and, apart from not giving up, the conductor is not necessarily obliged to 'do something'.

At times the conductor is aware of a major event, such as a recent attempted suicide of one of the members, which is being avoided at the expense of 'safer' topics. In this situation the issue should usually be raised at some time during the meeting.

Another common event is the repeated questioning of the conductor by one or more group members; this poses a problem, because although it is often appropriate to give direct answers, an excess of this type of interaction fosters dependency and impairs group communication. It may be necessary for the conductor to say that a question will be answered later in another setting, or that an excess of questions and answers is unhelpful in group meetings. However, it is rarely appropriate to completely ignore a question.

Group members may try and strike up a special relationship with the conductor, perhaps by imparting 'confidential' information between meetings, but the conductor should usually make it clear that he/she is not able to accept information on this basis and that if it is confided, the right to bring it to the attention of the group will be reserved. There are many ways in which members attempt to manipulate the conductor to carry out inappropriate actions.

The overtalkative group member who monopolizes meetings is another common problem. Often group pressures and firm interventions by the conductor are effective, but in the case of hypomanic patients in inpatient units, temporary exclusion may be necessary.

Negative effects

A negative effect has been defined as a lasting deterioration in a patient, directly attributable to therapy; however transient effects may also be important (Hadley & Strupp, 1976).

Existing problems may be magnified, for example, the inability of the dependent patient to refuse unreasonable demands may be exploited by group members, the paranoid patient may consistently evoke hostility that strengthens his/her beliefs, and social phobias may be intensified in a group that lacks cohesion, concern and support. Psychotic patients or those with limited intelligence may not be able to join in, thus compounding a feeling of inadequacy, while exposure to an emotionally charged situation may exacerbate a psychosis in vulnerable individuals. Also, maladaptive defence mechanisms and behaviour patterns may be reinforced; for example, the withdrawn individual may become more socially isolated, or the group may provide an opportunity to display undue aggression.

New problems may also arise. A system of defence mechanisms can represent the best possible way of coping and, if these are challenged, decompensation may result in further impairment of the patient's adjustment, perhaps involving depression, anxiety or excessive dependence on the group. In addition, new defences may develop that are even more maladaptive than the originals. Symptom substitution may occur; for example a preoccupation with somatic complaints may be replaced by the overt development of a previously covert paranoid delusion. The setting of unrealistic goals will lead to frustration, disappointment and loss of hope for both the patient and therapist, while for some patients the pursuit of 'therapy' can become an unproductive end in itself, which protects the individual from the need to face up to immediate problems. Breaches of confidentiality may occasionally have serious consequences, for example if they involve extramarital relationships or criminal activity, while for some patients a relapse in the severity of their disorder, perhaps involving suicidal intent, may not be recognized in a group setting.

Emotional arousal may have several harmful effects; heightened emotions can give rise to destructive or antisocial 'acting out' behaviour, such as taking an overdose, and can occasionally precipitate a relapse of manic-depressive or schizophrenic features in patients who are predisposed to these disorders.

The conductor must monitor the group sessions for harmful effects and take active steps to stop their development. If necessary a patient should be excluded, either temporarily or permanently, for his/her own good or to prevent harm to others. If meetings are consistently characterized by anger, distrust and lack of concern, the disadvantages will probably outweigh any advantages, and disbanding the group should be considered. However, this should not be necessary with an experienced conductor and careful selection of patients.

Finally, the development of a sexual relationship between two group members may occur, usually with adverse consequences, especially if the male patient has pronounced antisocial personality traits. This potential problem should be anticipated when selecting the group members.

Training and supervision for group conductors

A group conductor should have certain attributes of personality, a degree of self-awareness, and some theoretical knowledge and experience.

Self-awareness and theoretical knowledge can be acquired in various ways, which often include a meeting of trainee conductors with their supervisor in a group setting. In this group, the same phenomena that are found in psychotherapeutic groups may occur; for example, the trainees may show resistance by avoiding discussion of certain aspects of their work, or by an inability to monitor group processes. Trainees' counter-transferences to the group members may be apparent to other members of the supervision group; for instance, a trainee conductor may inappropriately feel that the problems of a group member have a bad prognosis. A transference on the part of the trainee to the supervisor may show itself in an excessive need for approval, an unresolved hostility to authority, or intense rivalry with fellow trainees.

Varieties of group psychotherapy

Various types of group psychotherapy, with different degrees of structure, can be organized within a psychiatric service. Some groups may cater for outpatients alone, or the conductor may select a relatively homogeneous group with regard to PD diagnosis or to treatment goals. Although some group activities for outpatients may involve little more than social contact and a cup of tea, others may have goals which include significant personality change. These are often closed but 'open' formats may also be used. Each session may last for between 60 and 150 minutes and may occur weekly, perhaps for about 12–18 months for closed groups. Sometimes groups may be selected with regard to the homogeneity of presenting problems such as social phobia, agoraphobia, alcoholism, drug addiction or sociopathy. Groups for sociopathic individuals should be in the context of a specialist institution or service. Other groups may target couples with marital difficulties, the relatives of patients, or several members of one family.

Additional varieties of group occur outside the setting of a psychiatric service. 'Marathon' groups have been described, lasting for between 6 and 48 hours, and peer self-help groups such as Alcoholics Anonymous and

Depressives Anonymous may not include a professional conductor. The use of so-called alternate sessions involve the patient/client members of an outpatient group meeting on their own, alternately with conventional sessions.

Group psychotherapy and borderline personality disorder

Overview

It has been widely accepted that group treatment, in particular relatively structured groups, can be useful for the management of patients with borderline PD, although concurrent individual sessions are usually recommended. But it is important to note the high drop-out rate from treatment.

Clinical practice has mainly developed on the basis of the opinions of experienced clinicians, although there is some evidence that supports the provision of weekly, task-orientated groups for patients who all have a borderline PD diagnosis, running in parallel with individual treatment sessions from a different therapist (Horwitz, 1987).

Waldinger & Gunderson (1984), in a retrospective study of 790 patients with borderline PD, noted that they generally ended treatment earlier than recommended. In relation to group treatments, Kretsch, Goren & Wasserman (1987) looked at the effects of a combination of individual and group therapy over several years and concluded that the group element had been useful. But the best evidence for the use of groups for those with borderline PD comes from Linehan and colleagues (1991), who compared a combination of individual therapy and weekly group therapy with 'treatment as usual'. The weekly group lasted $2\frac{1}{2}$ hours and had a structured, educational format, focussing on the teaching of behavioural skills such as managing interpersonal interactions, distress tolerance, accepting reality and regulating emotional expression.

If patients drop out of treatment early, or have to be discharged because of lack of benefit, it can be useful to present this to the patient as a failure of the treatment to be helpful, rather than a failure of the patient to cooperate. This can be combined with an offer to consider a re-referral to rejoin a treatment programme at a later date.

Positive ingredients

Gunderson (1984) considered that groups can exert a socializing influence on those with borderline PD, while Macaskill (1982) found that patients who had experienced group treatment reported that increased self-under-standing and the opportunity to try and help others had been the most valued aspects. Also, groups may be a unique way of helping those individuals who cannot tolerate or agree to individual psychotherapy (Grobman, 1980).

If a group is selected with a view to an unstructured explorative approach, it may be appropriate to limit the number of members with a borderline PD to two, because of the danger of the development of uncontrolled aggression in an unstructured group in which all members have a borderline PD (Pines, 1990). In this situation, it has been suggested that the same therapist should also be involved in providing parallel individual sessions (Wong, 1980).

It often seems that a patient's peers in a group are better able than clinicians to confront maladaptive and impulsive behaviour, as their comments are accepted more readily. Another advantage of a group compared with individual sessions is that some patients are able to identify dependent and manipulative behaviour in others, which can be a first step in recognizing these aspects in themselves. Also, a group can provide a forum in which to practise communication of feelings and the development of empathy for others, while confrontation by peer pressure can be balanced by support.

But perhaps the main advantages that a group can offer compared with individual psychotherapy alone, is to dilute, or avoid, the intense feelings (transference) of either idealization or devaluation that usually occur when the patient with features of borderline or dependent PD is being seen regularly by an individual clinician only. A group reduces the danger of an uncontrolled escalation of childlike feelings of anger and dependence (regression), which can lead to severe or repeated episodes of self-harm. This is a particular risk for some patients with borderline PD who receive frequent (once or twice weekly) long-term individual psychotherapy of an unstructured, explorative nature, if they are not able to tolerate this demanding intervention. Such a risk can be reduced by limiting the frequency and duration of individual sessions, and by giving priority to the discussion of external, current problems, as well as by arranging for concurrent group therapy.

In general, an unstructured format is considered to be inadvisable for those groups whose members all have a diagnosis of borderline PD, as regression and self-destructiveness may dominate the picture. For such patients, relatively structured groups can be used to promote reality testing, self-esteem and skills for interpersonal relationships. Specific tasks can be given, such as the discussion of decision making, problem solving, collaboration with others, discharge planning, development of daily living or improvement of social skills (Goldstein, 1990). Also, current external problems should be a frequent topic of discussion, for example, the situations that led to recent crises.

Multimodal treatments for borderline PD (and some other PDs)

Group psychotherapy is often part of several concurrent or sequential treatment interventions in psychiatric practice, and combining treatments is important in relation to borderline PD. Group therapy has often been used as part of a treatment 'package' which, over time, may involve hospital admission, long-term residential treatment, day care, night care, and outpatient treatment. Group methods may play a part in management in all these settings.

The importance of the social environment (or milieu) in psychiatric hospitals and other institutions has long been recognized, and Main (1946) introduced the term 'therapeutic community', which has come to imply frequent group meetings, an emphasis on problems involving social relationships, good interpersonal communication, flattening of the pyramid of institutional authority, free emotional expression and examination of institutional roles (Clark & Myers, 1970). However, this type of organization produces its own problems (Zeitlyn, 1967).

Considerable and relatively exclusive emphasis on these principles results in the therapeutic community 'proper', and has been advocated for some long-stay wards of psychiatric hospitals and for some specialist units catering for those with antisocial or borderline PDs and for those who abuse drugs and alcohol. But this approach is not suitable for a typical short-stay psychiatric 'admission' unit, which must cater for a wide range of psychiatric disorders. However, principles derived from the therapeutic community 'proper' are of considerable value in psychiatric 'admission' units. A variety of group activities should be available, the patients are encouraged to assume as much responsibility for themselves and their fellow patients as is possible, while staff of all disciplines should be willing to consider constructive and informed criticism, taking decisions in consultation with their colleagues. However, in the case of disagreement, it should be recognized that it is the responsibility of the psychiatrist to make the final decision regarding the medical aspects of treatment or management. Staff and patients of an admission unit may meet regularly for an unstructured 'community meeting', which may involve up to 30 people for 45 minutes, but the patients should know that they are free to choose not to attend. Although daily meetings of this type have been advocated, these can be limited to the beginning and end of the week, with various structured communal activities scheduled for other days.

A 'large group' has been defined as a meeting that includes more than 30 people (Kreeger, 1975), and Schiff & Glassman (1969) have described the consequences of increasing group size: a higher proportion of patients are silent, subgrouping increases, the participation of the less active members is reduced, and the contribution of the conductor and staff is increased.

There is some overlap between the activities of community meetings in an admission unit and group psychotherapy, but the former should focus on day-to-day problems in the ward and administrative matters. Community meetings also enable the staff to identify the main management problems of the ward and assess a large number of patients in a short time. All the staff who attend should be urged to participate, although not necessarily in every meeting, and one of their members is designated as the conductor.

Various forms of structured group activity should contribute to an admission unit's programme; for example, a weekly review meeting chaired by a member of the nursing staff can discuss non-confidential aspects of treatment, considering each patient in turn, but if patients prefer not to participate, this wish should be respected. Administrative arrangements, including those for weekend leave, can also be clarified. Other forms of structured group activity may involve art, music, psychodrama, and various forms of recreation.

Staff members require their own group activities, although there is a danger that an excess of time is spent in this way. Inexperienced staff who are involved in group psychotherapy can be supervised in weekly meetings and all staff in a group can spend about 15 minutes after each meeting discussing the session. The overall staff effectiveness in an admission unit depends to a significant extent on adequate communication, and all staff should meet regularly for an administrative meeting. This can be structured, with a chairperson and an agenda.

If hospital care is required for borderline PD it is usually short-term (i.e. less than 4 weeks) and precipitated by a crisis. The aim may be to reduce self-destructive and antisocial behaviour or to reduce the intensity of the transference relationship if the patient is receiving individual psychotherapy. Also, the ground may be prepared for future outpatient treatment. But for the most severely-affected individuals, for instance those who show repeated episodes of self-harm, longer-term residential care may be indicated, although there is a risk that an intense dependence will develop, with severe regression. If possible, less intensive long-term treatment should be considered, such as day (or night) care.

When a patient with borderline PD is in an hospital or residential setting (including day care), it has been generally recommended that, apart from formal treatment sessions, the 'milieu' should have as much structured activity as possible. Also, a balance has to be struck, particularly in relation to borderline PD, between setting limits and being supportive and tolerant. Clinicians and other staff must be as clear and consistent as possible with regard to expectations, limits and sanctions. But it must be expected that patients will display their maladaptive behaviour in treatment settings.

Many patients with PD can benefit from self-help groups such as those provided by Alcoholics Anonymous (AA), Narcotics Anonymous, and organizations concerned with eating disorders. In some cases, a support group is backed-up by a 24-hour/day phone support.

The design of a multimodal treatment programme for each individual patient is usually a matter of judgement. For those with borderline PD, a crisis admission to hospital may be followed by individual outpatient sessions running concurrently with attendance at weekly group therapy. Subsequently, one or other of these interventions may be discontinued and, if individual sessions remain, their duration and frequency may be gradually reduced.

Karterud *et al.* (1992) described a day hospital therapeutic community programme for patients with various PDs, including borderline PD. The mean time in treatment was 6 months and the dropout rate for schizotypal and borderline PD patients was 38%. 'Cluster C' PD did best, and results were rated as 'modest' for borderline PD and 'very modest' for schizotypal PD. However, it appeared that the 'containing capacity' of this regime is considerable, and may reduce the need for long-term inpatient care for the minority who would require this if an alternative is not available.

9

Management of offenders with personality disorders

A. T. GROUNDS

Personality disorders in offender populations

The frequency of PDs amongst people who commit criminal offences is difficult to determine. A high proportion of criminal offences are unreported, and in only a minority of reported cases are the suspects apprehended. Only some of these result in criminal proceedings, and a smaller proportion again will be cautioned or convicted. In the UK it is estimated that only 3% of crimes result in cautions or convictions. Thus, by the time a potential population of offenders becomes identifiable and accessible for research purposes they are unlikely to be representative of offenders as a whole. Populations of prisoners, on whom most epidemiological research has been carried out, are an even more highly selected group.

Figures from the UK British Crime Survey and from UK annual criminal statistics indicate that about 15 million criminal offences are committed annually in England and Wales with a population of around 50 million, of which half are reported to the police. In 1992, the number of people cautioned or convicted of criminal offences was 1.8 million and the number of people sentenced to imprisonment was 58 000 in 1992 (Home Office, 1993*a*).

A further difficulty in assessing rates of PD amongst offenders lies in the variety of definitions and research instruments for identifying PD. In offender populations, in whom antisocial behaviour is of particular importance, a variety of diagnostic approaches have been used. Dolan & Coid (1993) summarized the main contemporary systems, including the ICD-10 diagnosis of dissocial PD (World Health Organization, 1992), the DSM-III-R diagnosis of antisocial PD (American Psychiatric Association, 1987), and the Hare Psychopathy Checklist (Hare, 1991).

The most recent major study of the prevalence of psychiatric disorder in

321

the sentenced prison population of England and Wales was carried out by Gunn, Maden & Swinton (1991), and reported that 7.3% of sentenced adult men and 8.4% of sentenced adult women had primary diagnoses of PD. But these were clinical diagnoses based on interviews conducted by research psychiatrists who did not employ standardized diagnostic instruments, and the researchers' limited access to comprehensive information probably led, as they acknowledge, to an underestimate of true prevalence rates. Coid (1993*a*) reviewed the epidemiological studies that have employed standardized diagnostic instruments for antisocial PD, and noted that studies of North American prison samples have found prevalence rates varying between 39% and 76% of subjects. These figures compare with a lifetime prevalence rate for DSM-III-R antisocial PD of 2.6% (4.5% for men and 0.8% for women) in the US Epidemiological Catchment Area study (Robins *et al.*, 1984; Robins & Regier, 1991). It is important to note that although there is a strong association between criminality and antisocial PD, the two are distinct, as a substantial amount of criminality is committed by people who would not qualify for the diagnosis of antisocial PD (Robins, 1993).

In clinical practice a careful and rigorous approach must be taken to the diagnosis of PD among offenders who are seen within psychiatric services, and a history of criminal offending, however heinous, does not in itself justify a diagnosis of PD. The broad diagnostic principles outlined in ICD-10 or the DSM-IV should be followed, and it must be kept in mind that the basic feature of a PD is longstanding abnormality of personality that adversely affects several domains of a person's life, and that has a disabling effect on social functioning.

Particular care must be taken to avoid making unwarranted diagnoses of PD amongst people with histories of psychoses, such as schizophrenia, who later engage in recurrent offending behaviour. There is now good evidence from cohort studies that serious mental illness is associated with increased risk of criminal offending, and, in relation to schizophrenia, criminal careers of such patients are likely to commence at a later age than in most offenders (Hodgins, 1992). Not uncommonly, people with a diagnosis of psychosis in early adult life may present subsequently with problems that are dominated by troublesome offending behaviour in the absence of prominent psychotic features. A careful history will often establish that the behaviour represents a deterioration from the person's pre-morbid level of functioning, and if this is the case the proper diagnosis is likely to be of chronic psychosis rather than of primary PD.

Clinical assessment for treatment

Offenders with PDs may often be referred for psychiatric assessment because they or the referring agency hope that psychiatric treatment will be effective in achieving psychological change, but referrals may also be made in a wider range of situations.

Defendants charged with offences and awaiting trial may be referred for assessments by courts, the probation service or lawyers. Also, when faced with the stress and crisis of court proceedings, defendants may turn to primary care physicians who may then request psychiatric assessment and support. Later on in the criminal process, offenders facing sentencing may be referred for assessment in order to provide courts with advice about specific treatment options that may be available as an alternative to a custodial sentence. In addition, sentenced prisoners may need evaluation of their treatment needs in prison or their suitability for transfer to hospital for treatment during sentence. On release they may be referred for psychiatric follow-up, and, in a few cases, psychiatric supervision may be made a condition of a parole licence.

While most offenders with PDs will not receive a medical 'disposal' from the courts, in England and Wales the Mental Health Act 1983 contains equivalent powers in relation to 'psychopathic disorder' and 'mental illness'. But there is the proviso, in the case of patients with 'psychopathic disorder', that treatment is likely to alleviate or prevent deterioration of the person's condition. In practice, however, only a small minority of offenders with PDs are recommended for 'hospital orders'. Such individuals tend to have committed grave offences and require detention in a secure hospital setting and restrictions on discharge. When conditionally discharged from hospital they are likely to be subject to statutory psychiatric supervision.

It is important to have a clear understanding of the context and purpose of the psychiatric assessment in the case of an offender with PD, and the person being assessed should also appreciate the uses to which the assessment may be put. A patient referred by a primary care physician may be willing to disclose more than would be the case if a report has been requested by a court. If there is a possibility that a court report will be requested at a later stage, the patient should be made aware of this, and separate consent to prepare such a report should be obtained.

Assessment of offenders requires the identification of the range of the patient's psychiatric and social difficulties. Patients with PDs may have multiple, severe and chronic disabilities, and also suffer from episodes of other psychiatric disorders, particularly in situations of stress. Usually, psychiatric management will require agreement and commitment by the patient, and a realistic approach has to be taken in assessing the prospects of success and in setting goals that are achievable. Motivation should be carefully evaluated, but its absence at a particular time should not necessarily result in no help being offered. Some patients will require life-long support, which will be provided by intermittent contact with a psychiatric service over many years, during which they seek help when they wish.

When preparing reports for courts in cases where psychiatric support and treatment may provide an alternative to a prison sentence, it is particularly important to ensure that the court clearly understands the nature and likely success of the treatment, and the extent to which treatment may or may not influence re-offending risk. In cases where the clinical opinion is that treatment should be provided, but it will not necessarily prevent further offending, this needs to be carefully explained.

For most offenders with PDs, treatment is an enterprise that involves the offender working in partnership with clinicians; such treatment cannot be compelled and major short-term improvement is not to be expected. As with any patient who has chronic disabilities, the aim of treatment is long-term and rehabilitative in approach, with a focus on measures that promote and maintain the person's best possible level of functioning within their limits, together with extra support in times of crisis or deterioration.

Range of interventions

A wide range of treatment interventions may be considered in the management of offenders with PDs. These include a variety of psychotherapies, social support and, in a minority of cases, medication. Also, counselling for problems of drug or alcohol abuse may be needed. The treatment setting will usually be outpatient-based, with brief admission to hospital as a possible option at times of crisis. In a minority of cases longer-term specialized inpatient treatment may be indicated, but such facilities are scarce. In the UK, the Henderson Hospital provides 'therapeutic community' treatment in an open hospital setting, while offenders convicted of grave offences who are facing sentencing may be considered for treatment in 'special hospitals' if they meet the criterion for admission to maximum security, namely that they constitute a grave and immediate danger to the public. However, there must be careful consideration about what treatment is proposed, its availability and the prospects for success.

People convicted of sexual offences may or may not merit a diagnosis of

PD or other psychiatric disorders, but convicted sex offenders receiving non-custodial sentences may be considered for community-based treatment programmes, which, in the UK, are usually organized by the probation service. Residential group-based treatment in the UK is provided at the Gracewell Clinic, Birmingham. Programmes for sentenced prisoners serving 4 years or more have been established in a number of UK prisons, and the 'special hospitals' also provide treatment for some patients with histories of sexual offending.

Community and outpatient settings

The clinical management of offenders with PDs will often involve working jointly with other agencies, particularly the probation service in the UK, and as Joseph (1992) stressed, psychiatrists also need to work in close partnership with primary care physicians. In psychiatric outpatient settings, the medium through which care and treatment are provided is the relationship with the patient, and attention must be given to how the relationship is established and maintained. From the outset efforts should be made to ensure that the patient feels understood, and that there is shared agreement about realistic treatment objectives and mutual expectations. Offenders with diagnoses of antisocial or psychopathic personality disorders are particularly likely to have early histories of deprivation and impaired early relationships, sometimes associated with rejection or victimization of the child (Luntz & Widom, 1994). In adult life the patient may therefore be abnormally sensitive to perceived provocation or rejection, and particular vigilance and care is required at the outset in handling the first interview.

The adoption of a realistic attitude towards treatment goals is important clinically in order to ensure that the clinician and the patient commence with appropriate expectations of each other. It is also consistent with the available research evidence on the efficacy of treatment for psychopathic and antisocial personality disorders. As West (1983) emphasizes in his excellent brief review, treatment and rehabilitation programmes for offenders have generally not shown strongly beneficial effects in terms of reducing recidivism. However, he cautions against the adoption of a nihilistic attitude by clinicians towards antisocial offenders. As he notes, antisocial behaviour and delinquency cannot be separated from their social context, and it is social and educational intervention that is primarily needed. Thus, the relatively poor results of treatment programmes do not necessarily imply that offenders have not benefited individually, but they illustrate the fact that crime is overwhelmingly socially determined. Psychological changes in the individual may therefore have a relatively small overall influence on likelihood of reoffending. Nevertheless, continuing psychiatric interest and involvement in trying to help antisocial offenders should be maintained. As West (1983) suggests, a careful diagnostic approach is needed to ensure that any organic disorders and learning disability are identified. The secondary consequences of antisocial behaviour, including substance abuse, relationship and family disturbances, and any co-morbid psychiatric disorders need attention, and clinicians should work in close liaison with social and criminal justice agencies:

A developed anti-sociality syndrome is a serious maladjustment and an unhappy state of affairs for society and for the family as well as for the individual concerned (West, 1983).

The recent review of the effectiveness of treatment for psychopathic and antisocial PD by Dolan & Coid (1993) reached similar conclusions. They summarized the lack of good studies of the outcome of treatment in this area, although they noted some positive effects from studies of cognitive/behavioural psychotherapies, community supervision, and, in particular, therapeutic community approaches. Overall they concluded that: 'there is still no convincing evidence that psychopaths can or cannot be successfully treated' (Dolan & Coid, 1993). They urged caution in readily accepting the view that these patients are 'untreatable', noting that: 'the "untreatability of psychopaths" may, in part, result from the professionals' inadequate assessment in the first place, followed by an inability to develop, describe, research and adequately demonstrate the efficacy of treatment strategies' (Dolan & Coid, 1993).

Health care services have responsibilities to provide care and treatment for patients with PDs, and, in the UK, there has been an increasing emphasis during recent years on the adoption of the 'Care Programme Approach' (CPA) to the care of patients referred to psychiatric services. The key elements are: first, systematic assessment of health and social care needs; second, an agreed care plan; third, the allocation of a key worker to ensure the programme of care is delivered; and fourth, the regular review of the patient's progress and needs (Department of Health, 1990). The CPA has been recommended in the management of certain patients with PDs (Department of Health, 1994a), and such patients are also specifically included in the requirements on health authorities in the UK to establish, from October 1994, 'supervision registers' for patients who are at significant risk of suicide, severe self-neglect or of causing serious violence to others. The purpose of supervision registers is to identify and prioritize these patients, to provide care plans for them, and to ensure careful monitoring and planning for their care. The circular introducing these arrangements notes that: 'Mental illness in this context includes people with a diagnosed personality disorder, including psychopathic disorders, who are receiving treatment from specialist psychiatric services' (Department of Health, 1994*b*).

Providing a supportive relationship is of central importance in the management of offenders with PD. This needs to be consistent, tolerant and potentially long-term. Patients with disorganized and unstable lifestyles may have difficulty in maintaining regular outpatient attendance, and such patients may best be managed by an open-ended commitment to see them again on request at times of crisis. Contact may therefore be intermittent over a long period, and it will be necessary to make a fresh assessment on each occasion, and to work on any new problems that have arisen. Relatively dependent patients may need to be seen regularly over a very long period, and the management of such a relationship can be difficult. Limits may have to be set to ensure that the frequency and duration of contact is kept within reasonable bounds, but without losing an attitude of acceptance, 'professional friendship' and a willingness to increase support at times of crisis. For some patients, the relationship with the clinician may be the only long-term, confiding relationship that they have, and its importance should not be underestimated. A long-term perspective on the part of a clinician is required; over short- and medium-term time scales, support in a series of crises may be needed in the context of little change in the underlying PD, but over a few years the emotional and social stability of some offender patients can show unexpected improvement.

Psychodynamic psychotherapy

There is a consensus that engaging in psychodynamic psychotherapy with personality-disordered offenders on an outpatient basis should be approached with great caution; first, because of limited evidence of the efficacy of this approach, and second, because of an increased risk of disturbed behaviour. Malan (1979) recommended careful scrutiny of the individual's history when assessing the suitability for such psychotherapy because of the possibility that the most disturbed behaviour the person has exhibited in the past might be re-enacted during the therapeutic process. Main (1957) and Shapiro (1978) have provided good descriptions of the pathological transference and counter-transference relationships that patients with features of borderline PD may engender, with oscillation between extreme idealization and denigration of the therapist, and promotion of splitting and division between clinical staff (Kernberg, 1984).

Whilst most offenders with PDs are not suitable for individual 'psychodynamic psychotherapy' as described in Chapter 7, the clinician should retain an awareness of psychodynamic issues for three reasons. First, psychodynamic theories may be necessary in order to develop a proper psychological understanding of the patient's behaviour and the organization of his or her emotional life. Second, because the relationship with the patient is the medium through which the clinician works, and the dynamics of that relationship need to be recognised and understood. The emotions and attributions exhibited by the patient towards the therapist, and vice versa, need to be considered in terms of what they reveal about the patient's history and emotional life. Not uncommonly, patients who in early life have been subjected to cruelty or rejection develop similar pathological patterns of relating in adult life and these may begin to feature in the therapeutic relationship with the clinician. Care needs to be taken to recognize this and to avoid re-enacting rejection or punitiveness in the clinical relationship and attitudes to the patient. Third, offenders with personality disorders may sometimes present with a genuine desire for insight and self-understanding. They may be confused and distressed by their destructive behaviour, the chaos of their lives, and their inability to change. In taking the initial psychiatric history the clinician is likely to see links and continuities between patients' early life experiences and their problems as adults. Spending time over a limited number of sessions, taking the patient in detail through his or her life history, may help them see for the first time parallels between past and present. In reconstructing their biographies, patients can experience relief and illumination through recognizing the experiences that shaped their adult expectations and views of their social world. For example, suspiciousness and paranoid sensitivity in adult life, with a tendency to perceive threat and provocation in others and to react explosively, may have understandable links with childhood experiences of living in an early environment of genuine fear and threat of unpredictable violence. Patients can be helped to see the parallels between the way they view other people in their adult lives, and the way they experienced significant others as children, and thus how their distorted attributions and inappropriate responses arise. Although from a psychoanalytic perspective this work is superficial, it may, nonetheless, be safe and useful: it can be carried out over a limited period of time, it need not involve the development of difficult and dependent transference relationships, and its limited nature means that it is not too psychologically demanding of the patient.

However, it can also enable careful testing of the patient's capacity to accept interpretations and to see links between past and present, and in some cases this may help identify those patients who might benefit from long-term and more demanding psychodynamic psychotherapy. An important UK national centre specializing in outpatient individual and group psychoanalytic treatment of offenders is the Portman Clinic, Hampstead, London.

Cognitive psychotherapy and behaviour therapy

Short-term cognitive and behavioural treatments, focussed on specific symptoms or problem behaviours, may have a useful part to play in the outpatient management of some offenders with PDs. But such interventions should be seen as an adjunct rather than an alternative to long-term support. Clinical judgement is needed when considering such treatments, as more empirical evidence is still required for their efficacy in the management of offenders with antisocial PDs (Dolan & Coid, 1993).

Common problem-areas to which cognitive and behavioural treatments may have a contribution to make include social anxiety with avoidance, repeated aggression and violence, sexual offending and paranoid sensitivity. Specific problem-behaviours such as repeated shoplifting and compulsive gambling may also be helped by these approaches (Gudjonson, 1980; Greenberg & Rankin, 1982). The application of these techniques to problems of violence and sexual offending will be briefly outlined (also see Chapter 7).

In a cognitive-behavioural approach to anger management, patients can initially learn to identify the circumstances in which responses of rage occur and to keep records of their experiences. They can then be taught to view the onset of these situations as tasks to be worked through, rather than intolerable provocations, and they learn a variety of coping skills, including relaxation training. Their skills are then progressively tested.

Community-based treatment programmes for convicted sex offenders have been established in recent years by the probation service in many areas of the UK, while some sexual offenders (or non-offenders with deviant sexual behaviour) may be referred to psychiatrists. Treatment programmes (as described in more detail in Chapter 7) may focus on four problem areas: firstly, changing deviant sexual arousal; secondly, changing cognitive distortions about offending and its impact on victims; thirdly, improving social skills deficits; and fourthly, developing strategies for relapse prevention.

Sexual offenders may have a variety of distorted cognitions about sexual behaviour, sexual offending and the role of victims. Offenders against children, for example, may have fixed beliefs that their behaviour is an expression of affection or a harmless educational experience for the child. Kennedy & Grubin (1992) distinguished several different patterns of denial amongst imprisoned men convicted of sexual offences (see Chapter 7). The treatment of such cognitive distortions may involve individual sessions or be carried out in a group setting, and challenges may be particularly powerful in the group context. In view of this, the individual's capacity to cope with such pressure should be considered before embarking on such treatment.

Deficits in social skills may also be addressed in the context of group therapy, for example, using role-play, and may involve teaching appropriate assertiveness and social interaction skills.

Strategies for relapse prevention are also considered. Offenders are taught to identify the circumstances and events that may precede re-offending, and they may learn coping strategies for avoiding and coping with situations of risk. Offenders learn what constitutes a lapse in their individual case (e.g. use of alcohol or the onset of a deviant fantasy), and their task is to prevent this becoming a relapse. This approach is likely to be strengthened if it is carried out in the context of long-term supervision in which there is an expectation of open reporting by the offender, and the supervisor and offender work in close partnership in devising agreed strategies for the avoidance of re-offending.

It should not be assumed that a generic treatment programme can be devized that is suitable for all sexual offenders, as such individuals are heterogeneous in their sexual arousal patterns, cognitive sets, social skills, and motivation to change. They may also have a variety of other associated psychiatric difficulties. Other treatment methods may also help in some cases, for example the use of antiandrogen medication, particularly in older men who are distressed by high sexual drive, and whose consent and willingness to accept the medication is unequivocal. Careful assessment of the offender's needs, deficits and skills should be carried out in each individual case.

Statutory supervision in the community

In the UK, psychiatrists may be involved in the statutory outpatient supervision of two groups of offenders: sentenced prisoners released on parole, and conditionally discharged patients who had been detained in hospital under the provisions of mental health legislation (Restriction orders made under section 41, Mental Health Act, 1983).

Prisoners released on parole are under the supervision of a probation officer until the period of parole ends, and a condition of psychiatric supervision may be attached to the parole licence. Normally, the probation officer will have an informal discussion with the relevant psychiatrist as to whether psychiatric supervision would be appropriate and available before the decision to grant parole with a condition of psychiatric supervision is made, and the psychiatrist will liaise closely with the probation officer during the supervision period.

Life-sentenced prisoners released on licence in the UK may also have a condition of psychiatric supervision, or may be referred by a probation officer for voluntary psychiatric help in relation to a complex range of social and psychological difficulties following release from a long period in custody. Most life-sentenced prisoners in the UK are sentenced for homicide offences, and their victims are commonly partners or other close acquaintances. Family break-up as a consequence of their offences or the long-term imprisonment is common. Sapsford (1978) found that wives and girlfriends of male 'lifers' had nearly all lost contact by the end of the fifth year of sentence. Over half had no contact at all after conviction except to serve divorce papers. Life-sentenced prisoners are also a group with high rates of mental disorders (Smith, 1979; Taylor, 1986), and they have to face major problems of adjustment after prolonged detention. As is the case with other groups who have experienced prolonged captivity (Herman, 1992), they may present with chronic features of dysphoria, sleep disturbance, difficulties in coping with intimate relationships and loss of a sense of purpose for the future.

Ex-prisoners have a variety of social needs in areas of accommodation, employment, finance, social isolation, family difficulties and alcohol and drug use, and it is likely that the ex-prisoner's social situation has a significant impact on the likelihood of re-offending. A stable situation with family support and constructive activities, in other words a situation in which the individual has positive links with the community, probably helps reduce the risk of recidivism (Haines, 1990).

In England and Wales, mentally disordered offenders who are detained in secure hospitals under 'restriction orders' are likely to leave hospital in due course either on trial leave or by being conditionally discharged by a Mental Health Review Tribunal (or the responsible government minister, who is the Home Secretary). The total number of 'restricted' patients in hospitals in England and Wales was 2333 at the end of 1992, of whom just under a fifth (419) came within the Mental Health Act category of 'psychopathic disorder'. Two-thirds of these had committed offences of personal violence (including sexual offences). Just over half of all 'restricted' patients in England and Wales are detained in maximum-security hospitals (Home Office, 1994). In recent years approximately 200 'restricted' patients have been discharged to the community annually (Home Office, 1994). Conditionally-discharged 'restricted' patients remain liable to recall to hospital, and the conditions of discharge are likely to include supervision by a psychiatrist and a probation officer (or social worker), and there may also be conditions about accommodation and the continuation of treatment. The careful planning of community supervision and after-care for this group is particularly important. Close liaison between the psychiatric and social supervisors has to be maintained, and regular reports are submitted to the appropriate government department, known as the C3 Division of the Home Office. This is the administrative unit that specializes in mental health matters, and much of its work is concerned with the close monitoring of conditionally discharged 'restricted' patients. As a matter of good practice, the supervisors of restricted patients should keep in close touch with the Home Office officials in C3, who may often be able to give helpful information and advice. The Home Office also issues a useful set of guidance notes for supervising psychiatrists (Home Office/Department of Health and Social Security, 1987).

In terms of reconvictions, conditionally discharged patients with 'psychopathic disorder' have higher reoffending rates than patients with other forms of mental disorder (Home Office, 1993*b*). Bailey & MacCulloch (1992) followed up a series of 112 patients discharged from England's Park Lane secure 'special hospital' between 1974 and 1989. The follow-up periods varied between 9 months and 14 years, (mean 6 years). During the follow-up period, 13 of the 50 patients with 'psychopathic disorder' (26%) were reconvicted of a serious criminal offence, compared with six of the 61 patients with mental illness (10%). MacCulloch and his colleagues reviewed in detail the cases of serious reoffending (MacCulloch *et al.*, 1993*a*, 1993*b*, 1994) and drew particular attention to the lack of individual treatment programmes during the hospital admissions, aimed at deviant sexual behaviour, in those patients who were reconvicted of serious sexual offences.

Inpatient settings

Crisis admissions

While treatment and support for personality-disordered offenders is primarily outpatient based, short-term admissions may have a useful role to play in the management of crises. Short hospital admissions can be a useful safety net when individuals are seriously at risk. These patients may need admission when suffering from severe situationally determined depressive reactions, for example.

Brief admissions for assessment may also be appropriate when personality-disordered offenders are seen urgently at the request of the police or criminal courts. The offences may be the culmination of serious social and psychological difficulties and the offender may present in severe distress, sometimes associated with suicidal ideation and substance abuse. There may be a complex array of problems and it may not be possible to make an accurate assessment of the individual's needs, including whether there is a significant psychiatric disorder, without a period of observation in hospital. In England and Wales, a remand for assessment order (section 35 of the Mental Health Act, 1983) may be used in such cases, but recommendations for local hospital admission should take account of the nature of the alleged offence, to ensure that the admission is acceptably safe and not associated with a serious risk of absconding.

Inpatient therapeutic community treatment

Specialist inpatient treatment using a therapeutic community model is provided in the UK at the Henderson Hospital, Sutton, Surrey. The unit has 29 places for adults, and admission has to be on a voluntary basis following a selection interview. The ability to verbalize feelings and problems and to engage in a group setting are important for selection. The majority of the patients admitted have histories of drug abuse, alcohol abuse or criminal convictions, and the maximum length of stay is a year. Residents are expected to participate in a highly structured programme of therapeutic groups, community meetings, practical tasks and other activities, with the aim of achieving 'a therapeutic mixture of supportive containment and "reality confrontation" ...' (Norton, 1992).

Secure units and UK 'special' hospitals

Personality-disordered offenders constitute a minority of admissions to secure units and 'special hospitals' in the UK, and those who are admitted are generally sent by the criminal courts. Such individuals may be remanded by the courts for assessment (section 35 of the Mental Health Act, 1983), or for treatment under an hospital order (section 37 of the Mental Health Act, 1983). Those admitted to secure hospitals with the legal category of 'psychopathic disorder' have generally committed serious offences, and will have additional restriction orders (section 41, Mental Health Act, 1983). Some patients with 'psychopathic disorder' who are ready to be discharged from 'special hospitals' will be transferred to 'regional secure units' as a first step towards gradual rehabilitation in the community.

The question of whether offenders with serious PDs should be recommended for hospital and restriction orders under the provisions of mental health legislation as an alternative to sentences of imprisonment is controversial (Mawson, 1983; Grounds, 1987; Dell & Robertson, 1988; Chiswick, 1992). Although when grave offences are committed in the context of certain serious mental disorders such as schizophrenia, detention in a secure hospital is often generally accepted as an appropriate way of providing treatment that will reduce the risk of re-offending, in the case of PDs, the prospects of effective treatment are usually uncertain. This makes the selection of personality-disordered offenders for admission to a secure hospital very problematic. In practice, younger patients with significant anxiety, depression and distress, and who appear motivated to change, tend to be judged as most suitable, but there is little satisfactory empirical evidence about the factors that predict good and bad responses to clinical interventions. But the specific treatment programmes that have been developed use psychological methods that require the patient's active participation and commitment, so that motivation and capacity for psychological work is therefore an important practical consideration. Grounds *et al.* (1987) described the work of one unit in Broadmoor Hospital (a UK 'special hospital') specializing in the treatment of young men with 'psychopathic disorder'. The unit provides individual and group psychotherapy using psychodynamic and cognitive/behavioural principles, and a central focus is on seeking psychological understanding of the patient's offence.

The general criterion for admission to a secure 'special hospital' is that the patient constitutes a 'grave and immediate' danger to the public, and that the patient could not be safely managed in less than maximum security. In the UK each of the 'special hospitals' (Broadmoor, Rampton and Ashworth Hospitals) covers a particular geographical region, and applications for admission are considered by an admissions panel in each hospital.

Prisons

In the UK, it has been recommended that mentally-disordered offenders who need treatment should generally receive this in facilities that are outside the criminal justice system (Home Office, 1990). Imprisonment does not have treatment as its primary purpose, and psychiatrists and sentencers cannot assume that specific treatment will be provided if an offender is sentenced to imprisonment. The amount of psychiatric input to prison establishments is highly variable. Some prison health service doctors have psychiatric experience and some establishments have visiting psychiatrists, but many do not.

The frequency of violent and aggressive behaviour amongst prisoners is related, in part, to the character of the prison regime (Bottoms, 1992), and special prison units with radically different regimes have been developed in the UK with the aim of dealing in a more humane and effective way with 'disruptive' prisoners, for example the 'Barlinnie Unit' in Scotland. In England, Grendon Underwood Prison provides a specialist regime using a therapeutic community approach in which prisoners engage in demanding, confrontative group therapy. Although evidence is lacking that Grendon has a substantial impact on re-offending rates, it has been argued that for some well-motivated men the experience of Grendon does provide a unique opportunity for change (Robertson & Gunn, 1987).

Sexual offenders are a group particularly likely to be victimized in prison and may be isolated from other prisoners for their own protection. In recent years new efforts have been made in the UK to introduce treatment programmes for sex offenders, but only for those serving sentences of 4 years or more, and these programmes are available only in a limited number of establishments (Home Office, 1991). Prisoners serving less than 4 years may not receive any specialist help.

Assessments and reports for legal proceedings

The principles to be adopted when making assessments and writing reports for legal proceedings are essentially the same, irrespective of the particular issue being considered. The patient should be advised at the outset about the purpose of the assessment, the uses to which it may be put and the likely circulation of the report. The person should understand that what is said in the interview may not remain strictly confidential because the report may be seen by a variety of parties in the legal proceedings. Participation in the assessment has to be voluntary.

It is essential that any report is based on full information. If the patient is facing criminal proceedings, the reporting psychiatrist should see all the prosecution witness statements. The patient's background history should also be corroborated, if possible, by an independent informant. Reports should not be undertaken if all relevant information is not disclosed. In the criminal courts, if a report is based solely on what the defendant says without account being taken of other evidence, the report is unlikely to carry weight or credibility.

Reports should be clear and well organized in their layout and content. Customarily there is an introductory paragraph outlining the purpose and information sources of the report, followed by a summary of the relevant background history, the findings on psychiatric examination, and, finally, the concluding opinion on the questions at issue. Accuracy, clarity, and avoidance of technical vocabulary or emotive statements are necessary. The concluding opinions should be substantiated with a clear explanation of the reasons for the conclusions.

Psychiatric reports on personality-disordered offenders may be needed for a variety of purposes. Most commonly, reports will be requested for use in criminal proceedings when questions are raised about the person's state of mind at the time of the alleged offence, or when advice is sought in relation to a 'treatment disposal'. In England and Wales, reports may have to be prepared for Mental Health Review Tribunals, and in such cases the key questions are likely to be whether the patient still suffers from any form of mental disorder warranting continued detention in hospital for treatment, and whether they would pose a risk to others if discharged. Risk is also likely to be a key issue when reporting in other contexts on people with histories of offending, for example, for the parole board or for social services departments in child protection cases.

In serious criminal cases the judgement about whether to recommend a hospital order for subjects with PDs is, as noted above, a difficult one. If the offender is regarded as being within the legal category of 'psychopathic disorder', the requirement that treatment is likely to alleviate or prevent a deterioration in their condition has to be fulfilled if an hospital order is to be made. While, from a clinical viewpoint, motivation for psychological treatment is clearly important, it should be recognized that the courts may interpret a 'treatability' criterion more broadly than many clinicians. In the 'Andrews' case in the UK (R. v. Cannons Park Mental Health Review Tribunal. The Times Law Report 2 March 1994) it was suggested that the legal criterion of treatability would be fulfilled provided that hospital treatment would prevent deterioration. It would not have to alleviate the condition. Also, the absence of a patient's willingness to accept a specific form of treatment would not prevent the patient being regarded as 'treatable', if there was a reasonable prospect of benefit from treatment at some point in the future.

In cases of doubt, one possibility is to recommend an interim hospital order (under section 38 of the Mental Health Act, 1983), which would allow a trial period in hospital for 3 or 6 months before the court has to make a final decision about whether to impose a 'hospital order' under the provision of section 37 of the Mental Health Act, 1983.

Psychiatrists should also be aware of the possible consequences of reporting that a personality-disordered offender is not treatable and therefore unsuitable for a Mental Health Act order. Psychiatric evidence of untreatable PD may be used by sentencers as a reason for considering a longer-than-normal custodial sentence under the provisions of the Criminal Justice Act 1991 for offenders convicted of violent or sexual offences. In the most serious offences, such evidence may be used as an argument for a life sentence. The Court of Appeal has confirmed that the life sentence should be reserved for people who have committed offences of substantial gravity and who appear to be suffering from some disorder of personality or instability of character that makes them likely to commit grave offences in the future if left at large or released from a fixed term of imprisonment. (See R. v. Hodgson (1968) 52 Cr. App. R. 113, and R. v. Billam (1986) Cr. App. R. (S.) 347.)

In reports considering possible discharge from secure hospitals of offenders with 'psychopathic disorder', three aspects merit particular attention. Firstly, any current evidence of disorder and how much the patient has changed psychologically. Secondly, if the patient was detained because of a serious offence, there should be consideration of how well the offence is psychologically understood, and how much insight the patient has into the important factors that contributed to the offence. Thirdly, how 'supervisable' will the patient be? Do they recognize their need for supervision? Are they likely to disclose openly how they are managing and any problems that may arise? Do they recognize the difficulties that may lie ahead and will they use the supervisory relationship well?

Assessment of risk depends predominantly on history. There needs to be a thorough and detailed understanding of the patient's past history of offending, the context in which it arose, its precursors and the patient's psychiatric condition at the time. In looking to the future, and to the task of ongoing supervision, what should be looked for is the likelihood of any repetition of the context in which past offending occurred. The precise factors of importance will vary in individual cases. For example, in one case a key factor may be heavy alcohol intake, while in another it may be the establishment of a sexual relationship in which pathological jealousy begins to develop.

A useful checklist of key questions for the clinician when assessing the risk of future violent behaviour was given by Monahan (1981):

1. Is it a prediction of violent behaviour that is being requested?
2. Am I professionally competent to offer an estimate of the probability of future violence?
3. Are any issues of personal or professional ethics involved in this case?
4. Given my answers to the above questions, is this case an appropriate one in which to offer a prediction?
5. What events precipitated the question of the person's potential for violence being raised, and in what context did these events take place?
6. What are the person's relevant demographic characteristics?
7. What is the person's history of violent behaviour?
8. What is the base rate of violent behaviour among individuals of this person's background?
9. What are the sources of stress in the person's current environment?
10. What cognitive and affective factors indicate that the person may be predisposed to cope with stress in a violent manner?
11. What cognitive and affective factors indicate that the person may be predisposed to cope with stress in a non-violent manner?
12. How similar are the contexts in which the person has used violent coping mechanisms in the past to the contexts in which the person will be likely to function in the future?
13. In particular, who are the likely victims of the person's violent behaviour, and how available are they?
14. What means does the person possess to commit violence?

Social management

One of the key features of PDs, in particular when criminal offences are involved, is their damaging and disabling effects on social functioning. Both in their past histories and current situations, personality-disordered patients may have serious difficulties in their family and social relationships, and the clinical management has to include consideration of the social context. Interventions may be needed to try to facilitate the patient's social stability and, if possible, to prevent and mitigate socially damaging outcomes.

Relatives and partners may find the patient's behaviour intolerable or inexplicable, and they may also have unrealistic hopes or expectations about the person's ability to change, and the influence of treatment. They often need to be provided with explanation and support to develop a realistic appraisal of the nature of the patient's disability, together with guidance about how to manage difficulties and to protect themselves. Parents may have particular problems of unrealistic guilt and self-blame in relation to their children and they need sensitive advice and reassurance.

In cases where families and partners have been victims of violence, it is vital that they are given advice about possible future risks, and where this is significant they may need information about obtaining legal assistance and about places of refuge.

Patients with PDs may also pose problems for other agencies such as employers and housing authorities. The loss of stable accommodation and employment may put some patients at increased risk of depressive symptoms, of offending or of other disturbed behaviour, and it may be important to invest time in liaising with, and providing support to, these agencies, provided that the patient gives permission for disclosure of the relevant personal information. Residential provision may be difficult to secure when there are worries about the possibility of unstable and hazardous behaviour, but the knowledge that psychiatric backup with rapid intervention (for example, by a short crisis admission) will be provided may assist in securing suitable residential placements.

The most disorganized and chaotic individuals with PDs are likely to have recurrent breakdowns in their relationships, work and accommodation, and clinical staff need to maintain an attitude that combines realism and continuing commitment. Failure should not necessarily be greeted with surprise and refusal of further help. A long-term perspective should be maintained, as it is unrealistic to expect major short-term psychological change, but even when there is slow improvement over one or two decades, and clinical interventions over that time have helped to avoid serious harm to the patient or others, much will have been achieved.

References

Abraham, K. (1921). Contributions to the theory of the anal character. In: K. Abraham, *On Character and Libido Development*. New York: Basic Books, published in 1966.

Abraham, K. (1924). The influence of oral eroticism on character formation. In: *Selected Papers of Karl Abraham*, trans. D. Bryan & A. Strachy. New York: Basic Books, published in 1948.

Adler, D.A., Drake, R.E. & Teague, G.B. (1990). Clinicians' practices in personality assessment. *Comprehensive Psychiatry*, **31**, 125–33.

Adler, G. (1981). The borderline-narcissistic personality disorder continuum. *American Journal of Psychiatry*, **138**, 46–50.

Adler, G. (1985). *Borderline Psychopathology and its Treatment*. New York: Jason Aronson.

Adler, G. & Buie, D.H. (1979). Aloneness and borderline psychopathology: the possible relevance of child development issues. *International Journal of Psychoanalysis*, **60**, 83–96.

Akhtar, S. (1987). Schizoid personality disorder: a synthesis of developmental, dynamic, and descriptive features. *American Journal of Psychotherapy*, **41**, 499–518.

Akhtar, S. & Thomson, J.A. (1982). Overview: narcissistic personality disorder. *American Journal of Psychiatry*, **139**, 12–19.

Akiskal, H.S. (1983). Dysthymic disorder: psychopathology of proposed chronic depressive subtypes. *American Journal of Psychiatry*, **140**, 11–20.

Akiskal, H.S. (1991). Chronic depression. *Bulletin of the Menninger Clinic*, **55**, 156–71.

Akiskal, H.S., Hirschfeld, R.M.A. & Yerevanian, B.I. (1983). The relationship of personality to affective disorders: a critical review. *Archives of General Psychiatry*, **40**, 801–10.

Akiskal, H.S., Rosenthal, T.L. & Haykal, R.F. (1980). Characterological depressions. Clinical and sleep EEG findings separating subaffective dysthymias from character spectrum disorders. *Archives of General Psychiatry*, **37**, 777–83.

Alden, L. (1989). Short-term structured treatment for avoidant personality disorder. *Journal of Consulting and Clinical Psychology*, **56**, 756–64.

Alexander, F. (1930). The neurotic character. *International Journal of Psychoanalysis*, **11**, 291–311.

340

Allebeck, P. & Allgulander, C. (1990*a*). Psychiatric diagnoses as predictors of suicide. *British Journal of Psychiatry*, **157**, 339–44.

Allebeck, P. & Allgulander, C. (1990*b*). Suicide among young men: psychiatric illness, deviant behaviour and substance abuse. *Acta Psychiatrica Scandinavica*, **81**, 565–70.

Allebeck, P., Allgulander, C. & Fisher, L.D. (1988). Predictors of completed suicide in a cohort of 50 465 young men: role of personality and deviant behaviour. *British Medical Journal*, **297**, 176–8.

Allport, G.W. (1937). *Personality: A Psychological Interpretation*. New York: Holt.

Alm, P.O., Alm, M., Humble, K. *et al.* (1994). Criminality and platelet monoamine oxidase activity in former juvenile delinquents as adults. *Acta Psychiatrica Scandinavica*, **89**, 41–5.

Alnaes, R. & Torgersen, S. (1988*a*). DSM-III symptom disorders (Axis I) and personality disorders (Axis II) in an outpatient population. *Acta Psychiatrica Scandinavica*, **78**, 348–55.

Alnaes, R. & Torgersen, S. (1988*b*). The relationship between DSM-III symptom disorders (Axis I) and personality disorders (Axis II) in an outpatient population. *Acta Psychiatrica Scandinavica*, **78**, 485–92.

Alnaes, R. & Torgersen, S. (1990). DSM-III personality disorders among patients with major depression, anxiety disorders and mixed conditions. *Journal of Nervous and Mental Disease*, **178**, 693–8.

Alnaes, R. & Torgersen, S. (1991). Personality and personality disorders among patients with various affective disorders. *Journal of Personality Disorders*, **5**, 107–21.

American Psychiatric Association (1952). *Diagnostic and Statistical Manual of Mental Disorders*, 1st edn. Washington DC: American Psychiatric Association.

American Psychiatric Association (1968). *Diagnostic and Statistical Manual of Mental Disorders*, 2nd edn. (DSM-II). Washington DC: American Psychiatric Association.

American Psychiatric Association (1980). *Diagnostic and Statistical Manual of Mental Disorders*, 3rd edn. (DSM-III). Washington DC: American Psychiatric Association.

American Psychiatric Association (1987). *Diagnostic and Statistical Manual of Mental Disorders*, 3rd edn, revised, (DSM-III-R). Washington DC: American Psychiatric Association.

American Psychiatric Association (1994). *Diagnostic and Statistical Manual of Mental Disorders*, 4th edn. Washington DC: American Psychiatric Association.

Andreoli, A., Gressot, G. & Aapro, N. (1989). Personality disorders as a predictor of outcome. *Journal of Personality Disorders*, **3**, 307–20.

Andrews, G. (1991). The evaluation of psychotherapy. *Current Opinion in Psychiatry*, **4**, 379–83.

Andrews, G. (1993). The essential psychotherapies. *British Journal of Psychiatry*, **162**, 447–51.

Andrews, G., Neilson, M., Hunt, C. *et al.* (1990). Diagnosis, personality and the long-term outcome of depression. *British Journal of Psychiatry*, **157**, 13–18.

Andy, O.J. (1975). Thalamotomy for psychopathic behaviour. *Southern Medical Journal*, **68**, 437–42.

Argyle, M., Bryant, B.M. & Trower, P. (1974). Social skills training and

psychotherapy: a comparative study. *Psychological Medicine*, **4**, 435–43.
August, G.J., Steward, M.A. & Holmes, C.S. (1983). A four-year follow-up of hyperactive boys with and without conduct disorder. *British Journal of Psychiatry*, **143**, 192–8.
Baer, L., Jenike, M.A., Black, D.W. *et al.* (1992). Effect of axis II diagnoses on treatment outcome with clomipramine in 55 patients with obsessive-compulsive disorder. *Archives of General Psychiatry*, **49**, 862–6.
Baer, L., Jenike, M.A., Ricciardi, J.N. *et al.* (1990). Standardized assessment of personality disorders in obsessive-compulsive disorder. *Archives of General Psychiatry*, **47**, 826–30.
Bailey, J. & MacCulloch, M. (1992). Characteristics of 112 cases discharged directly to the community from a new special hospital and some comparisons of performance. *Journal of Forensic Psychiatry*, **3**, 91–112.
Bardenstein, K.K. & McGlashan, T.H. (1988). The natural history of a residentially treated borderline sample: Gender differences. *Journal of Personality Disorders*, **2**, 69–83.
Barley, W.D., Buie, S.E., Peterson, E.W. *et al.* (1993). Development of an inpatient cognitive-behavioral treatment program for borderline personality disorder. *Journal of Personality Disorders*, **7**, 232–40.
Barnard, M.A. (1993). Needle sharing in context: patterns of sharing among men and women injectors and HIV risks. *Addiction*, **88**, 805–12.
Baron, M. (1981). *Schedule for Interviewing Borderlines*. New York: New York State Psychiatric Institute.
Baron, M., Gruen, R., Asnis, L. & Lord, S. (1985). Familial transmission of schizotypal and borderline personality disorders. *American Journal of Psychiatry*, **142**, 927–34.
Bass, C. & Benjamin, S. (1993). The management of chronic somatisation. *British Journal of Psychiatry*, **162**, 472–80.
Bateman, A.W. (1993). Personality disorders. *Current Opinion in Psychiatry*, **6**, 205–9.
Beattie, J.O., Day, R.E., Cockburn, F. & Gary, R.A. (1983). Alcohol and the fetus in the west of Scotland. *British Medical Journal*, **287**, 17–20.
Beck, A.T. & Freeman, A. (1990). *Cognitive Therapy of Personality Disorders (with associates)*. New York: The Guilford Press.
Bellak, L. (1985). ADD psychosis as a separate entity. *Schizophrenia Bulletin*, **11**, 523–7.
Benjamin, J., Silk, K.R., Lohr, N.E. & Westen, D. (1989). The relationship between borderline personality disorder and anxiety disorders. *American Journal of Ortho-psychiatry*, **59**, 461–7.
Bentall, R.P., Claridge, G.S. & Slade, P.D. (1989). The multidimensional nature of schizotypal traits: a factor analytic study with normal subjects. *British Journal of Psychology*, **28**, 363–75.
Berelowitz, M. & Tarnopolsky, A. (1993). The validity of borderline personality disorder: an updated review of recent research. In: *Personality Disorder Reviewed*, ed. P. Tyrer & G. Stein, pp. 90–112. London: Gaskell.
Bergeman, C.S., Plomin, R., McClearn, G.E. *et al.* (1988). Genotype–environment interaction in personality development: identical twins reared apart. *Psychology and Aging*, **3**, 399–406.
Berlin, F.S. & Meinecke, C.F. (1981). Treatment of sex offenders with antiandrogenic medication. *American Journal of Psychiatry*, **138**, 601–7.
Bernstein, D. (1993). Childhood precursors of adolescent personality disorders.

Paper presented at the *Third International Congress on the Disorders of Personality*. Cambridge, Mass.

Berrios, G.E. (1993). European views on personality disorders: a conceptual history. *Comprehensive Psychiatry*, **34**, 14–30.

Beumont, P.J.V., George, G.C.W. & Smart, D.F. (1976). 'Dieters' and 'vomiters and purgers' in anorexia nervosa. *Psychological Medicine*, **6**, 617–22.

Bezirganian, S., Cohen, P. & Brook, J.S. (1993). The impact of mother–child interaction on the development of borderline personality disorder. *American Journal of Psychiatry*, **150**, 1836–42.

Biederman, J. (1988). Pharmacologic treatment of adolescents with Affective Disorders and Attention Deficit Disorder. *Psychopharmacology Bulletin*, **24**, 81–7.

Biederman, J., Faraone, S.V., Spencer, T. *et al.* (1993). Patterns of psychiatric comorbidity, cognition, and psychosocial functioning in adults with attention deficit hyperactivity disorder. *American Journal of Psychiatry*, **150**, 1792–8.

Biederman, J., Newcorn, J. & Sprich, S. (1991). Comorbidity of attention deficit hyperactivity disorder with conduct, depressive, anxiety and other disorders. *American Journal of Psychiatry*, **148**, 564–77.

Bion, W.R. (1961). *Experiences in Groups and Other Papers*. London: Tavistock Publications.

Birtchnell, J. (1991). The measurement of dependence by questionnaire. *Journal of Personality Disorders*, **5**, 281–95.

Black, D.W., Bell, S. & Hulbert, J. (1988). The importance of Axis II in patients with major depression. *Journal of Affective Disorders*, **14**, 115–22.

Black, D.W., Noyes, R., Pfohl, B. *et al.* (1993). Personality disorder in obsessive-compulsive volunteers, well comparison subjects, and their first-degree relatives. *American Journal of Psychiatry*, **150**, 1226–32.

Black, D.W., Yates, W.R., Noyes, R. *et al.* (1989). DSM-III personality disorder in obsessive-compulsive study volunteers. A controlled study. *Journal of Personality Disorders*, **3**, 58–62.

Blackburn, R. (1968). Personality in relation to extreme aggression in psychiatric offenders. *British Journal of Psychiatry*, **114**, 821–8.

Blackburn, R. (1971). Personality types among abnormal homicides. *British Journal of Criminology*, **11**, 14–31.

Blackburn, R. (1975). An empirical classification of psychopathic personality. *British Journal of Psychiatry*, **127**, 456–60.

Blackburn, R. (1984). The person and dangerousness. In: *Psychology and Law*, ed. D.J. Muller, D.E. Blackman & A.J. Chapman, pp. 102–11. Chichester: Wiley.

Blackburn, R. (1986). Patterns of personality deviation amongst violent offenders: replication and extension of an empirical taxonomy. *British Journal of Criminology*, **26**, 254–69.

Blackburn, R. (1988). On moral judgements and personality disorders. The myth of psychopathic personality revisited. *British Journal of Psychiatry*, **153**, 505–12.

Blackburn, R. (1989). Psychopathy and personality disorder in relation to violence. In: *Clinical Approaches to Violence*, ed. K. Howells & C.R. Hollin, pp. 61–88. Chichester: John Wiley & Sons.

Blackburn, R. (1992). Clinical programmes with psychopaths. In: *Clinical Approaches to the Mentally Disordered Offender*, ed. K. Howells & C.

Hollin. Chichester: John Wiley.

Blackburn, R. (1993). Biological Correlates of Antisocial Behaviour. In: *The Psychology of Criminal Conduct*, pp. 136–59. Chichester: John Wiley & Sons.

Bland, R.C., Newman, S.C. & Orn, H. (1988). Lifetime prevalence of psychiatric disorders in Edmonton. *Acta Psychiatrica Scandinavica*, 77 (suppl. 338), 24–32.

Blashfield, R., Sprock, J., Pinkston, K. & Hodgin, J. (1985). Exemplar prototypes of personality disorder diagnoses. *Comprehensive Psychiatry*, **26**, 11–21.

Blazer, D., George, L.K., Landerman, R. *et al.* (1985). Psychiatric disorders. A rural/urban comparison. *Archives of General Psychiatry*, **42**, 651–6.

Bleuler, E. (1908). *Textbook of Psychiatry*, trans. A.A. Brill. New York: The Macmillan Company, published in 1924.

Bleuler, E. (1911). *Dementia Praecox or the Group of Schizophrenias*. New York: IUP, published in 1950.

Bloch, S. (1979). Group psychotherapy. In: *An Introduction to the Psychotherapies*, ed. S. Bloch. Oxford: Oxford University Press.

Blum, H.M. & Marziali, E. (1988). Time-limited, group psychotherapy for borderline patients. *Canadian Journal of Psychiatry*, **33**, 364–9.

Blumer, D. & Heilbronn, M. (1982). Chronic pain as a variant of depressive disease. The pain-prone disorder. *Journal of Nervous and Mental Disease*, **170**, 381–406.

Blumstein, A. & Cohen, J. (1979). Estimation of individual crime rates from arrest records. *Journal of Criminal Law and Criminology*, **70**, 561–85.

Bodlund, O., Kullgren, G., Sundbom, E. & Höjerback, T. (1993). Personality traits and disorders among trans-sexuals. *Acta Psychiatrica Scandinavica*, **88**, 322–7.

Bohman, M., Cloninger, R., Sigvardsson, S. & Von-Knorring, A.L. (1987). The genetics of alcoholism and related disorders. *Journal of Psychiatric Research*, **21**, 447–52.

Bonnet, K.A. & Redford, H.R. (1982). Levodopa in borderline disorders. *Archives of General Psychiatry*, **39**, 862.

Bornstein, R.F., Klein, D.N., Mallon, J.C. & Slater, J.F. (1988). Schizotypal personality disorder in an outpatient population: incidence and clinical characteristics. *Journal of Clinical Psychology*, **44**, 322–5.

Bottoms, A.E. (1992). Violence and disorder in long-term prisons: the influence of institutional environments. *Criminal Behaviour and Mental Health*, **2**, 126–36.

Bouchard, T.J., Lykken, D.T., McGue, M. *et al.* (1990). Sources of human psychological differences: the Minnesota study of twins reared apart. *Science*, **250**, 223–8.

Bowden, P. (1991). Treatment: use, abuse and consent. *Criminal Behaviour and Mental Health*, **1**, 130–41.

Boyce, P., Hadzi-Pavlovic, D., Parker, G. *et al.* (1989). Depressive type and state effects on personality measures. *Acta Psychiatrica Scandinavica*, **81**, 197–200.

Boyce, P., Parker, G., Barnett, B. *et al.* (1991). Personality as a vulnerability factor to depression. *British Journal of Psychiatry*, **159**, 106–14.

British Association of Psychotherapists (1993). Information leaflet. 37, Mapesbury Road, London NW2 4HJ, UK.

Bronisch, T. & Klerman, G.L. (1991). Personality functioning: change and stability in relationship to symptoms and psychopathology. *Journal of Personality Disorders*, **5**, 307–17.

Brooks, R.B., Baltazar, P.L., McDowell, D.E. *et al.* (1991). Personality disorders co-occurring with panic disorder with agoraphobia. *Journal of Personality Disorders*, **5**, 328–36.

Brooks, R.B., Baltazar, P.L. & Munjack, D.J. (1989). Co-occurrence of personality disorders with panic disorder, social phobia, and generalized anxiety disorder: a review of the literature. *Journal of Anxiety Disorders*, **3**, 259–85.

Brooner, R.K., Bigelow, G.E., Strain, E. & Schmidt, C.W. (1990). Intravenous drug abusers with antisocial personality disorder: increased HIV risk behavior. *Drug and Alcohol Dependence*, **26**, 39–44.

Brooner, R.K., Greenfield, L., Schmidt, C.W. & Bigelow, G.E. (1993). Antisocial personality disorder and HIV infection among intravenous drug abusers. *American Journal of Psychiatry*, **150**, 53–8.

Brooner, R.K., Schmidt, C.W., Felch, L.J. & Bigelow, G.E. (1992). Antisocial behaviour of intravenous drug abusers: implications for diagnosis of antisocial personality disorder. *American Journal of Psychiatry*, **149**, 482–7.

Brown, G.W. & Harris, T.O. (1978). *Social Origins of Depression: A Study of Psychiatric Disorders in Women*. London: Tavistock Publications.

Brown, S.L., Svrakic, D.M., Przybeck, T.R. & Cloninger, C.R. (1992). The relationship of personality to mood and anxiety states: a dimensional approach. *Journal of Psychiatric Research*, **26**, 197–211.

Brownstone, D.Y. & Swaminath, R.S. (1989). Violent behaviour and psychiatric diagnosis in female offenders. *Canadian Journal of Psychiatry*, **34**, 190–4.

Burchard, J.D. & Wood, T.W. (1982). Crime and delinquency. In: *International Handbook of Behaviour Modification and Therapy*, ed. A.S. Bellack, M. Herson & A.E. Kazdin. New York: Plenum.

Burnham, D.L., Gladstone, A.I. & Gibson, R.W. (1969). *Schizophrenia and the Need-Fear Dilemma*. New York: International Universities Press.

Bursten, B. (1989). The relationship between narcissistic and antisocial personalities. *Psychiatric Clinics of North America*, **12**, 571–84.

Buss, A.H. & Durkee, A. (1957). An inventory for assessing different kinds of hostility. *Journal of Consulting Psychology*, **21**, 343–9.

Buss, A.H. & Plomin, R. (1986) The EAS approach to temperament. In: *The Study of Temperament: Changes, Continuities and Challenges*, ed. R. Plomin & J. Dunn. Hillside NJ: Lawrence Erlbaum.

Buydens-Branchey, L., Branchey, M.H. & Noumair, D. (1989). Age of alcoholism onset. Relationship to psychopathology. *Archives of General Psychiatry*, **46**, 225–30.

Cadoret, R.J. (1978). Psychopathology in adopted-away offspring of biologic parents with antisocial behaviour. *Archives of General Psychiatry*, **35**, 176–84.

Cadoret, R.J., O'Gorman, T.W., Troughton, E. & Heywood, E. (1985). Alcoholism and antisocial personality. Interrelationships, genetic and environmental factors. *Archives of General Psychiatry*, **42**, 161–7.

Cadoret, R.J. & Stewart, M.A. (1991). An adoption study of attention deficit/hyperactivity/aggression and their relationship to adult antisocial personality. *Comprehensive Psychiatry*, **32**, 73–82.

Cadoret, R.J., Troughton, E., Bagford, J. & Woodworth, G. (1990). Genetic and environmental factors in adoptee antisocial personality. *European Archives of Psychiatry and Neurological Science*, **239**, 231–40.

Cappe, R.F. & Alden, L.E. (1986). A comparison of treatment strategies for clients functionally impaired by extreme shyness and social avoidance. *Journal of Consulting and Clinical Psychology*, **54**, 796–801.

Carney, F.L. (1977). Outpatient treatment of the aggressive offender. *American Journal of Psychotherapy*, **31**, 265–74.

Carroll, K.M. & Rounsaville, B.J. (1993). History and significance of childhood attention deficit disorder in treatment-seeking cocaine abusers. *Comprehensive Psychiatry*, **34**, 75–82.

Casey, P. (1988). The epidemiology of personality disorder. In: *Personality Disorders*, ed. P. Tyrer, pp. 74–81. London: Wright.

Casey, P.R., Dillon, S. & Tyrer, P.J. (1984). The diagnostic status of patients with conspicuous psychiatric morbidity in primary care. *Psychological Medicine*, **14**, 673–81.

Casey, P.R. & Tyrer, P.J. (1986). Personality, functioning and symptomatology. *Journal of Psychiatric Research*, **20**, 363–74.

Casey, P.R. & Tyrer, P. (1990). Personality disorder and psychiatric illness in general practice. *British Journal of Psychiatry*, **156**, 261–5.

Casper, R.C., Eckert, F.D., Halmi, K.A. *et al.* (1980). Bulimia. *Archives of General Psychiatry*, **37**, 1030–5.

Castaneda, R. & Franco, H. (1985). Sex and ethnic distribution of borderline personality disorder in an inpatient sample. *American Journal of Psychiatry*, **142**, 1202–3.

Cavior, H.E. & Schmidt, A.A. (1978). Test of the effectiveness of a differential treatment strategy at the Robert F. Kennedy Centre. *Criminal Justice and Behaviour*, **5**, 131–9.

Chambless, D.L., Renneberg, B., Goldstein, A. & Gracely, E.J. (1992). MCMI-diagnosed personality disorders among agoraphobic outpatients. *Journal of Anxiety Disorders*, **6**, 193–211.

Chandrasekaran, R., Goswami, U. & Sivakumar, C. (1994). Hysterical neurosis – a follow-up study. *Acta Psychiatrica Scandinavica*, **89**, 78–80.

Chaplin, W.F., John, O.P. & Goldberg, L.R. (1988). Conceptions of states and traits: Dimensional attributes with ideals as prototypes. *Journal of Personality and Social Psychology*, **54**, 541–57.

Chapman, L.J., Chapman, J.P. & Raulin, M.L. (1978). Body-image aberration in schizophrenia. *Journal of Abnormal Psychology*, **87**, 399–407.

Chiswick, D. (1992). Compulsory treatment of patients with psychopathic disorder: an abnormally aggressive or seriously irresponsible exercise? *Criminal Behaviour and Mental Health*, **2**, 106–13.

Christiansen, K.O. (1974). The genesis of aggressive criminality. Implications of a study of crime in a Danish twin study. In: *Determinants and Origins of Aggressive Behaviour*, ed. J. de Wit & W.W. Hartup. The Hague: Mouton.

Christiansen, K.O. (1977). A preliminary study of criminality among twins. In *Biosocial Bases of Criminal Behavior*, ed. S.A. Mednick & K.O. Christiensen. New York: Gardiner Press.

Claridge, G.S. & Broks, P. (1984). Schizotypy and hemisphere function. I. Theoretical considerations and the measurement of schizotypy. *Personality and Individual Differences*, **5**, 633–48.

Clark, D.H. & Myers, K. (1970). Themes in a therapeutic community. *British Journal of Psychiatry*, **117**, 389–93.

Clark, L.A. (1989). *Preliminary Manual for the Schedule for Normal and Abnormal Personality (SNAP)*. Dallas TX: Department of Psychology, Southern Methodist University.

Clark, L.A. (1992). Resolving taxonomic issues in personality disorders: the value of large-scale analyses of symptom data. *Journal of Personality Disorders*, **6**, 360–76.

Cleckley, H. (1941). *The Mask of Sanity*. London: Henry Kimpton.

Cleckley, H. (1976). *The Mask of Sanity*, 5th edn, St. Louis, MO: Mosby.

Cloninger, C.R. (1978). The link between hysteria and sociopathy. In: *Psychiatric Diagnosis: Exploration of Biological Predictors*, ed. H.S. Akiskal & W.L. Webb, pp. 189–218. New York: Spectrum Press.

Cloninger, C.R. (1986). A unified biosocial theory of personality and its role in the development of anxiety states. *Psychiatric Developments*, **4**, 167–226.

Cloninger, C.R. (1987a). A systematic method for clinical description and classification of personality variants. *Archives of General Psychiatry*, **44**, 573–88.

Cloninger, C.R. (1987b). *Tridimensional Personality Questionnaire (TPQ)*. Department of Psychiatry and Genetics, Washington University School of Medicine, The Jewish Hospital of St. Louis: 216 S. Kingshighway Blvd. PO Box 14109, St. Louis, MO 63178.

Cloninger, C.R. (1987c). Neurogenetic adaptive mechanisms in alcoholism. *Science*, **236**, 410–6.

Cloninger, C.R., Christiansen, K.O., Reich, T. & Gottesman, I.I. (1978). Implications of sex differences in the prevalence of antisocial personality, alcoholism, and criminality for familial transmission. *Archives of General Psychiatry*, **35**, 941–51.

Cloninger, C.R. & Gottesman, I.I. (1987). Genetic and environmental factors in antisocial behaviour disorders. In: *The Causes of Crime: New Biological Approaches*, ed. S.A.Mednick, T.F. Moffitt & S.A. Stack, pp. 92–109. Cambridge: Cambridge University Press.

Cloninger, C.R. & Guze, S.B. (1970). Psychiatric illness and female criminality: the role of sociopathy and hysteria in the antisocial woman. *American Journal of Psychiatry*, **127**, 303–11.

Cloninger, C.R., Martin, R.L., Guze, S.B. & Clayton, P. (1985). Diagnosis and prognosis in schizophrenia. *Archives of General Psychiatry*, **42**, 15–25.

Cloninger, C.R., Sigvardsson, S., Gilligan, S.B. et al. (1988). Genetic heterogeneity and the classification of alcoholism. *Advances in Alcohol and Substance Abuse*, **7**, 3–16.

Cloninger, C.R., Svrakic, D.M. & Przybeck, T.R. (1993). A psychobiological model of temperament and character. *Archives of General Psychiatry*, **50**, 975–90.

Coccaro, E.F., Siever, L.J., Klar, H. et al. (1989). Serotonergic abnormalities in patients with affective and personality disorders correlate with suicidal and impulsive aggressive behavior. *Archives of General Psychiatry*, **46**, 587–99.

Cohen, G.H., Garey, R.E., Evans, A. & Wilchinsky, M. (1980). Treatment of heroin addicts: is the client–therapist relationship important? *International Journal of Addiction*, **15**, 207–14.

Cohn, L.D. (1991). Sex differences in the course of personality development: a meta-analysis. *Psychological Bulletin*, **109**, 252–66.

Coid, J.W. (1991). Psychiatric profiles of difficult/disruptive prisoners. In: *Special Units for Difficult Prisoners*, ed. K. Bottomley & W. Hay. Hull: Centre for

Criminology and Criminal Justice, University of Hull.

Coid, J.W. (1992). DSM-III diagnosis in criminal psychopaths: a way forward. *Criminal Behaviour and Mental Health*, **2**, 78–94.

Coid, J.W. (1993*a*). Current concepts and classifications of psychopathic disorder. In: *Personality Disorder Reviewed*, ed. P. Tyrer & G. Stein, pp. 113–164. London: Gaskell.

Coid, J.W. (1993*b*). An affective syndrome in psychopaths with borderline personality disorder? *British Journal of Psychiatry*, **162**, 641–50.

Coid, J., Allolio, B. & Rees, L.H. (1983). Raised plasma metenkephalin in patients who habitually mutilate themselves. *Lancet*, **2**, 545–6.

Coid, J.W., Wilkins, J. & Coid, B. (1992). Self-mutilation in female remanded prisoners II: a cluster analytic approach towards identification of a behavioural syndrome. *Criminal Behaviour and Mental Health*, **2**, 1–14.

Conte, H., Plutchik, R. & Karasu, T. (1980). A self-report borderline scale: discriminative validity and preliminary norms. *Journal of Nervous and Mental Disease*, **168**, 428–35.

Conte, H.R., Plutchik, R., Picard, S. & Karasu, T.B. (1991). Can personality traits predict psychotherapy outcome? *Comprehensive Psychiatry*, **32**, 66–72.

Cornelius, J.R., Soloff, P.H., Perel, J.M. & Ulrich, R.F. (1991). A preliminary trial of fluoxetine in refractory borderline patients. *Journal of Clinical Psychopharmacology*, **11**, 116–20.

Cornelius, J.R., Soloff, P.H., Perel, J.M. & Ulrich, R.F. (1993). Continuation pharmacotherapy of borderline personality disorder with haloperidol and phenelzine. *American Journal of Psychiatry*, **150**, 1843–8.

Copas, J.B. & Whiteley, J.S. (1976). Predicting success in the treatment of psychopaths. *British Journal of Psychiatry*, **129**, 388–92.

Coryell, W., Winokur, G., Shea, T. *et al.* (1994). The long-term stability of depressive subtypes. *American Journal of Psychiatry*, **151**, 199–204.

Coryell, W.H. & Zimmerman, M. (1989). Personality disorder in the families of depressed, schizophrenic and never-ill probands. *American Journal of Psychiatry*, **146**, 496–502.

Costa, P. (1993). Some implications of longitudinal personality research for the study of personality disorders. Paper presented at the *Third International Congress on the Disorders of Personality*. Cambridge, Mass.

Costa, P.T. & McCrae, R.R. (1992). The five-factor model of personality and its relevance to personality disorders. *Journal of Personality Disorders*, **6**, 343–59.

Cowdrey, R.W. & Gardner, D.L. (1988). Pharmacotherapy of borderline personality disorder: alprazolam, carbamazapine, trifluoperazine and tranylcypromine. *Archives of General Psychiatry*, **45**, 111–9.

Craft, M.J. (1965*a*). *Ten Studies into Psychopathic Personality*. Bristol: John Wright.

Craft, M. (1965*b*). The natural history of psychopathic disorder. *British Journal of Psychiatry*, **115**, 39–44.

Craig, A.R., Franklin, J.A. & Andrews, G. (1984). A rating scale to measure locus of control of behaviour. *British Journal of Medical Psychology*, **57**, 173–80.

Creed, F. & Guthrie, E. (1993). Techniques for interviewing the somatising patient. *British Journal of Psychiatry*, **162**, 467–71.

Crow, J.J. (1986). The continuum of psychosis and its implications for the structure of the gene. *British Journal of Psychiatry*, **149**, 419–29.

Crowe, R.R. (1972). The adopted offspring of women criminal offenders – a study of their arrest records. *Archives of General Psychiatry*, **27**, 600–3.

Crowell, J.A., Waters, E., Kring, A. & Riso, L.P. (1993). The psychosocial etiologies of personality disorders: what is the answer like? *Journal of Personality Disorders*, Spring suppl., 118–28.

Cutting, J. (1985). *The Psychology of Schizophrenia*. London: Churchill Livingstone.

Cutting, J., Cowen, P.J., Mann, A.H. & Jenkins, R. (1986). Personality and psychosis: use of the Standardized Assessment of Personality. *Acta Psychiatrica Scandinavica*, **73**, 87–92.

Dahl, A.A. (1993). The personality disorders: a critical review of family, twin and adoption studies. *Journal of Personality Disorders*, Spring suppl. 86–99.

Dalén, P. & Hays, P. (1990). Aetiological heterogeneity of schizophrenia: the problem and the evidence. *British Journal of Psychiatry*, **157**, 119–22.

Dalgaard, O.S. & Kringlen, E. (1976). A Norwegian study of criminality. *British Journal of Criminology*, **16**, 213–32.

Dalkin, T., Murphy, P., Glazebrook, C. *et al.* (1994). Premorbid personality in first-onset psychosis. *British Journal of Psychiatry*, **164**, 202–7.

Davidson, P.R. (1984). Behavioral treatment for incarcerated sex offenders: post-release outcome. Paper presented at *Conference on Sex Offender Assessment and Treatment*, Kingston, Ontario. March.

Davies, W. (1989). The prevention of assault on professional helpers. In: *Clinical Approaches to Violence*, ed. K. Howells & C.R. Hollin, pp. 311–28. New York: John Wiley & Sons Inc.

De Jong, J., Virkkunen, M. & Linnoila, M. (1992). Factors associated with recidivism in a criminal population. *Journal of Nervous and Mental Disease*, **180**, 543–50.

Delito, J.A. & Stam, M. (1989). Psychopharmacological treatment of avoidant personality disorder. *Comprehensive Psychiatry*, **30**, 498–504.

Dell, S. & Robertson, G. (1988). *Sentenced to Hospital*. Oxford: Oxford University Press.

de Maré, P.B. & Kreeger, L.C. (1974). *Introduction to Group Treatments in Psychiatry*. London: Butterworths.

Department of Health (1990). 'Caring for people': The care programme approach for people with a mental illness referred to the specialist psychiatric services. *Health Circular (90) 23/LASSL (90) 11*. London: Department of Health.

Department of Health (1994*a*). *Draft guidance on the discharge of mentally disordered people from hospital and their continuing care in the community*. London: Department of Health.

Department of Health (1994*b*). Introduction of supervision registers for mentally ill people from 1st April 1994. *Health Service guidelines (94) 5*. London: Department of Health.

Department of Health and Social Security (1985). Mental Illness Hospitals and Units in England. Results from the Mental Health Enquiry. *Statistical Bulletin*, Government Statistical Service. London: HMSO.

Dieckmann, G., Schneider-Jonietz, B. & Schneider, M. (1988). Psychiatric and neuropsychological findings after stereotactic hypothalamotomy, in cases of extreme sexual aggressivity. *Acta Neurochirurgica*, Suppl. 44, 163–6.

Digman, J.M. (1990). Personality structure: emergence of the five-factor model. *Annual Review of Psychology*, **41**, 417–40.

Dinwiddie, S.H., Reich, T. & Cloninger, C.R. (1992). Psychiatric comorbidity and suicidality among intravenous drug users. *Journal of Clinical Psychiatry*, **53**, 364–9.

Dinwiddie, S.H., Zorumski, C.F. & Rubin, E.H. (1987). Psychiatric correlates of chronic solvent abuse. *Journal of Clinical Psychiatry*, **48**, 334–7.

Docherty, J.P., Fiester, S.J. & Shea, T. (1986). Syndrome diagnosis and personality disorder. In: *Psychiatry Update*, vol. 5, ed. A.J. Frances & R.E.Halls, pp. 315–55. Washington, DC: American Psychiatric Press.

Dolan, B. & Coid, J. (1993). *Psychopathic and Antisocial Personality Disorders*. London: Gaskell.

Dolan, B., Evans, C. & Norton, K. (1994). Disordered eating behaviour and attitudes in female and male patients with personality disorders. *Journal of Personality Disorders*, **8**, 17–27.

Dowson, J.H. (1977). The phenomenology of severe obsessive-compulsive neurosis. *British Journal of Psychiatry*, **131**, 75–82.

Dowson, J.H. (1987). MAO inhibitors in mental disease: their current status. *Journal of Neural Transmission*, suppl. **23**, 121–38.

Dowson, J.H. (1992*a*). DSM-III-R narcissistic personality disorder evaluated by patients' and informants' self-report questionnaires. *Comprehensive Psychiatry*, **33**, 397–406.

Dowson, J.H. (1992*b*). Assessment of DSM-III-R personality disorders by self-report questionnaires: the role of informants and a screening test for co-morbid personality disorders (STCPD). *British Journal of Psychiatry*, **161**, 344–52.

Dowson, J.H. (1992*c*). Associations between self-induced vomiting and personality disorder in patients with a history of anorexia nervosa. *Acta Psychiatrica Scandinavica*, **86**, 399–404.

Dowson, J.H. (1994). DSM-III-R self-defeating personality disorder criteria evaluated by self-report questionnaire. *Acta Psychiatrica Scandinavica*, **90**, 32–7.

Dowson, J.H. & Berrios, G.E. (1991). Factor structure of DSM-III-R personality disorders shown by self-report questionnaire: implications for classifying and assessing personality disorders. *Acta Psychiatrica Scandinavica*, **84**, 555–60.

Dubro, A., Wetzler, S. & Kahn, M.W. (1988). A comparison of three self-report questionnaires for the diagnosis of DSM-III personality disorders. *Journal of Personality Disorders*, **2**, 256–66.

Duggan, C.F., Lee, A.S. & Murray, R.M. (1990). Does personality predict long-term outcome in depression? *British Journal of Psychiatry*, **157**, 19–24.

Easser, B. & Lesser, S. (1965). Hysterical character and psychoanalysis. *Psychoanalytic Quarterly*, **34**, 390–405.

Editorial (1994). Attention Deficit Hyperactivity Disorder in adults. *American Journal of Psychiatry*, **151**, 633–7.

Edwards, J.G. & Goldie, A. (1987). A ten-year follow-up study of Southampton opiate addicts. *British Journal of Psychiatry*, **151**, 679–83.

Elkin, L., Shea, T. & Watkins, J.T. (1989). National Institute of Mental Health treatment of depression collaborative research program. General effectiveness of treatments. *Archives of General Pychiatry*, **46**, 971–82.

Ellison, J.M. & Adler, D.A. (1990). A strategy for the pharmacotherapy of personality disorders. In: *Treating Personality Disorders*, ed. D.A. Adler, pp. 43–64. San Francisco: Jossey-Bass Inc.

Endicott, J. & Shea, M.T. (1989). Measurement of change in personality disorders. *Psychopharmacology Bulletin*, **25**, 572–7.

Ennis, J., Barnes, R. & Spenser, H. (1985). Management of the repeatedly suicidal patient. *Canadian Journal of Psychiatry*, **30**, 535–8.

Evans, C. & Lacey, J.H. (1992). Multiple self-damaging behaviour among alcoholic women. *British Journal of Psychiatry*, **161**, 643–7.

Eysenck, H.J. (1982). *Personality, Genetics and Behavior*. New York: Prager.

Eysenck, H.J. & Eysenck, S.B.G. (1964). *Manual of the Eysenck Personality Inventory*. London: University of London Press.

Eysenck, H.J. & Eysenck, S.B.G. (1975). *The EPQ*. London: University of London Press.

Fahy, T.A., Eisler, I. & Russell, G.F.M. (1993). Personality disorder and treatment response in bulimia nervosa. *British Journal of Psychiatry*, **162**, 765–70.

Faltus, F.J. (1984). The positive effect of alprazolam in the treatment of three patients with borderline personality disorder. *American Journal of Psychiatry*, **141**, 802–3.

Famularo, R., Kinscherff, R. & Fenton, T. (1991). Post-traumatic stress disorder among children clinically diagnosed as borderline personality disorder. *Journal of Nervous and Mental Disease*, **179**, 428–31.

Famularo, R., Kinscherff, R. & Fenton, T. (1992). Psychiatric diagnoses of abusive mothers. *Journal of Nervous and Mental Disease*, **180**, 658–61.

Farrington, D.P. (1978). The family backgrounds of aggressive youths. In: *Aggression and Antisocial Disorder in Children*, ed. M. Berger & D. Schaffer, pp. 98–122. London: Pergamon Press.

Favazza, A.R. & Conterio, K. (1989). Female habitual self-mutilators. *Acta Psychiatrica Scandinavica*, **79**, 283–9.

Fawcett, J. & Siomopouloo, J. (1971). Dextroamphetamine response as a possible predictor of improvement with tricyclic therapy in depression. *Archives of General Psychiatry*, **25**, 244–7.

Fenton, W.C. & McGlashan, T.H. (1989). Risk of schizophrenia in character disordered patients. *American Journal of Psychiatry*, **146**, 1280–84.

Ferguson, B. & Tyrer, P. (1988). Classifying personality disorder. In: *Personality Disorders: Diagnosis, Management and Course*, ed. P. Tyrer, pp. 12–32. London: Wright.

Ferguson, B. & Tyrer, P. (1989). Personality disorders. In: *The Instruments of Psychiatric Research*, ed. C. Thompson. Chichester: John Wiley & Sons.

Ferguson, B. & Tyrer, P. (1991). Personality disorder: the flamboyant group. *Current Opinion in Psychiatry*, **4**, 200–4.

Feshbach, S. & Price, J. (1984). The development of cognitive competencies and the control of aggression. *Aggressive Behaviour*, **10**, 185–200.

Fiester, S.J. (1991). Self-defeating personality disorder: a review of data and recommendations for DSM-IV. *Journal of Personality Disorders*, **5**, 194–209.

Fiester, S.J. & Gay, H. (1991). Sadistic personality disorder: a review of data and recommendations for DSM-IV. *Journal of Personality Disorders*, **5**, 376–85.

Foerster, A., Lewis, S., Owen, M. & Murray, R. (1991). Premorbid adjustment and personality in psychosis. Effects of sex and diagnosis. *British Journal of Psychiatry*, **158**, 171–6.

Ford, M.R. & Widiger, T.A. (1989). Sex bias in the diagnosis of histrionic and antisocial personality disorders. *Journal of Consulting and Clinical Psychology*, **57**, 301–5.

Foulkes, S.H. & Anthony, E.J. (1965). *Group Psychotherapy*, 2nd edn. Harmondsworth UK: Penguin Books.

Frances, A. (1982). Categorical and dimensional systems of personality diagnosis: a comparison. *Comprehensive Psychiatry*, **23**, 516–526.

Frances, A.J., Widiger, T.A. & Fyer, M.R. (1990). The influence of classification methods on comorbidity. In: *Comorbidity of Mood and Anxiety Disorders*, ed. J.D. Maser & C.R. Cloninger, pp. 41–59. Washington, DC: American Psychiatric Press.

Frank, J.D. (1974). The restoration of morale. *American Journal of Psychiatry*, **131**, 271–5.

Frank, J.D. (1979). What is psychotherapy? In: *An Introduction to the Psychotherapies*, ed. S. Bloch. Oxford: Oxford University Press.

Frankenburg, F.R. & Zanarini, M.C. (1993). Clozapine treatment of borderline patients: a preliminary study. *Comprehensive Psychiatry*, **34**, 402–5.

Frederiksen, L.W. & Rainwater, N. (1981). Explosive behaviour: a skill development approach to treatment. In: *Violent Behaviour: Social Learning Approaches to Prediction, Management and Treatment*, ed. R.B. Stuart, pp. 211–34. New York: Brunner/Mazel.

Freeman, C. & Tyrer, P. (1989). *Research Methods in Psychiatry*, ed. C. Freeman & P. Tyrer. London: Gaskell (Royal College of Psychiatrists).

Freud, S. (1955). On narcissism: an introduction. In: *Complete Psychological Works*, standard edn. pp. 135–243. London, UK: Hogarth.

Freud, S. (1957). *The Economic Problem of Masochism*, standard edn. vol. 14. London, UK: Hogarth Press.

Freud, S. (1959). Character and anal-eroticism. In: *The Standard Edition of the Complete Psychological Works of Sigmund Freud*, vol. 9, trans. J. Strachey. London: Hogarth Press (original work published in 1908).

Freud, S. (1961). *Complete Psychological Works*, standard edn. vol. 19. London, UK: Hogarth Press (original work published in 1924).

Freud, S. (1962). Introductory Lectures on Psychoanalysis. Lecture 21. In: *The Complete Works of Sigmund Freud*, vol. 16, pp. 320–338. London: Hogarth Press.

Freund, L.S., Reiss, A.L., Hagerman, R. & Vinogradov, S. (1992). Chromosome fragility and psychopathology in obligate female carriers of the fragile X chromosome. *Archives of General Psychiatry*, **49**, 54–60.

Furby, L., Weinrott, M.R. & Blackshaw, L. (1989). Sex offender recidivism: a review. *Psychological Bulletin*, **155**, 3–30.

Gabbard, G.O. & Coyne, L. (1987). Predictors of response of antisocial patients to hospital treatment. *Hospital and Community Psychiatry*, **38**, 1181–5.

Gardner, D.L., Leibenluft, E., O'Leary, K.M. & Cowdry, R.W. (1991). Self-ratings of anger and hostility in borderline personality disorder. *Journal of Nervous and Mental Diseases*, **179**, 157–61.

Gardner, D.L., Lucas, P.B. & Cowdry, R.W. (1990). CSF metabolites in borderline personality disorder compared with normal controls. *Biological Psychiatry*, **28**, 247–54.

Garfinkel, P.E., Moldofsky, H. & Garner, D.M. (1980). The heterogeneity of anorexia nervosa. *Archives of General Psychiatry*, **37**, 1036–40.

Gartner, A.F., Marcus, R.N., Halmi, K. & Loranger, A.W. (1989). DSM-III-R personality disorder in patients with eating disorders. *American Journal of Psychiatry*, **146**, 1585–91.

Gelder, M., Gath, D. & Mayou, R. (1983). *Oxford Textbook of Psychiatry*.

Oxford: Oxford University Press.

George, A. & Soloff, P.H. (1986). Schizotypal symptoms in patients with borderline personality disorders. *American Journal of Psychiatry*, **143**, 212–15.

Gill, K., Nolimal, D. & Crowley, T.J. (1992). Antisocial personality disorder, HIV risk behavior amd retention in methadone maintenance therapy. *Drug Alcohol Dependence*, **30**, 247–52.

Glenn, S.W. & Nixon, S.J. (1991). Applications of Cloninger's subtypes in a female alcoholic sample. *Alcohol Clinical Experimental Research*, **15**, 851–7.

Goldberg, D.P. (1972). The detection of psychiatric illness by questionnaire. *Institute of Psychiatry Maudsley Monographs*, no. 21. London: Oxford University Press.

Goldberg, S.C., Schulz, S.C., Schulz, P.M. *et al.* (1986). Borderline and schizotypal personality disorders treated with low-dose thiothixene vs placebo. *Archives of General Psychiatry*, **43**, 680–6.

Goldfried, M.R. & Goldfried, A.P. (1975). Cognitive change methods. In: *Helping People Change*, ed. F.H. Kaufer & A.P. Goldstein. New York: Pergamon Press.

Goldman, R.G., Skodol, A.E., McGrath, P.J. & Oldham, J.M. (1994). Relationship between the tridimensional personality questionnaire and DSM-III-R personality traits. *American Journal of Psychiatry*, **151**, 274–6.

Goldman, S.J., D'Angelo, E.J. & De Maso, D.R. (1993). Psychopathology in the families of children and adolescents with borderline personality disorder. *American Journal of Psychiatry*, **150**, 1832–5.

Goldstein, E.G. (1990). *Borderline Disorders: Clinical Models and Techniques*. New York: The Guilford Press.

Goldstein, J.M. & Tsuang, M.T. (1990). Gender and schizophrenia: an introduction and synthesis of findings. *Schizophrenia Bulletin*, **16**, 179–83.

Gordon, A.M. (1983). Drugs and delinquency. *British Journal of Psychiatry*, **142**, 169–73.

Gough, H.G. (1969). *Manual for the California Psychological Inventory*. Palo Alto, CA: Consulting Psychologists Press.

Greenberg, D. & Rankin, H. (1982). Compulsive gamblers in treatment. *British Journal of Psychiatry*, **140**, 364–6.

Griggs, S.M.L.B. & Tyrer, P.J. (1981). Personality disorder, social adjustment and treatment outcome in alcoholics. *Journal of Studies in Alcohol*, **42**, 802–5.

Grinker, R., Werble, B. & Drye, R.C. (1968). *The Borderline Syndrome*. New York: Basic Books.

Grobman, J. (1980). The borderline patient in group psychotherapy: a case report. *International Journal of Group Psychotherapy*, **30**, 299–318.

Grounds, A.T. (1987). Detention of 'psychopathic disorder' patients in special hospitals: critical issues. *British Journal of Psychiatry*, **151**, 474–8.

Grounds, A.T., Quayle, M.T., France, J. *et al.* (1987). A unit for psychopathic disorder patients in Broadmoor Hospital. *Medical Science and Law*, **27**, 21–31.

Grove, W.M. & Tellegen, A. (1991). Problems in the classification of personality disorders. *Journal of Personality Disorders*, **5**, 31–41.

Grueneich, R. (1992). The borderline personality disorder diagnosis. *Journal of Personality Disorders*, **6**, 197–212.

Gudjonsson, G.H. (1980). Psychological and psychiatric aspects of shoplifting.

Medicine, Science and Law, **30**, 45–51.

Gunderson, J.G. (1984). *Borderline Personality Disorder*. Washington DC: American Psychiatric Press.

Gunderson, J.G. & Elliott, G.R. (1985). The interface between borderline personality disorder and affective disorder. *American Journal of Psychiatry*, **142**, 277–88.

Gunderson, J.G., Frank, A.F., Katz, H.M. *et al.* (1984). Effects of psychotherapy in schizophrenia: II. Comparative outcome of two forms of treatment. *Schizophrenia Bulletin*, **10**, 564–98.

Gunderson, J.G. & Kolb, J.E. (1978). Discriminating features of borderline patients. *American Journal of Psychiatry*, **135**, 792–6.

Gunderson, J., Kolb, J. & Austin, V. (1981). The diagnostic interview for borderline patients. *American Journal of Psychiatry*, **138**, 896–903.

Gunderson, J.G. & Phillips, K.A. (1991). A current view of the interface between borderline personality disorder and depression. *American Journal of Psychiatry*, **148**, 967–75.

Gunderson, J.G., Ronningstam, E. & Bodkin, A. (1990). The diagnostic interview for narcissistic patients. *Archives of General Psychiatry*, **47**, 676–80.

Gunderson, J.G., Ronningstam, E. & Smith, L.E. (1991a). Narcissistic personality disorder: a review of data on DSM-III-R descriptions. *Journal of Personality Disorders*, **5**, 167–77.

Gunderson, J. & Sabo, A.N. (1993a). Treatment of borderline personality disorder: A critical review. In: *Borderline Personality Disorder*, ch.18, ed. J. Paris, pp. 385–406. Washington DC: American Psychiatric Press Inc.

Gunderson, J.G. & Sabo, A.N. (1993b). The phenomenological and conceptual interface between borderline personality disorder and PTSD. *American Journal of Psychiatry*, **150**, 19–27.

Gunderson, J.G. & Singer, M.T. (1975). Defining borderline patients: an overview. *American Journal of Psychiatry*, **132**, 1–10.

Gunderson, J.G. & Zanarini, M.C. (1987). Current overview of the borderline diagnosis. *Journal of Clinical Psychiatry*, **48**, 5–11.

Gunderson, J.G., Zanarini, M.C. & Kisiel, C.L. (1991b). Borderline personality disorder: a review of data on DSM-III-R descriptions. *Journal of Personality Disorders*, **5**, 340–52.

Gunn, J., Maden, T. & Swinton, M. (1991). *Mentally Disordered Prisoners*. London: Home Office.

Gunn, J. & Robertson, G. (1976). Drawing a criminal profile. *British Journal of Criminology*, **16**, 156–60.

Gunn, J., Robertson, G., Dell, S. & Way, C. (1978). *Psychiatric Aspects of Imprisonment*. London: Academic Press.

Gurman, A.S. & Gustafson, J.P. (1976). Patients' perceptions of the therapeutic relationship and group therapy outcome. *American Journal of Psychiatry*, **133**, 1290–5.

Guze, S.B. (1976). *Criminality and Psychiatric Disorders*. New York: Oxford University Press.

Guze, S.B., Wolfgram, E.D. & McKinney, J.K. (1967). Psychiatric illness in the families of convicted criminals: a study of 519 first-degree relatives. *Diseases of the Nervous System*, **28**, 651–9.

Guze, S.B., Woodruff, R.A. & Clayton, P.J. (1971a). A study of conversion symptoms in psychiatric outpatients. *American Journal of Psychiatry*, **128**,

643–6.
Guze, S.B., Woodruff, R.A. & Clayton, P.J. (1971*b*). Hysteria and antisocial behavior: further evidence of an association. *American Journal of Psychiatry*, **127**, 957–60.
Hadley, H. & Strupp, H.H. (1976). Contemporary views of negative effects in psychotherapy. *Archives of General Psychiatry*, **33**, 1291–5.
Haines, K. (1990). *After-care Services for Released Prisoners: A Review of the Literature*. Cambridge: Institute of Criminology.
Hall, C.S. & Lindsey, G. (1978). *Theories of Personality*, 3rd edn. New York: Wiley.
Halperin, J.M., Sharma, V., Siever, L.J. *et al.* (1994). Serotonergic function in aggressive nonaggressive boys with attention deficit hyperactivity disorder. *American Journal of Psychiatry*, **151**, 243–8.
Hamberger, L.K. & Hastings, J. (1988). Characteristics of male spouse abusers consistent with personality disorders. *Hospital and Community Psychiatry*, **39**, 763–70.
Hare, R.D. (1970). *Psychopathy: Theory and Research*. New York: Wiley.
Hare, R.D. (1980). A research scale for the assessment of psychopathy in criminal populations. *Personality and Individual Differences*, **1**, 111–17.
Hare, R. (1985). Comparison of procedures for the assessment of psychopathy. *Journal of Consulting and Clinical Psychology*, **53**, 7–16.
Hare, R.D. (1991). *The Hare Psychopathy Checklist – Revised*. Toronto: Multi-Health Systems.
Hare, R.D., Hart, S.D. & Harpur, T.J. (1991). Psychopathy and the DSM-IV criteria for antisocial personality disorder. *Journal of Abnormal Psychology*, **100**, 391–8.
Hare, R.D. & McPherson, L.M. (1984). Violent and aggressive behaviour by criminal psychopaths. *International Journal of Law and Psychiatry*, **7**, 35–50.
Hare, R.D., McPherson, L.M. & Forth, A.E. (1988). Male psychopaths and their criminal careers. *Journal of Consulting and Clinical Psychology*, **56**, 710–14.
Hart, S.D., Dutton, D.G. & Newlove, T. (1993). The prevalence of personality disorder among wife assaulters. *Journal of Personality Disorders*, **7**, 329–41.
Hechtman, L. (1991). Resilience and vulnerability in long-term outcome of attention deficit hyperactive disorder. *Canadian Journal of Psychiatry*, **36**, 415–21.
Heilbrun, A.B. (1982). Cognitive models of criminal violence based on intelligence and psychopathy levels. *Journal of Consulting and Clinical Psychology*, **50**, 546–57.
Heilbrun, A.B. & Heilbrun, M.R. (1985). Psychopathy and dangerousness: comparison, integration and extension of two psychopathic typologies. *British Journal of Clinical Psychology*, **24**, 181–95.
Henderson, D.K. (1939). *Psychopathic States*. New York: Norson.
Henderson, M. (1982). An empirical classification of convicted violent offenders. *British Journal of Criminology*, **22**, 1–20.
Henderson, M. (1989). Behavioural approaches to violent crime. In: *Clinical Approaches to Violence*, ed. K. Howells & C.R. Hollin, pp. 25–38. Chichester: John Wiley & Sons.
Herman, J.L. (1992). *Trauma and Recovery*. New York: Basic Books.
Herman, J.L., Perry, J.C. & Van der Kolk, B.A. (1989). Childhood trauma in borderline personality disorder. *American Journal of Psychiatry*, **146**, 490–95.

Herzog, D.B., Keller, M.B., Lavori, P.W. *et al.* (1992). The prevalence of personality disorders in 210 women with eating disorder. *Journal of Clinical Psychiatry*, **53**, 147–52.

Higgitt, A. & Fonagy, P. (1992). Psychotherapy in borderline and narcissistic personality disorder. *British Journal of Psychiatry*, **161**, 23–43.

Hill, D.C. (1970). Outpatient management of passive-dependent women. *Hospital and Community Psychiatry*, **21**, 38–41.

Hill, J., Harrington, R., Fudge, H. *et al.* (1989). Adult personality functioning assessment (APFA). *British Journal of Psychiatry*, **155**, 24–35.

Hinde, R.A. & Stevenson-Hinde, J. (1986). Relating childhood relationships to individual characteristics. In: *Relationships and Development*, ed. W.W. Hartup & Z. Rubin. Hillsdale, NJ: Lawrence Erlbaum.

Hirschfeld, R.M.A. & Holzer, C.E. (1994). Depressive Personality Disorder: clinical implications. *Journal of Clinical Psychiatry*, **55**, 10–17.

Hirschfeld, R.M.A., Klerman, G.L., Gough, H.G. *et al.* (1977). A measure of interpersonal dependency. *Journal of Personality Assessment*, **41**, 610–8.

Hirschfeld, R.M.A. & Shea, M.T. (1992). Personality. In: *Handbook of Affective Disorders*, 2nd edn, ed. E.S. Paykel, pp. 185–94. Edinburgh: Churchill Livingstone.

Hirschfeld, R.M.A., Shea, M.T. & Weiss, R. (1991). Dependent personality disorder: perspectives for DSM-IV. *Journal of Personality Disorders*, **5**, 135–49.

Hodges, J. & Tizard, B. (1989). IQ and behavioural adjustment of ex-institutional adolescents. *Journal of Child Psychology and Psychiatry and Allied Disciplines*, **30**, 53–75.

Hodgins, S. (1992). Mental disorder, intellectual deficiency and crime: Evidence from a birth cohort. *Archives of General Psychiatry*, **49**, 476–83.

Hoffart, A. & Martinsen, E.W. (1993). The effect of personality disorders and anxious-depressive comorbidity on outcome in patients with unipolar depression and with panic disorder and agoraphobia. *Journal of Personality Disorders*, **7**, 304–11.

Hoffart. A., Thornes, K., Hedley. L.M. & Strand, J. (1994). DSM-II-R Axis I and II disorders in agoraphobic patients with and without panic disorder. *Acta Psychiatrica Scandinavica*, **89**, 186–91.

Hollander, E., Stein, D.J., De Caria, C.M. *et al.* (1994). Serotonergic sensitivity in borderline personality disorder: preliminary findings. *American Journal of Psychiatry*, **151**, 277–80.

Home Office (1990). *Provision for Mentally Disordered Offenders* (Circular 66/90). London: Home Office.

Home Office (1991). *Treatment Programmes for Sex Offenders in Custody: a Strategy*. London: Home Office.

Home Office (1993*a*). *Criminal Statistics England and Wales 1992*. London: HMSO.

Home Office (1993*b*). *Life Licensees and Restricted Offenders Reconvictions: England and Wales 1990*. Home Office Statistical Bulletin 03/93. London: Home Office Research and Statistics Department.

Home Office (1994). *Statistics of Mentally Disordered Offenders: England and Wales 1992*. Home Office Statistical Bulletin 04/94. London: Home Office Research and Statistics Department.

Home Office/Department of Health and Social Security. (1975). *Report of the Committee on Abnormal Offenders*. London: HMSO.

Home Office/Department of Health and Social Security. (1987). *Mental Health*

Act 1983. Supervision and After-Care of Conditionally Discharged Restricted Patients: Notes for the Guidance of Supervising Psychiatrists. London: Home Office.

Horney, K. (1945). *Our Inner Conflicts*. New York: Norton.

Horney, K. (1950). *Neurosis and Human Growth*. New York: Norton.

Horowitz, M.J. (1989). Clinical phenomenology of narcissistic pathology. *Psychiatric Clinics of North America*, **12**, 531–9.

Horowitz, M., Marmar, C. & Weiss, D. (1986). Comprehensive analysis of change after brief dynamic psychotherapy. *American Journal of Psychiatry*, **143**, 582–9.

Horwitz, L. (1987). Indications for group psychotherapy with borderline and narcissistic patients. *Bulletin of the Menninger Clinic*, **51**, 248–60.

Howland, R.H. & Thase, M.E. (1993). A comprehensive review of cyclothymic disorder. *Journal of Nervous and Mental Disease*, **181**, 485–93.

Huesmann, L.R., Eron, L.D., Lefkowitz, M.M. & Walder, L.O. (1984). Stability of aggression over time and generations. *Developmental Psychology*, **20**, 1120–34.

Hull, J.W., Clarkin, J.F. & Alexopoulos, J. (1992). Time series analysis of interventive effects, fluoxetine therapy as a case illustration. *Journal of Nervous and Mental Disease*, **181**, 48–53.

Hunt, C. & Andrews, G. (1992). Measuring personality disorder: the use of self-report questionnaires. *Journal of Personality Disorders*, **6**, 125–33.

Hurt, S., Clarkin, J., Widiger, T. *et al.* (1988). DSM-III and borderline personality disorder: Decision rules and their implications. Paper presented at the *First International Congress on the Disorders of Personality*, Copenhagen.

Hurt, S.W., Clarkin, J.F., Widiger, T.A. *et al.* (1990). Evaluation of DSM-III decision rules for case detection using joint conditional probability structures. *Journal of Personality Disorders*, **4**, 121–30.

Hutchings, B. & Mednick, S.A. (1975). Registered criminality in the adopted and biological parents of registered male adoptees. In: *Genetics, Environment and Psychopathology*, ed. S.A. Mednick, F. Schulzinger & J. Higgins. Amsterdam: Elsevier.

Hwe, H.F., Yeh, E.K. & Chang, L.Y. (1989). Prevalence of psychiatric disorders in Taiwan defined by the Chinese Diagnostic Interview Schedule. *Acta Psychiatrica Scandinavica*, **79**, 136–47.

Hyler, S.E., Rieder, R.O., Williams, J.B.W. *et al.* (1988). The Personality Diagnostic Questionnaire: Development and preliminary results. *Journal of Personality Disorders*, **2**, 229–37.

Hyler, S.E., Reider, R.O., Williams, J.B.W. *et al.* (1989). A comparison of clinical and self-report diagnoses of DSM-III personality disorders in 552 patients. *Comprehensive Psychiatry*, **30**, 170–8.

Hyler, S.E., Skodol, A.E., Kellman, H.D. *et al.* (1990). Validity of the personality diagnostic questionnaire-revised: comparison with two structured interviews. *American Journal of Psychiatry*, **147**, 1043–8.

Inman, D.J., Bascue, L.O. & Skoloda, T. (1985). Identification of borderline personality disorders among substance abuse inpatients. *Journal of Substance Abuse and Treatment*, **2**, 229–32.

Jackson, H.J., Whiteside, H.L., Bates, G.W. *et al.* (1991). Diagnosing personality disorders in psychiatric inpatients. *Acta Psychiatrica Scandinavica*, **83**, 206–13.

Jaspers, K. (1946). *Allgemeine Psychopathologie*, 4th edn. Berlin: Springer.

Jenike, M.A., Baer, L., & Minichiello, W.E. (1986). Concomitant obsessive-compulsive disorder and schizotypal personality disorder. *American Journal of Psychiatry*, **143**, 530–2.

Jensen, J. (1988). Pain in non-psychotic psychiatric patients: life events, symptomatology and personality traits. *Acta Psychiatrica Scandinavica*, **78**, 201–7.

Joffe, R.T. & Regan, J.J. (1988). Personality and depression. *Journal of Psychiatric Research*, **22**, 279–86.

Joffe, R.T., Swinson, R.P. & Regan, J.J.(1988). Personality features of obsessive-compulsive disorder. *American Journal of Psychiatry*, **145**, 1127–9.

Johnson, C., Tobin, D. & Dennis, A. (1990). Differences in treatment outcome between borderline and nonborderline bulimics at one year follow-up. *International Journal of Eating Disorders*, **9**, 617–27.

Jordan, B.K., Swartz, M.S., George, L.K. *et al.* (1989). Antisocial and related disorders in a southern community. *Journal of Nervous and Mental Disease*, **177**, 529–32.

Joseph, P. (1992). Non custodial treatment: Can psychopaths be treated in the community? *Criminal Behaviour and Mental Health*, **2**, 192–200.

Joyce, P.R., Mulder, R.T. & Cloninger, C.R. (1994a). Temperament and hypercortisolemia in depression. *American Journal of Psychiatry*, **151**, 195–8.

Joyce, P.R., Mulder, R.T. & Cloninger, C.R. (1994b). Temperament predicts clomipramine and disipramine response in major depression. *Journal of Affective Disorders*, **30**, 35–46.

Judd, P.H. & Ruff, R.M. (1993). Neuropsychological dysfunction in borderline personality disorder. *Journal of Personality Disorders*, **7**, 275–84.

Kagan, J. & Moss, H.A. (1962). *Birth to Maturity*. New York: Wiley.

Kagan, J., Reznick, J.S. & Snidman, N. (1986). Temperamental inhibition in early childhood. In: *The Study of Temperament: Changes, Continuities and Challenges*, ed. R. Plumin & J. Dunn. Hillsdale, NJ: Lawrence Erlbaum.

Kagan, J., Reznick, J.S. & Snidman, N. (1988). Biological bases of childhood shyness. *Science*, **239**, 167–71.

Kahn, E. (1928). Psychopathic personalities. In: *Bumke's Handbook of Mental Diseases*, vol. 5, p. 227. Berlin: Springer.

Kaminsky, M. & Slavney, P. (1983). Hysterical and obsessional features in patients with Briquet's syndrome (somatization disorder). *Psychological Medicine*, **13**, 111–20.

Kandel, E., Brennan, P.A., Mednick, S.A. & Michelson, N.M. (1989). Minor physical anomalies and recidivistic adult violent criminal behavior. *Acta Psychiatrica Scandinavica*, **79**, 103–7.

Kandel, E., Mednick, S.A., Kirkegaard-Sorensen, L. *et al.* (1988). IQ as a protective factor for subjects at high risk for antisocial behavior. *Journal of Consulting and Clinical Psychology*, **56**, 224–6.

Karno, M., Golding, J.M. & Sorenson, S.B. (1988). The epidemiology of obsessive-compulsive disorder in five US communities. *Archives of General Psychiatry*, **45**, 1094–9.

Karpman, B. (1948). The myth of the psychopathic personality. *American Journal of Psychiatry*, **104**, 523–34.

Karterud, S., Vaglum, S., Friis, S. *et al.* (1992). Day hospital therapeutic community treatment for patients with personality disorders. *Journal of Nervous and Mental Disease*, **180**, 238–43.

Kass, F., MacKinnon, R.A. & Spitzer, R.L. (1986). Masochistic personality: An empirical study. *American Journal of Psychiatry*, **143**, 216–8.

Kass, F., Skodol, A. & Charles, E. (1985). Scaled ratings of DSM-III personality disorders. *American Journal of Psychiatry*, **142**, 627–30.

Kass, F., Spitzer, R.L. & Williams, J.B.W. (1983). An empirical study of the issue of sex bias in the diagnostic criteria of DSM-III Axis II personality disorders. *American Psychologist*, **38**, 799–801.

Kass, F., Spitzer, R.L., Williams, J.B.W. & Widiger, T. (1989). Self-defeating personality disorder and DSM-III-R: Development of the diagnostic criteria. *American Journal of Psychiatry*, **146**, 1022–6.

Kay, S.R., Wolkenfeld, F. & Murrill, L.M. (1988a). Profiles of aggression among psychiatric patients. *Journal of Nervous and Mental Disease*, **176**, 539–46.

Kay, S.R., Wolkenfeld, F. & Murrill, L.M. (1988b). Profiles of aggression among psychiatric patients. II. Covariates and predictors. *Journal of Nervous and Mental Disease*, **176**, 547–57.

Kayser, A., Robinson, D.S., Nies, A. & Howard, D. (1985). Response to phenelzine among depressed patients with features of hysteroid dysphoria. *American Journal of Psychiatry*, **142**, 486–8.

Kendell, R.E. (1983). The principles of classification in relation to mental disease. In: *Handbook of Psychiatry*, vol. 1, ed. M. Shepherd & O.L. Zangwill, pp. 191–8. Cambridge: Cambridge University Press.

Kendler, K.S. (1985). Diagnostic approaches to schizotypal personality disorder: a historical perspective. *Schizophrenia Bulletin*, **11**, 538–53.

Kendler, K.S. (1988). Familial aggregation of schizophrenia and schizophrenia spectrum disorders: evaluation of conflicting results. *Archives of General Psychiatry*, **45**, 377–83.

Kendler, K.S. & Eaves, L.J. (1986). Models for the joint effect of genotype and environment on liability to psychiatric illness. *American Journal of Psychiatry*, **143**, 279–89.

Kendler, K.S. & Gruenberg, A.M. (1984). An independent analysis of the Danish adoption study of schizophrenia. VI. The relationship between psychiatric disorders as defined by DSM-III in the relatives and adoptees. *Archives of General Psychiatry*, **41**, 555–64.

Kendler, K.S., Gruenberg, A.M. & Strauss, J.S. (1981). An independent analysis of the Copenhagen sample of the Danish adoption study of schizophrenia. II. The relationship between schizotypal personality disorder and schizophrenia. *Archives of General Psychiatry*, **38**, 982–4.

Kendler, K.S., Lieberman, J.A. & Walsh, D. (1989). The Structured Interview for Schizotypy (SIS): a preliminary report. *Schizophrenia Bulletin*, **15**, 559–71.

Kendler, K.S., Masterson, C.C., Ungaro, R. & Davis, K.L. (1984). A family history study of schizophrenia-related personality disorders. *American Journal of Psychiatry*, **141**, 424–7.

Kendler, K.S., McGuire, M., Gruenberg, A.M. *et al.* (1993a). The Roscommon Family Study. I. Methods, diagnosis of probands, and risk of schizophrenia in relatives. *Archives of General Psychiatry*, **50**, 527–40.

Kendler, K.S., McGuire, M., Gruenberg, A.M. *et al.* (1993b). The Roscommon Family Study. Schizophrenia-related personality disorders in relatives. *Archives of General Psychiatry*, **50**, 781–8.

Kendler, K.S., Neale, M.C., Kessler, R.C. *et al.* (1993c). A longitudinal twin study of personality and major depression in women. *Archives of General*

Psychiatry, **50**, 853–62.

Kendler, K.S., Ochs, A.L., Gorman, A.M. *et al.* (1991). The structure of schizotypy: a pilot multitrait twin study. *Psychiatry Research*, **36**, 19–36.

Kennedy, H.G. & Grubin, D.H. (1992). Patterns of denial in sex offenders. *Psychological Medicine*, **22**, 191–6.

Kernberg, O. (1967). Borderline personality organisation. *Journal of the American Psychoanalytic Association*, **15**, 641–85.

Kernberg, O. (1977). The structural diagnosis of borderline personality organization. In: *Borderline Personality Disorder*, ed. P. Hartocoullis. New York: International University Press.

Kernberg, O.F. (1984). *Severe Personality Disorders*. New Haven: Yale University Press.

Kernberg, O.F., Burstein, E., Coyne, L. *et al.* (1972). Psychotherapy and psychoanalysis: final report of the Menninger Foundation's psychotherapy research project. *Bulletin of the Menninger Clinic*, **36**, 1–275.

Khouri, P.J., Haier, R.J., Reider, R.O. & Rosenthal, D. (1980). A symptom schedule for the diagnosis of borderline schizophrenia. A first report. *British Journal of Psychiatry*, **137**, 140–7.

Kilzieh, N. & Cloninger, C.R. (1993). Psychophysiological antecedents of personality. *Journal of Personality Disorders*, Suppl. Spring, 100–17.

Kjelsberg, E., Eikeseth, P.H. & Dahl, A.A. (1991). Suicide in borderline patients – predictive factors. *Acta Psychiatrica Scandinavica*, **84**, 283–7.

Klassen, D. & O'Connor, W.H. (1988). A prospective study of predictors of violence in adult male mental health admissions. *Law and Human Behavior*, **12**, 143–58.

Klein, D.F. & Davis, J.M. (1969). The diagnosis of affective disorders. In: *Diagnosis and Treatment of Psychiatric Disorders*, 1st edn, ed. D.F. Klein & J.M. Davis. Baltimore: Williams & Wilkins.

Klein, M. (1985). *Wisconsin Personality Inventory (WISPI)*, Department of Psychiatry, 600 Highland Ave., Madison, WI 53792, USA.

Klein, R.G. & Mannuzza, S. (1991). Long-term outcome of hyperactive children: a review. *Journal of the American Academy of Child and Adolescent Psychiatry*, **30**, 383–87.

Kleinman, P.H., Miller, A.B., Millman, R.B. *et al.* (1990). Psychotherapy among cocaine abusers entering treatment. *Journal of Nervous and Mental Disease*, **178**, 442–7.

Klerman, G.L., Endicott, J. & Spitzer, R. (1979). Neurotic depression: a systematic analysis of multiple criteria and meanings. *American Journal of Psychiatry*, **136**, 57–61.

Klerman, G.L. & Hirschfeld, R.M.A. (1988). Personality as a vulnerability factor: with special attention to clinical depression. In: *Handbook of Social Psychiatry*, ed. Henderson & Burrows, pp. 41–53. Amsterdam: Elsevier.

Klinteberg, B.af., Schalling, D., Edman, G. *et al.* (1987). Personality correlates of platelet monoamine oxidase (MAO) activity in female and male subjects. *Neuropsychobiology*, **18**, 89–96.

Knight, R.P. (1953). Borderline states. *Bulletin of the Menninger Clinic*, **17**, 1–12.

Koch, J.L.A. (1891). *Die Psychopathischen Minderwertigkeiten*. Ravensburg: Dorn.

Kohut, H. (1968). The psychoanalytic treatment of narcissistic personality disorders. *Psychoanalytic Study of the Child*, **23**, 86–113.

Kohut, H. (1977). *The Restoration of Self*. New York: International Universities

Press.

Kolb, J.E. & Gunderson, J.G. (1990). Psychodynamic psychotherapy of borderline patients. *International Review of Psycho-Analysis*, **17**, 515–6.

Kolb, L. (1982). Assertive traits fostering social adaptation and creativity. *Psychiatric Journal of the University of Ottawa*, **7**, 219–25.

Korn, M.L., Botsis, A.J. Kotler, M. *et al.* (1992). The suicide and aggression survey: a semistructured instrument for the measurement of suicidality and aggression. *Comprehensive Psychiatry*, **33**, 359–65.

Kraepelin, E. (1905). *Lectures on Clinical Psychiatry*, 2nd edn, trans. T. Johnstone. London: Baillière Tindall & Co.

Kraepelin, E. (1921). *Manic-Depressive Insanity and Paranoia*, trans. R.M. Barclay, ed. G.M. Robertson. Edinburgh: E. & S. Livingstone.

Krafft-Ebing, R. (1901). *Psychopathia Sexualis: A Medico-Forensic Study*. New York: Pioneer Publications (published in 1950).

Krarup, G., Nielsen, B., Rask, P. & Petersen, P. (1991). Childhood experiences and repeated suicidal behavior. *Acta Psychiatrica Scandinavica*, **83**, 16–19.

Kreeger, L. (1975). *The Large Group*, ed. L. Kreeger. London: Constable.

Kretchmer, E. (1918). *Der Sensitive Beziehungswahn*. Berlin: Springer.

Kretchmer, E. (1922). *Korperban und Charakter*. Berlin: Springer.

Kretchmer, E. (1925). *Physique and Character*. New York: Harcourt Brace; London: Kegan-Paul, Trench & Trabner.

Kretsch, R., Goren, Y. & Wasserman, A. (1987). Change patterns of borderline patients in individual and group therapy. *International Journal of Group Psychotherapy*, **37**, 95–112.

Kroll, J.L., Carey, K.S. & Sines, L.K. (1985). Twenty-year follow-up of borderline personality disorder: a pilot study. In: *IV World Congress of Biological Psychiatry*, vol. 3, ed. C. Stragass. New York: Elsevier.

Krupnick, J.L. & Pincus, H.A. (1992). The cost-effectiveness of psychotherapy: a plan for research. *American Journal of Psychiatry*, **149**, 1295–1305.

Kullgren, G. (1988). Factors associated with completed suicide in borderline personality disorder. *Journal of Nervous and Mental Disease*, **176**, 40–4.

Kumar, H.V., McMahon, K.J., Allman, K.M. *et al.* (1989). Pericentric inversion chromosome 9 and personality disorder. *British Journal of Psychiatry*, **155**, 408–10.

Kune, G., Kune, S., Watson, L.F. & Bahnson, C.B. (1991). Personality as a risk factor in large bowel cancer: data from the Melbourne Colorectal Cancer Study. *Psychological Medicine*, **21**, 29–41.

Lacey, J.H. (1984). Moderation of bulimia. *Journal of Psychosomatic Research*, **28**, 397–402.

Lahmeyer, H.W., Reynolds, C.F., Kupfer, D.J. & King, R. (1989). Biologic markers in borderline personality disorder: a review. *Journal of Clinical Psychiatry*, **50**, 217–25.

Laitinen, L.V. (1988). Psychosurgery today. *Acta Neurochirurgica*, Suppl. 44, 158–62.

Lane, P.J. & Kling, J. (1979). Construct validity of the overcontrolled hostility scale of the MMPI. *Journal of Consulting and Clinical Psychology*, **47**, 781–2.

Lazare, A. (1971). The hysterical character in psychoanalytic theory. *Archives of General Psychiatry*, **25**, 131–7.

Lazare, A., Klerman, G. & Armor, D.J. (1966). Oral, obsessive and hysterical personality patterns. *Archives of General Psychiatry*, **14**, 624–30.

Lazare, A., Klerman, G. & Armor, D.J. (1970). Oral, obsessive and hysterical personality patterns: replications of factor analysis in an independent sample. *Journal of Psychiatric Research*, 7, 275–9.

Leff, J.P. & Isaacs, A.D. (1990). History-taking: The personal background. In: *Psychiatric Examination in Clinical Practice*, 3rd edn, pp. 13–26. Oxford: Blackwell Scientific Publications.

Leonhard, K. (1968). *Akzentuierte Persönlichkeiten*. Berlin: Verlag Volk und Gesundheit.

Lesieur, H.R. & Blume, S.B. (1987). The South Oaks Gambling Screen (SOGS). *American Journal of Psychiatry*, 144, 1184–8.

Levitt, A.J., Joffe, R.T., Ennis, J. *et al.* (1990). The prevalence of cyclothymia in borderline personality disorder. *Journal of Clinical Psychiatry*, 51, 335–9.

Lewis, G. & Appleby, L. (1988). Personality disorder: the patients psychiatrists dislike. *British Journal of Psychiatry*, 153, 44–49.

Lewis, S.J. & Harder, D.W. (1991). A comparison of four measures to diagnose DSM-III-R borderline personality disorder in outpatients. *Journal of Nervous and Mental Disease*, 179, 329–37.

Liberman, R.P. & Eckman, T. (1981). Behaviour therapy vs insight-orientated therapy for repeated suicide attempters. *Archives of General Psychiatry*, 38, 1126–30.

Lie, N. (1992). Follow-ups of children with attention deficit hyperactivity disorder (ADHD). *Acta Psychiatrica Scandinavica*, suppl. 85, 1–40.

Liebowitz, M.R. & Klein, D.F. (1979). Hysteroid dysphoria. *Psychiatric Clinics of North America*, 2, 555–75.

Liebowitz, M.R. & Klein, D.F. (1981). Interrelationship of hysteroid dysphoria and borderline personality disorder. *Psychiatric Clinics of North America*, 4, 67–87.

Lilienfeld, S., Van Volkenburg, C., Larntz, K. & Akiskal, H. (1986). The relationship of histrionic personality disorder to antisocial personality and somatization disorder. *American Journal of Psychiatry*, 143, 718–22.

Linehan, M.M. (1987). Dialectical behavioral therapy: a cognitive behavioral approach to parasuicide. *Journal of Personality Disorders*, 1, 328–33.

Linehan, M.M., Heard, H.L. & Armstrong, H.E. (1993). Naturalistic follow-up of a behavioral treatment for chronically parasuicidal borderline patients. *Archives of General Psychiatry*, 50, 971–4.

Linehan, M.M., Hubert, A.E., Suarez, A. *et al.* (1991). Cognitive-behavioral treatment of chronically parasuicidal borderline patients. *Archives of General Psychiatry*, 48, 1060–4.

Links, P. (1993). Seven Year Follow-Up Study of Borderline Personality Disorder: Factors Predicting Persistence. Paper presented at *Third International Congress on the Disorders of Personality*. Cambridge, Mass.

Links, P.S., Mitton, J.E. & Steiner, M. (1990). Predicting outcome for borderline personality disorder. *Comprehensive Psychiatry*, 31, 490–8.

Linnoila, V.M.I. & Virkkunen, M. (1992). Aggression, suicidality and serotonin. *Journal of Clinical Psychiatry*, 53(10 Suppl.), 46–51.

Liskow, B., Powell, B.J., Nickel, E.J. & Penick, E. (1990). Diagnostic subgroups of antisocial alcoholics: outcome at 1 year. *Comprehensive Psychiatry*, 31, 549–56.

Livesley, W.J. (1991). Classifying personality disorders: ideal types, prototypes, or dimensions? *Journal of Personality Disorders*, 5, 52–9.

Livesley, W.J. & Jackson, D.N. (1992). Guidelines for developing, evaluating and revising the classification of personality disorders. *Journal of Nervous and*

Mental Disease, **180**, 609–18.

Livesley, W.J., Jong, K.L., Jackson, D.N. & Vernon, P.A. (1993). Genetic and environmental contributions to dimensions of personality disorder. *American Journal of Psychiatry*, **150**, 1826–31.

Livesley, W.J. & Schroeder, M.L. (1990). Dimensions of personality disorder. *Journal of Nervous and Mental Disease*, **178**, 627–35.

Livesley, W.J. & Schroeder, M.L. (1991). Dimensions of personality disorder. The DSM-III-R cluster B diagnosis. *Journal of Nervous and Mental Disease*, **179**, 320–8.

Livesley, W.J., Schroeder, M.L. & Jackson, D.N. (1990). Dependent personality disorder and attachment problems. *Journal of Personality Disorders*, **4**, 232–40.

Loeber, R. (1990). Development and risk factors of juvenile antisocial behaviour and delinquency. *Clinical Psychology Review*, **10**, 1–41.

Lofgren, D.P., Bemporad, J., King, J. *et al.* (1991). A prospective follow-up study of so-called borderline children. *American Journal of Psychiatry*, **148**, 1541–7.

Loranger, A.W., Hirschfeld, R.M.A., Sartorius, N. & Regier, D.A. (1991). The WHO/ADAMHA international pilot study of personality disorders: background and purpose. *Journal of Personality Disorders*, **5**, 296–306.

Loranger, A.W., Lenzenweger, M.F., Gartner, A.F. *et al.* (1991). Trait-state artifacts and the diagnosis of personality disorders. *Archives of General Psychiatry*, **48**, 720–8.

Loranger, A., Oldham, J. & Tullis, E. (1982). Familial transmission of DSM-III borderline personality disorder. *Archives of General Psychiatry*, **39**, 795–9.

Loranger, A., Susman V., Oldham, J. & Russaroff, L.M. (1987). The personality disorder examination: a preliminary report. *Journal of Personality Disorders*, **1**, 1–13.

Luborsky, L. (1984). *Principles of Psychoanalytic Psychotherapy. A Manual for Supportive-Expressive Treatment*. New York: Basic.

Lucas, P.B., Gardner, D.L., Wolkowitz, O.M. & Cowdry, R.W. (1987). Dysphoria associated with methylphenidate infusion in borderline personality disorder. *American Journal of Psychiatry*, **144**, 1577–9.

Luntz, B.K. & Widom, C.S. (1994). Antisocial personality disorder in abused children grown up. *American Journal of Psychiatry*, **151**, 670–4.

Lykouras, E., Markianos, M. & Moussas, G. (1989). Platelet monoamine oxidase, plasma dopamine β-hydroxylase activity, dementia and family history of alcoholism in chronic alcoholics. *Acta Psychiatrica Scandinavica*, **80**, 487–91.

Macaskill, N.D. (1982). Therapeutic factors in group therapy with borderline patients. *International Journal of Group Psychotherapy*, **32**, 61–74.

MacCulloch, M., Bailey, J., Jones, C. & Hunter, C. (1993a). Nineteen serious reoffenders who were discharged direct to the community from a special hospital: 1. General characteristics. *Journal of Forensic Psychiatry*, **4**, 237–48.

MacCulloch, M., Bailey, J., Jones, C. & Hunter, C. (1993b). Nineteen serious reoffenders who were discharged direct to the community from a special hospital: 2. Illustrated clinical issues. *Journal of Forensic Psychiatry*, **3**, 451–70.

MacCulloch, M., Bailey, J., Jones, C. & Hunter, C. (1994). Nineteen serious reoffenders who were discharged direct to the community from a special hospital: 3. Illustrated administrative issues. *Journal of Forensic Psychiatry*, **5**, 63–82.

Maden, T., Swinton, M. & Gunn, J. (1994). Psychiatric disorder in women serving a prison sentence. *British Journal of Psychiatry*, **164**, 44–54.

Maier, W., Lichtermann, D., Klingler, T. *et al.* (1992). Prevalence of personality disorders (DSM-III-R) in the community. *Journal of Personality Disorders*, **6**, 187–96.

Main, T.F. (1946). The hospital as a therapeutic institution. *Bulletin of the Menninger Clinic*, **10**, 66–71.

Main, T.F. (1957). The ailment. *British Journal of Medical Psychology*, **30**, 129–45.

Malan, D.H. (1973). The outcome problem in psychotherapy research. *Archives of General Psychiatry*, **29**, 719–23.

Malan, D.H. (1979). *Individual Psychotherapy and the Science of Psychodynamics*. London: Butterworth.

Malan, D.H., Balfour, F.H.G., Hood, V.G. & Shooter, M.N. (1976). Group psychotherapy. *Archives of General Psychiatry*, **33**, 1303–9.

Malloy, R., Noel, N., Longabaugh, R. & Beattie, M. (1990). Determinants of neuropsychological impairment in antisocial substance abusers. *Addictive Behavior*, **15**, 431–8.

Malow, R.M., West, J.A., Williams, J.L. & Sutker, P.B. (1989). Personality disorders classifications and symptoms in cocaine and opioid addicts. *Journal of Consulting and Clinical Psychology*, **57**, 765–7.

Mann, A.H., Jenkins, R., Cutting, J.C. & Cowen, P.T. (1981). The development and use of a standardized assessment of abnormal personality. *Psychological Medicine*, **11**, 839–47.

Mann, J. (1973). *Time-Limited Psychotherapy*. Cambridge, MA: Harvard University Press.

Mannuzza, S., Klein, R.G., Bessler, A. *et al.* (1993). Adult outcome of hyperactive boys: educational achievement, occupational rank, and psychiatric status. *Archives of General Psychiatry*, **50**, 565–76.

Mannuzza, S., Klein, R.G., Boragura, N. *et al.* (1991). Hyperactive boys almost grown up. Replication of psychiatric status. *Archives of General Psychiatry*, **48**, 77–83.

Mannuzza, S., Klein, R.G., Konig, P.H. & Giampino, T.L. (1989). Hyperactive boys almost grown up. *Archives of General Psychiatry*, **46**, 1073–9.

Marchand, A. & Wapler, M. (1993). The effect of personality disorders on the efficacy of behavioral cognitive therapy of panic disorders with agoraphobia. *Canadian Journal of Psychiatry*, **38**, 163–6.

Marin, D.B., Kocsis, J.H., Frances, A.J. & Klerman, G.L. (1993). Personality disorders in dysthymia. *Journal of Personality Disorders*, **7**, 223–31.

Markowitz, J.C., Moran, M.E., Kocsis, J.H. & Frances, A.J. (1992). Prevalence and comorbidity of dysthymic disorder among psychiatric outpatients. *Journal of Affective Disorders*, **24**, 63–71.

Markowitz, P.J., Calabrese, J.R., Schulz, S.C. & Meltzer, H.Y. (1991). Fluoxetine in the treatment of borderline and schizotypal personality disorders. *American Journal of Psychiatry*, **148**, 1064–7.

Marmor, J. (1979). Short-term dynamic psychotherapy. *American Journal of Psychiatry*, **136**, 149–53.

Marshall, W.L. & Barbaree, H.E. (1989). Sexual violence. In: *Clinical Approaches to Violence*, ed. K. Howells & C.R. Hollin, pp. 205–49. Chichester: John

Wiley & Sons.

Martin, H.P. (1980). The consequences of being abused and neglected: how the child fares. In: *The Battered Child*, ed. L.H. Kempe & R.E. Helfer, pp. 347–365. Chicago: University of Chicago Press.

Martin, R.L. (1986). Excess mortality among psychiatric patients. The importance of unnatural death, substance abuse disorders, antisocial personality and homosexuality. *Acta Psychiatrica Belgica*, **86**, 553–4.

Martin, R.L., Cloninger, C.R. & Guze, S.B. (1982). The natural history of somatization and substance abuse in women criminals: a six year follow-up. *Comprehensive Psychiatry*, **23**, 528–37.

Marttunen, M.J., Aro, H.M., Henriksson, M.M. & Lönnqvist, J.K. (1994). Antisocial behaviour in adolescent suicide. *Acta Psychiatrica Scandinavica*, **89**, 167–73.

Marziali, E. (1992). The etiology of borderline personality disorder: developmental factors. In: *Borderline Personality Disorder*, ed. J.F. Clarkin, E. Marziali & H. Munroe-Blum, pp. 27–44. New York: Guilford Press.

Marzillier, J.S., Lambert, C. & Kellett, J. (1976). A controlled evaluation of systematic desensitization and social skills training for socially inadequate psychiatric patients. *Behaviour Research & Therapy*, **14**, 225–38.

Masterson, J.F. (1976). *Treatment of the Borderline Adult*. New York: Brunner-Mazel.

Masterson, J. (1981). *The Narcissistic and Borderline Disorders*. New York: Brunner-Mazel.

Matochik, J.A., Liebenauer, L.L., King, A.C. *et al.* (1994). Cerebral glucose metabolism in adults with attention deficit hyperactivity disorder after chronic stimulant treatment. *American Journal of Psychiatry*, **151**, 658–64.

Mattes, J.A. (1988). Carbamazepine v propranolol for rage outbursts. *Psychopharmacology Bulletin*, **24**, 179–82.

Maudsley, H. (1868). *A Physiology and Pathology of Mind*, 2nd edn. London: Macmillan.

Mavissakalian, M. (1990). The relationship between panic disorder/agoraphobia and personality disorders. *Psychiatric Clinics of North America*, **13**, 661–84.

Mavissakalian, M. & Hamann, M. (1986). DSM-III personality disorder and agoraphobia. *Comprehensive Psychiatry*, **27**, 471–9.

Mavissakalian, M., Hamann, M.S. & Jones, B. (1990*a*). A comparison of DSM-III personality disorders in panic/agoraphobia and obsessive-compulsive disorder. *Comprehensive Psychiatry*, **31**, 238–44.

Mavissakalian, M., Hamann, M.S. & Jones, B. (1990*b*). DSM-III personality disorders in obsessive-compulsive disorder: changes with treatment. *Comprehensive Psychiatry*, **31**, 432–7.

Mawson, D. (1983). 'Psychopaths' in special hospitals. *Bulletin of the Royal College of Psychiatrists*, **7**, 178–81.

Mawson, D., Grounds, A. & Tantam, D. (1985). Violence and Asperger's syndrome: A case study. *British Journal of Psychiatry*, **147**, 566–9.

Mazure, C.M., Nelson, J.C. & Jatlow, P.I. (1990). Predictors of hospital outcome without antidepressants in major depression. *Psychiatry Research*, **33**, 51–8.

McCann, U.D., Rossiter, E.M., King, R.J. & Agras, W.S. (1991). Nonpurging bulimia: a distinct subtype of bulimia nervosa. *International Journal of Eating Disorders*, **10**, 679–87.

McCarroll, J.E., Ursano, R.J. & Fullerton, C.S. (1993). Symptoms of posttraumatic stress disorder following recovery of war dead. *American*

Journal of Psychiatry, **150**, 1875–7.

McCord, W.M. (1983). *The Psychopath and Milieu Therapy*. New York: Academic Press.

McCormick, R.A., Taber, J., Kruedelbach, N. & Russo, A. (1987). Personality profiles of hospitalized pathological gamblers: the California Personality Inventory. *Journal of Clinical Psychology*, **43**, 521–7.

McCrae, R.R., Costa, P.T. & Arenberg, D. (1980). Constancy of adult personality structure in males: longitudinal, cross-sectional and times-of-measurement analysis. *Journal of Gerontology*, **35**, 877–83.

McElroy, S.L., Hudson, J.I., Pope, H.G. *et al.* (1992). The DSM-III-R impulse control disorders not elsewhere classified: Clinical characteristics and relationships to other psychiatric disorders. *American Journal of Psychiatry*, **149**, 318–27.

McGlashan, T.H. (1983). The borderline syndrome: is it a variant of schizophrenia or affective disorder? *Archives of General Psychiatry*, **40**, 1319–23.

McGlashan, T.H. (1986). The Chestnut Lodge follow-up study: III. Long-term outcome of borderline personality disorder. *Archives of General Psychiatry*, **43**, 20–30.

McGlashan, T.H. (1987). Testing DSM-III-R symptom criteria for schizotypal and borderline personality disorders. *Archives of General Psychiatry*, **44**, 143–8.

McGlashan, T.H. (1993). Implications of outcome research for the treatment of borderline personality disorder. In: *Borderline Personality Disorder*, ed. J. Paris, pp. 235–60. Washington, DC: American Psychiatric Press Inc.

McGlashan, T.H. & Heinssen, R.K. (1989). Narcissistic, antisocial and non-comorbid subgroups of borderline disorder: are they distinct entities by long-term clinical profile? *Psychiatric Clinics of North America*, **12**, 653–70.

McGuffin, P. & Gottesman, I.I. (1984). Genetic influences on normal and abnormal development. In: *Child Psychiatry: Modern Approaches*, 2nd edn, ed. M. Rutter & L. Hersov. London: Blackwell.

McGuffin, P. & Thapar, A. (1992). The genetics of personality disorder. *British Journal of Psychiatry*, **160**, 12–23.

McGuire, F.L. (1980). Heavy and light drinking – drivers as separate target groups for treatment. *American Journal of Drug and Alcohol Abuse*, **7**, 101–7.

McGurk, B. (1978). Personality types among normal homocides. *British Journal of Criminology*, **18**, 146–61.

McKay, J.R., Alterman, A.I., McLellan, A.T. & Snider, E.C. (1994). Treatment goals, continuity of care, and outcome in a day hospital substance abuse rehabilitation program. *American Journal of Psychiatry*, **151**, 254–9.

McMahon, R.C., Flynn, P.M. & Davidson, R.S. (1985). The personality and symptoms scales of the Millon Clinical Multiaxial Inventory: sensitivity to post-treatment outcomes. *Journal of Clinical Psychology*, **41**, 862–6.

Mednick, S.A., Gabrielli, W.F. & Hutchings, B. (1984). Genetic influences in criminal convictions: evidence from an adoption cohort. *Science*, **224**, 891–4.

Megargee, E.I. (1966). Undercontrolled and overcontrolled personality types in extreme antisocial aggression. *Psychological Monographs*, **80**, no. 611.

Mehlum, L., Friis, S., Irion, T. *et al.* (1991). Personality disorders 2–5 years after treatment: a prospective follow-up study. *Acta Psychiatrica Scandinavica*, **84**, 72–7.

Merikangas, K.R. & Weissman, M.H. (1986). Epidemiology of DSM-III Axis II personality disorders. In: *APA Annual Review*, ed. A.J. Frances & R.E. Hales (vol. 5, Psychiatry Update, pp. 258–78). Washington DC: American Psychiatric Press.

Merikangas, K.R., Wicki, W. & Angst, J. (1994). Heterogeneity of depression. *British Journal of Psychiatry*, **164**, 342–8.

Miller, L. (1988). Neuropsychological perspectives on delinquency. *Behavioral Sciences and the Law*, **6**, 409–28.

Millon, T. (1969). *Modern Psychopathology*. Philadelphia: Saunders.

Millon, T. (1981). *Disorders of Personality: DSM-III. Axis II*. New York: Wiley.

Millon, T. (1987). *Manual for the Millon Clinical Multi-axial Inventory II (MCM-II)*. Minnetonka: National Computer Systems.

Millon, T. (1991). Avoidant personality disorder: A brief review of issues and data. *Journal of Personality Disorders*, **5**, 353–62.

Mindham, R.H.S., Scadding, J.G. & Cawley, R.H. (1992). Diagnoses are not diseases. *British Journal of Psychiatry*, **161**, 686–91.

Minichiello, W.E., Baer, L. & Jenike, M.A. (1987). Schizotypal personality disorder: a poor prognostic indicator for behavior therapy in the treatment of obsessive-compulsive disorder. *Journal of Anxiety Disorders*, **1**, 273–6.

Modestin, J. & Emmenegger, P.A. (1986). Completed suicide and criminality: lack of a direct relationship. *Psychological Medicine*, **16**, 661–9.

Modestin, J., Foglia, A. & Toffler, G. (1989). Comparative study of schizotypal and schizophrenia patients. *Psychopathology*, **22**, 1–13.

Monahan, J. (1981). *The Clinical Prediction of Violent Behaviour*. Maryland: US Department of Health and Human Services.

Monroe, R.R. (1982). DSM-III style diagnoses for the episodic disorders. *Journal of Nervous and Mental Disease*, **170**, 664–9.

Montgomery, S.A. & Montgomery, D.D. (1982). Pharmacological prevention of suicidal behaviour. *Journal of Affective Disorders*, **4**, 291–8.

Moorey, S. (1991). Cognitive behaviour therapy. *Hospital Update*, September, 726–32.

Morey, L.C. (1988). The categorical representation of personality disorder: a cluster analysis of DSM-III-R personality features. *Journal of Abnormal Psychology*, **97**, 314–21.

Morey, L. & Ochoa, E. (1989). An investigation of adherence to diagnostic criteria: clinical diagnosis of the DSM-III personality disorders. *Journal of Personality Disorders*, **3**, 180–92.

Morey, L., Waugh, M. & Blashfield, R. (1985). MMPI scales for DSM-III personality disorders: their derivation and correlates. *Journal of Personality Assessment*, **49**, 245–51.

Morrison, J. (1989). Histrionic personality disorder in women with somatization disorder. *Psychosomatics*, **30**, 433–7.

Moyes, T., Tennent, T.G. & Bedford, A.P. (1985). Long-term follow-up study of a ward-based behaviour modification programme for adolescents with acting-out and conduct problems. *British Journal of Psychiatry*, **147**, 300–5.

Mulder, R.T. (1991). Personality disorders in New Zealand hospitals. *Acta Psychiatrica Scandinavica*, **84**, 197–202.

Mungas, D. (1988). Psychometric correlates of episodic violent behaviour. *British Journal of Psychiatry*, **152**, 180–7.

Murray, R.M. & O'Callaghan, E. (1991). Neurodevelopmental schizophrenia. *Schizophrenia Monitor*, **1**, 1–3.

Murthy, V.N. (1969). Personality and the nature of suicide attempts. *British Journal of Psychiatry*, **115**, 791–5.

Myers, J.K., Weissman, M.M., Tischler, G.L. *et al.* (1984). Six month prevalence of psychiatric disorders in three communities, 1980–1982. *Archives of General Psychiatry*, **41**, 959–67.

Nace, E.P. (1989). Substance use disorders and personality disorders: comorbidity. *Psychiatric Hospital*, **20**, 65–9.

Nace, E.P., Davis, C.W. & Gaspari, J.P. (1991). Axis II comorbidity in substance abusers. *American Journal of Psychiatry*, **148**, 118–20.

Nelson, J.C. & Charney, D.S. (1981). The symptoms of major depressive illness. *American Journal of Psychiatry*, **138**, 1–12.

Nestadt, G., Romanoski, A.J., Brown, C.H. *et al.* (1991). DSM-III compulsive personality disorder: an epidemiological survey. *Psychological Medicine*, **21**, 461–71.

Nestadt, G., Romanoski, A.J., Chahal, R. *et al.* (1990). An epidemiological study of histrionic personality disorder. *Psychological Medicine*, **20**, 413–22.

Nig, J., Silk, H.R., Ogata, S. *et al.* (1989). Sexual abuse and borderline personality disorder: a comparative study. Presented at the *142nd Annual Meeting, American Psychiatric Association*, San Francisco.

Norden, M.J. (1989). Fluoxetine in borderline personality disorder. *Progress in Neuropsychopharmacology and Biological Psychiatry*, **13**, 885–93.

Nordstrom, G. & Berglund, M. (1987). Type 1 and type 2 alcoholics have different patterns of successful long-term adjustment. *British Journal of Addiction*, **82**, 761–9.

North, C.S., Smith, E.M. & Spitznagel, E.L. (1993). Is antisocial personality a valid diagnosis among the homeless? *American Journal of Psychiatry*, **150**, 578–83.

Norton, K. (1992). Personality disordered individuals: The Henderson Hospital model of treatment. *Criminal Behaviour and Mental Health*, **2**, 180–91.

Noyes, R., Reich, J.H., Suelzer, M. & Christiansen, J. (1991). Personality traits associated with panic disorder: change associated with treatment. *Comprehensive Psychiatry*, **32**, 283–94.

Nurnberg, H.G., Raskin, M. & Levine, P.E. (1989). Borderline personality disorder as a negative prognostic factor in anxiety disorders. *Journal of Personality Disorders*, **3**, 205–16.

Nurnberg, H.G., Raskin, M., Levine, P.E. *et al.* (1991). The comorbidity of borderline personality disorder and other DSM-III-R Axis II personality disorders. *American Journal of Psychiatry*, **148**, 1371–7.

Nurnberg, H.G., Rifkin, A. & Doddi, S. (1993). A systematic assessment of the comorbidity of DSM-III-R personality disorders in alcoholic outpatients. *Comprehensive Psychiatry*, **34**, 447–54.

O'Brien, M.L. (1988). Further evidence of the validity of the O'Brien Multiphasic Narcissism Inventory. *Psychological Reports*, **62**, 879–82.

Ojehagen, A. & Berglund, M. (1986*a*). Early and late improvement in a two-year out-patient alcoholic treatment programme. *Acta Psychiatrica Scandinavica*, **74**, 129–36.

Ojehagen, A. & Berglund, M. (1986*b*). To keep the alcoholic in out-patient treatment. A differentiated approach through treatment contracts. *Acta Psychiatrica Scandinavica*, **73**, 68–75.

Oldham, J.M., Skodol, A.E., Kellman, H.D. *et al.* (1992). Diagnosis of DSM-III-R personality disorders by two structured interviews: patterns of comorbidity. *American Journal of Psychiatry,* **149**, 213–20.

O'Leary, K.M., Brouwers, P., Gardner, D.L. & Cowdry, R.W. (1991). Neuropsychological testing of patients with borderline personality disorder. *American Journal of Psychiatry*, **148**, 106–11.

Olweus, D. (1979). Stability of aggressive reaction patterns in males: a review. *Psychological Bulletin*, **86**, 852–75.

Overholser, J.C. (1989). Differentiation between schizoid and avoidant personalities: an empirical test. *Canadian Journal of Psychiatry*, **34**, 785–90.

Overholser, J.C., Kabakoff, R. & Norman, W.H. (1989). Personality characteristics in depressed and dependent psychiatric inpatients. *Journal of Personality Assessment*, **53**, 40–50.

Pallis, D.T. & Birtchnell, J. (1977). Seriousness of suicide attempts in relation to personality. *British Journal of Psychiatry*, **130**, 253–9.

Papp, L.A., Zitrin, C.M., Coplan, J. & Gorman, J.M. (1990). The role of personality in anxiety disorders. *Psychiatric Medicine*, **8**, 107–20.

Paris, J. (1993). Management of acute and chronic suicidality in patients with borderline personality disorder. In: *Borderline Personality Disorder*, ed. J. Paris, pp. 373–84. Washington DC: American Psychiatric Press Inc.

Paris, J., Brown R. & Nowlis, D. (1987). Long-term follow-up of borderline patients in a general hospital. *Comprehensive Psychiatry*, **28**, 530–5.

Paris, J., Nowlis, D. & Brown, R. (1989). Predictors of suicide in borderline personality disorder. *Canadian Journal of Psychiatry*, **34**, 8–9.

Paris, J., Zweig-Frank, H. & Guzder, H. (1993). The role of psychological risk factors in recovery from borderline personality disorder. *Comprehensive Psychiatry*, **34**, 410–3.

Parker, G., Hadzi-Pavlovic, D., Wilhelm, K. *et al.* (1994). Defining melancholia: properties of a refined sign-based measure. *British Journal of Psychiatry*, **164**, 316–26.

Parnas, J., Cannon, T.D., Jacobsen, B. *et al.* (1993). Lifetime DSM-III-R diagnostic outcomes in the offspring of schizophrenic mothers. *Archives of General Psychiatry*, **50**, 707–14.

Parsons, B., Quitkin, F.M., McGrath, P.J. *et al.* (1989). Phenelzine, imipramine and placebo in borderline patients meeting criteria for atypical depression. *Psychopharmacology Bulletin*, **25**, 524–34.

Pekarik, G., Jones, D.L. & Blodgett, C. (1986). Personality and demographic characteristics of dropouts and completers in a nonhospital residential alcohol treatment program. *International Journal of the Addictions*, **21**, 131–7.

Pelham, W.F., Bender, M.E., Caddell, J. *et al.* (1985). Methylphenidate and children with attention deficit disorder. *Archives of General Psychiatry*, **42**, 948–52.

Penick, E.C., Powell, B.J., Liskow, B.I. *et al.* (1988). The stability of coexisting psychiatric syndromes in alcoholic men after one year. *Journal of Studies in Alcohol*, **49**, 395–405.

Perkins, D. (1991). Clinical work with sex offenders in secure settings. In: *Clinical Approaches to Sex Offenders and their Victims*, ed. C.R. Hollin & K. Howells, pp. 151–78. Chichester: John Wiley & Sons.

Perkins, D.O., Davidson, E.J., Leserman, J. *et al.* (1993). Personality disorder in patients infected with HIV: a controlled study with implications for clinical care. *American Journal of Psychiatry*, **150**, 309–15.

Perry, J.C. (1990). Use of longitudinal data to validate personality disorders. In:

Personality Disorders: New Perspectives on Diagnostic Validity, ed. J.M. Oldham, pp. 23–40. Washington DC: American Psychiatric Press Inc.

Perry, J.C. (1992). Problems and considerations in the valid assessment of personality disorders. *American Journal of Psychiatry*, **149**, 1645–53.

Perry, J.C. (1993). Longitudinal studies of personality disorders. *Journal of Personality Disorders*, Spring suppl., 63–85.

Perry, J. & Klerman, G. (1980). Clinical features of borderline personality disorder. *American Journal of Psychiatry*, **137**, 165–73.

Perry, J.C., Lavori, P.W., Pagano, C.J. *et al.* (1992). Life events and recurrent depression in borderline and antisocial personality disorders. *Journal of Personality Disorders*, **6**, 394–407.

Peselow, E.D., Sanfilipo, M.P., Fieve, R.R. & Gulbenkian, G. (1994). Personality traits during depression and after clinical recovery. *British Journal of Psychiatry*, **164**, 349–54.

Peterson, C. & Seligman, M.E.P. (1984). Causal explanation as a risk factor for depression: theory and evidence. *Psychological Review*, **91**, 347–74.

Pfohl, B. (1991). Histrionic personality disorder: a review of available data and recommendations for DSM-IV. *Journal of Personality Disorders*, **5**, 150–66.

Pfohl, B., Barash, J., True, B. & Alexander, B. (1989). Failure of two Axis I measures to predict medication compliance among hypertensive patients. *Journal of Personality Disorders*, **3**, 45–52.

Pfohl, B. & Blum, N. (1991). Obsessive-compulsive personality disorder: a review of available data and recommendations for DSM-IV. *Journal of Personality Disorders*, **5**, 363–75.

Pfohl, B., Coryell, W., Zimmerman, M. & Stangl, D. (1987). Prognostic validity of self-report and interview measures of personality disorder in depressed inpatients. *Journal of Clinical Psychiatry*, **48**, 468–72.

Pfohl, B., Stangl, D. & Zimmerman, M. (1982). *The Structured Interview for DSM-III Personality Disorders (SIDP)*. Iowa City: University of Iowa Hospitals and Clinics.

Pfohl, B., Stangl, D. & Zimmerman, M. (1984). The implications for DSM-III personality disorders for patients with major depression. *Journal of Affective Disorders*, **7**, 309–18.

Phillips, K.A., Gunderson, J.G., Hirschfeld, R.M. & Smith, L.E. (1990). The depressive personality: a review. *American Journal of Psychiatry*, **147**, 830–7.

Pica, S., Edwards, J., Jackson, H.J. *et al.* (1990). Personality disorders in recent-onset bipolar disorder. *Comprehensive Psychiatry*, **31**, 499–510.

Pierce, D.W. (1977). Suicidal intent and self-injury. *British Journal of Psychiatry*, **130**, 377–85.

Pilgrim, J. & Mann, A. (1990). Use of the ICD-10 version of the Standardized Assessment of Personality to determine the prevalence of personality disorder in psychiatric in-patients. *Psychological Medicine*, **20**, 985–92.

Pilgrim, J.A., Mellers, J.D.. Boothby, H.A. & Mann, A.H. (1993). Inter-rater and temporal reliability of the Standardized Assessment of Personality and the influence of informant characteristics. *Psychological Medicine*, **23**, 779–86.

Pinel, P.H. (1809). *Traité Medico-Philosophique sur l'Aliénation Mentale*, 2nd edn. Paris, France: Brosson.

Pines, M. (1990). Group analytic psychotherapy and the borderline patient. In: *The Difficult Patient in Group Psychotherapy with Borderline and Narcissistic Disorders*, ed. B.E. Roth, W.N. Stone & H.D. Kibel, pp. 31–44. Madison,

Connecticut: International Universities Press Inc.

Piper, A. (1994). Multiple personality disorder. *British Journal of Psychiatry*, **164**, 600–12.

Piran, N., Lerner, P. & Garfinkel, P.E. (1988). Personality disorders in anorexic patients. *International Journal of Eating Disorders*, **7**, 589–99.

Plakun, E.M. (1989). Narcissistic personality disorder. A validity study and comparison to borderline personality disorder. *Psychiatric Clinics of North America*, **12**, 603–20.

Plakun, E.M. (1991). Prediction of outcome in borderline personality disorder. *Journal of Personality Disorders*, **5**, 93–101.

Plakun, E.M., Burkhardt, P.E. & Muller, J.P. (1985). 14-year follow-up of borderline and schizotypal personality disroders. *Comprehensive Psychiatry*, **26**, 448–55.

Pokorny, A.D., Miller, B.A. & Kaplan, H.B. (1972). The Brief MAST: a shortened version of the Michigan Alcoholism Screening Test. *American Journal of Psychiatry*, **129**, 342–5.

Pollack, J.M. (1979). Obsessive-compulsive personality: a review. *Psychological Bulletin*, **2**, 225–41.

Pollack, J. (1981). Hysterical personality: an appraisal in light of empirical research. *Genetic Psychology Monographs*, **104**, 71–105.

Pollack, J. (1987). Relationship of obsessive-compulsive personality to obsessive-compulsive disorder: a review of the literature. *Journal of Psychology*, **121**, 137–48.

Pollack, M.H., Otto, M.W., Rosenbaum, J.F. & Sachs, G.S. (1992). Personality disorders in patients with panic disorder. *Comprehensive Psychiatry*, **33**, 78–83.

Pollock, N., McBain, I. & Webster, C.D. (1989). Clinical decision making and the assessment of dangerousness. In: *Clinical Approaches to Violence*, ed. K. Howells & C.R. Hollin. Chichester: John Wiley & Sons.

Pope, H.G., Frankenburg, F.R., Hudson, J.I. *et al.* (1987). Is bulimia associated with borderline personality disorder? A controlled study. *Journal of Clinical Psychiatry*, **48**, 181–4.

Pope, H.G. & Lipinsky, J.F. (1978). Diagnosis in schizophrenia and manic depressive illness. *Archives of General Psychiatry*, **35**, 811–28.

Powell, B.J., Penick, E.C., Nickel, E.J. *et al.* (1992). Outcomes of comorbid alcoholic men: a 1-year follow-up. *Alcohol Clinical and Experimental Research*, **16**, 131–8.

Prentky, R.A. & Carter, D.L. (1984). The predictive value of the triad for sex offenders. *Behavioral Science and Law*, **2**, 341–54.

Prichard, J.C. (1835). *A Treatise of Insanity*. London, UK: Sherwood, Gilbert & Piper.

Prichard, J.C. (1837). *A treatise on insanity and other diseases affecting the mind.* Philadelphia: Harwell, Barrington & Harwell.

Quay, H.C. (1977). Measuring dimensions of deviant behaviour: The behavior problem checklist. *Journal of Abnormal Child Psychology*, **5**, 277–87.

Raczek, S.W. (1992). Childhood abuse and personality disorder. *Journal of Personality Disorders*, **6**, 109–16.

Rado, S. (1953). Dynamics and classification of disordered behaviour. *American Journal of Psychiatry*, **110**, 406–16.

Raine, A. & Allbutt, J. (1989). Factors of schizoid personality. *British Journal of Clinical Psychology*, **28**, 31–40.

Raine, A., Venables, P.H. & Williams, M. (1990). Relationships between central and autonomic measures of arousal at age 15 years and criminality at age 24 years. *Archives of General Psychiatry*, **47**, 1003–7.

Raskin, R. & Hall, C. (1979). A narcissistic personality inventory. *Psychological Reports*, **45**, 590–4.

Rasmussen, S.A. & Tsuang, M.T. (1986). Clinical characteristics and family history in DSM-III obsessive-compulsive disorder. *American Journal of Psychiatry*, **143**, 317–22.

Ratey, J.J., Morrill, R. & Oxenkrug, G. (1983). Use of propranolol for provoked and unprovoked episodes of rage. *American Journal of Psychiatry*, **140**, 1356–7.

Reese, W.G. (1979). A dog model for human psychopathology. *American Journal of Psychiatry*, **136**, 1168–72.

Regier, D.A., Boyd, J.H. & Burke, J.D. (1988). One-month prevalence of mental disorders in the United States. *Archives of General Psychiatry*, **45**, 977–86.

Reich, J. (1987). Sex distribution of DSM-III personality disorders in psychiatric outpatients. *American Journal of Psychiatry*, **144**, 485–8.

Reich, J. (1988). DSM-III personality disorders and the outcome of treated panic disorder. *American Journal of Psychiatry*, **145**, 1149–52.

Reich, J.H. (1989). Update on instruments to measure DSM-III and DSM-III-R personality disorders. *Journal of Nervous and Mental Disease*, **177**, 366–70.

Reich, J. (1990a). Familiality of DSM-III-R self-defeating personality disorders. *Journal of Nervous and Mental Disease*, **178**, 597–8.

Reich, J. (1990b). Relationship between DSM-III avoidant and dependent personality disorders. *Psychiatry Research*, **34**, 281–920.

Reich, J.H. (1990c). Effect of DSM-III personality disorders on outcome of tricyclic antidepressant-treated nonpsychotic outpatients with major or minor depressive disorder. *Psychiatry Research*, **32**, 175–81.

Reich, J. (1992). Measurement of DSM-III and DSM-III-R borderline personality disorder. In: *Borderline Personality Disorder: Clinical and Empirical Perspectives*, ed. J.F. Clarkin, E. Marziali & H. Munroe-Blum, pp. 116–48. New York: Guilford Press.

Reich, J., Boerstler, H., Yates, W. & Nduaguba, M. (1989). Utilization of medical resources in persons with DSM-III personality disorders in a community sample. *International Journal of Psychiatry in Medicine*, **19**, 1–9.

Reich, J.H. & Green, A.I. (1991). Effect of personality disorders on outcome of treatment. *Journal of Nervous and Mental Disease*, **179**, 74–82.

Reich, J., Nduaguba, M. & Yates, W. (1988). Age and sex distribution of DSM-III personality cluster traits in a community population. *Comprehensive Psychiatry*, **29**, 298–303.

Reich, J.H. & Noyes, R. (1987). A comparison of DSM-III personality disorders in acutely ill panic and depressed patients. *Journal of Anxiety Disorders*, **1**, 123–31.

Reich, J., Noyes, R., Hirschfeld, R. *et al.* (1987a). State and personality in depressed and panic patients. *American Journal of Psychiatry*, **144**, 181–7.

Reich, J.H., Noyes, R. & Troughton, E. (1987b). Dependent personality disorder associated with phobic avoidance in patients with panic disorder. *American Journal of Psychiatry*, **144**, 323–6.

Reich, J., Noyes, R. & Yates, W. (1989). Alprazolam treatment of avoidant personality traits in social phobic patients. *Journal of Clinical Psychiatry*, **50**, 91–5.

Reich, J.H. & Vasile, R.G. (1993). Effect of personality disorders on the treatment outcome of Axis I conditions: an update. *The Journal of Nervous and Mental Disease*, **181**, 475–84.

Remington, G.J. & Book, H. (1993). Discriminative validity of the borderline syndrome index. *Journal of Personality Disorders*, **7**, 312–9.

Renneberg, B., Goldstein, A.J., Phillips, D. & Chambless, D.L. (1990). Intensive behavioral group treatment of avoidant personality disorder. *Behavior Therapy*, **21**, 363–77.

Reus, N.D. & Markrow, S. (1984). Alprazolam in the treatment of borderline personality disorder. Paper presented at the 39th annual meeting of the Society of Biological Psychiatry, Los Angeles, CA.

Rey, J.M. (1993). Oppositional defiant disorder. *American Journal of Psychiatry*, **150**, 1769–78.

Rich, C.L., Fowler, R.C. & Fogarty, L.A. (1988). The San Diego Suicide Study III: relationships between diagnoses and stressors. *Archives of General Psychiatry*, **45**, 589–94.

Richman, J.A. & Flaherty, J.A. (1987). *Narcissistic Trait Scale (NTS)*, Department of Psychiatry, University of Illinois, College of Medicine, 912 S. Wood Street, Room 218, Chicago, IL. 60612, USA.

Rifkin, A., Quitkin, F. & Carrillo, C. (1972). Lithium carbonate in emotionally unstable character disorders. *Archives of General Psychiatry*, **27**, 519–23.

Rihmer, Z. (1990). Dysthymia – a clinician's perspective. In: *Dysthymic Disorder*, ed. S.W. Barton & H.S. Akiskal. London: Gaskell (Royal College of Psychiatrists).

Robertson, D.A.F., Ray, J., Diamond, I. & Edwards, J.G. (1989). Personality profile and affective state of patients with inflammatory bowel disease. *Gut*, **30**, 623–6.

Robertson, G. & Gunn, J. (1987). A ten-year follow-up of men discharged from Grendon Prison. *British Journal of Psychiatry*, **151**, 674–8.

Robins, E. & Guze, S.B. (1970). Establishment of diagnostic validity in psychiatric illness. Its application to schizophrenia. *American Journal of Psychiatry*, **126**, 983–8.

Robins, L.N. (1966). *Deviant Children Grown Up: A Sociological and Psychiatric Study of Sociopathic Personality*. Baltimore: Williams & Watkins.

Robins, L.N. (1978). Sturdy childhood predictors of adult antisocial behaviour: replications from longitudinal studies. *Psychological Medicine*, **8**, 611–22.

Robins, L.N. (1986). The consequences of conduct disorders in girls. In: *Development of Antisocial and Prosocial Behaviour. Research, Theories and Issues*, ed. D. Olwens, J. Block & M. Radke-Yarrow. Orlando: Academic Press.

Robins, L.N. (1993). Childhood conduct problems, adult psychopathology, and crime. In: *Mental Disorder and Crime*, ed. S. Hodgins. London: Sage.

Robins, L.N., Helzer J.E. & Weissman, M.M. (1984). Lifetime prevalence of specific psychiatric disorders in three sites. *Archives of General Psychiatry*, **41**, 949–58.

Robins, L.N. & Price, R.K. (1991). Adult disorders predicted by childhood conduct problems: results from the NIMH epidemiologic catchment area project. *Psychiatry*, **54**, 116–32.

Robins, L.N. & Regier, D.A. (1991). *Psychiatric Disorder in America. The ACA Study*. New York: Free Press.

Robins, L.N., Tipp, P. & Przybeck, T. (1991). Antisocial personality. In:

Psychiatric Disorder in America. The ECA Study, ed. L.N. Robins & D. Regier, pp. 258–290. New York: Free Press.

Robinson, A.D.T. & Duffy, J.C. (1989). A comparison of self-injury and self-poisoning from the Regional Poisoning Treatment Centre, Edinburgh. *Acta Psychiatrica Scandinavica*, **80**, 272–79.

Robinson, L.A., Berman, J.S. & Neimeyer, R.A. (1990). Psychotherapy for the treatment of depression: a comprehensive review of controlled outcome research. *Psychological Bulletin*, **108**, 77–84.

Ronningstam, E. (1988). Comparing three systems for diagnosing narcissistic personality disorder. *Psychiatry*, **51**, 300–11.

Ronningstam, E. & Gunderson, J. (1988). Narcissistic traits in psychiatric patients. *Comprehensive Psychiatry*, **29**, 545–9.

Ronningstam, E. & Gunderson, J. (1989). Descriptive studies on narcissistic personality disorder. *Psychiatric Clinics of North America*, **12**, 585–601.

Ronningstam, E. & Gunderson, J. (1990). Identifying criteria for narcissistic personality disorder. *American Journal of Psychiatry*, **147**, 918–22.

Ronningstam, E. & Gunderson, J. (1991). Differentiating borderline personality disorder from narcissistic personality disorder. *Journal of Personality Disorders*, **5**, 225–32.

Rosenvinge, J.H. & Mouland, S.O. (1990). Outcome and prognosis of anorexia nervosa. *British Journal of Psychiatry*, **156**, 92–7.

Ross, H.E., Glaser, F.B. & Germanson, T. (1988). The prevalence of psychiatric disorders in patients with alcohol and other drug problems. *Archives of General Psychiatry*, **45**, 1023–31.

Rossiter, E.M., Agras, W.S., Telch, C.F. & Schneider, J.A. (1993). Cluster B personality disorder characteristics predict outcome in the treatment of bulimia nervosa. *International Journal of Eating Disorders*, **13**, 349–57.

Rounsaville, B.J., Dolinsky, Z.S., Babor, T.F. & Meyer, R.E. (1987). Psychopathology as a predictor of treatment outcome in alcoholics. *Archives of General Psychiatry*, **44**, 505–13.

Rounsaville, B.J., Kosten, T.R. & Kleber, H.D. (1986). Long-term changes in current psychiatric diagnoses of treated opiate addicts. *Comprehensive Psychiatry*, **27**, 480–98.

Roy, A., Custer, R., Lorenz, V. & Linnoila, M. (1989*a*). Personality factors and pathological gambling. *Acta Psychiatrica Scandinavica*, **80**, 37–9.

Roy, A., De Jong, J. & Linnoila M. (1989*b*). Extraversion in pathological gamblers. *Archives of General Psychiatry*, **46**, 679–81.

Runeson, B. & Beskow, J. (1991). Borderline personality disorder in young Swedish suicides. *Journal of Nervous and Mental Disease*, **179**, 153–6.

Rushton, J.P., Fulker, D.W., Neale, M.C. *et al.* (1986). Altruism and aggression: the heritability of individual differences. *Journal of Personality and Social Psychology*, **50**, 1192–8.

Russ, M.J. (1992). Self-injurious behavior in patients with borderline personality disorder: biological perspective. *Journal of Personality Disorders*, **6**, 64–81.

Rutter, M. (1987). Temperament, personality and personality disorder. *British Journal of Psychiatry*, **150**, 443–58.

Rutter, M. & Giller, H. (1983). *Juvenile Delinquency: Trends and Perspectives.* Harmondsworth: Penguin.

Ryder, R.G. (1967). Birth to maturity revised: a canonical reanalysis. *Journal of Personality and Social Psychology*, **7**, 168–72.

Ryle, A. (1976). Group psychotherapy. *British Journal of Hospital Medicine*,

March, 239–43.

Ryle, A. (1989). *Cognitive-Analytic Therapy: Active Participation in Change.* London: John Wylie.

Sanderson, W.C., Wetzler, S., Beck, A.T. & Betz, F. (1992). Prevalence of personality disorders in patients with major depression and dysthymia. *Psychiatry Research*, **42**, 93–99.

Sanderson, W.C., Wetzler, S., Beck, A.T. & Betz, F. (1994). Prevalence of personality disorders among patients with anxiety disorders. *Psychiatry Research*, **51**, 167–74.

Sandler, J., Dare, C. & Holder, A. (1970). Basic psychoanalytic concepts: transference. *British Journal of Psychiatry*, **116**, 667–72.

Sandler, J. & Hazari, A. (1960). The 'obsessional'. On the psychological classification of obsessional character traits and symptoms. *British Journal of Medical Psychology*, **33**, 113–22.

Sandler, J., Holder, A. & Dare, C. (1970a). Basic psychoanaltyic concepts: the treatment alliance. *British Journal of Psychiatry*, **116**, 555–61.

Sandler, J., Holder, A. & Dare, C. (1970b). Basic psychoanalytic concepts: resistance. *British Journal of Psychiatry*, **117**, 215–9.

Sano, K. & Mayangi, Y. (1988). Posteromedial hypothalamotomy in the treatment of violent, aggressive behaviour. *Acta Neurochirurgica*, Suppl. 44, 145–51.

Sansone, R.A. & Fine, M.A. (1992). Borderline personality as a predictor of outcome in women with eating disorders. *Journal of Personality Disorders*, **6**, 176–86.

Sapsford, R.J. (1978). Life sentenced prisoners: psychological changes during sentence. *British Journal of Criminology*, **18**, 128–45.

Satel, S., Southwick, S. & Denton, C. (1988). Use of imipramine for attention deficit disorder in a borderline patient. *Journal of Nervous and Mental Disease*, **176**, 305–7.

Sato, T., Sakado, K. & Sato, S. (1993a). DSM-III-R personality disorders in outpatients with non-bipolar depression. *European Archives of Psychiatry and Clinical Neuroscience*, **242**, 273–8.

Sato, T., Sakado, K. & Sato, S. (1993b). Is there any specific personality disorder or personality disorder cluster that worsens the short-term treatment outcome of major depression? *Acta Psychiatrica Scandinavica*, **88**, 342–9.

Scadding, J.G. (1988). Health and disease: what can medicine do for philosophy. *Journal of Medical Ethics*, **14**, 118–24.

Scadding, J.G. (1990). The semantic problems of psychiatry. *Psychological Medicine*, **20**, 243–8.

Schalling, D., Asberg, M., Edman, G. & Oreland, L. (1987). Markers for vulnerability to psychopathology: temperament traits associated with platelet MAO activity. *Acta Psychiatrica Scandinavica*, **76**, 172–82.

Schiff, S.B. & Glassman, S.M. (1969). Large and small group therapy in a State mental health centre. *International Journal of Group Psychotherapy*, **19**, 2–10.

Schneider, K. (1923). *Die Psychopathischen Personlichkeiten.* Berlin: Springer.

Schneider, K. (1959). *Clinical Psychopathology*, trans. M.W. Hamilton. London: Grune & Stratton.

Schneier, F.R., Spitzer, R.L., Gibbon, M. *et al.* (1991). The relationship of social phobias subtypes and avoidant personality disorder. *Comprehensive Psychiatry*, **32**, 496–502.

Schroeder, M.L. & Livesley, W.J. (1991). An evaluation of DSM-III-R personality disorders. *Acta Psychiatrica Scandinavica*, **84**, 512–9.

Schuckit, M.A. (1985). The clinical implications of primary diagnostic groups among alcoholics. *Archives of General Psychiatry*, **42**(11), 1043–9.

Schulsinger, F., Parnas, J., Petersen, E.T. *et al.* (1984). Cerebral ventricular size in the offspring of schizophrenia mothers. *Archives of General Psychiatry*, **41**, 602–6.

Schulz, S.C., Cornelius, J., Schulz, P.M. & Soloff, P.H. (1988). The amphetamine challenge test in patients with borderline disorder. *American Journal of Psychiatry*, **145**, 809–14.

Schutz, W.C. (1958). In: *Firo: A Three-Dimensional Theory of Interpersonal Behaviour*. New York: Rinehart.

Sciuto, G., Diaferia, G., Battaglia, M. *et al.* (1991). DSM-III-R personality disorders in panic and obsessive-compulsive disorder: a comparison study. *Comprehensive Psychiatry*, **32**, 450–5.

Scott, J. (1993). Homelessness and mental illness. *British Journal of Psychiatry*, **162**, 314–24.

Seivewright, N. (1987). Relationship between life events and personality in psychiatric disorder. *Stress Medicine*, **3**, 163–8.

Shapiro, E.R. (1978). The psychodynamics and developmental psychology of the borderline patient: a review of the literature. *American Journal of Psychiatry*, **135**, 1305–15.

Shea, M.T. (1992). Some characteristics of the Axis II criteria sets and their implications for assessment of personality disorders. *Journal of Personality Disorders*, **6**, 377–81.

Shea, M.T. (1993). Psychosocial treatment of personality disorders. *Journal of Personality Disorders*, (Suppl.), 167–80.

Shea, M.T., Pilkonis, P.A., Beckham, E. *et al.* (1990). Personality disorders and treatment outcome in the NIMH treatment of depression collaborative research program. *American Journal of Psychiatry*, **147**, 711–8.

Sheard, M.H. (1971). Effect of lithium on human aggression. *Nature*, **230**, 113–4.

Sheard, M.H., Marini, J.L. & Bridges, C.I. (1976). The effect of lithium on unipolar aggressive behaviour in man. *American Journal of Psychiatry*, **133**, 1409–13.

Shearin, E.N. & Linehan, M.M. (1993). Dialectical behavior therapy for borderline personality disorder: Treatment goals, strategies and empirical support. In: *Borderline Personality Disorder*, ed. J. Paris, pp. 285–318. Washington DC: American Psychiatric Press Inc.

Shekim, W.O., Bylund, D.B. & Frankel, F. (1990). Platelet alpha 2 adrenergic receptor binding to ^{3}H yohimbine and personality variations in normals. *Psychiatry Research*, **32**, 125–34.

Sherwood, R.J., Funari, D.J. & Piekarski, A.M. (1990). Adapted character styles of Vietnam veterans with post-traumatic stress disorder. *Psychological Reports*, **66**, 623–31.

Sierles, F.S., Chen, J.J., McFarland, R.E. & Taylor, M.A. (1983). Posttraumatic stress disorder and concurrent psychiatric illness: a preliminary report. *American Journal of Psychiatry*, **140**, 1177–9.

Siever, L.J., Bernstein, D.P. & Silverman, J.M. (1991). Schizotypal personality disorder: a review of its current status. *Journal of Personality Disorders*, **5**, 178–93.

Siever, L.J. & Davis, K.L. (1991). A psychobiological perspective on the personality disorders. *American Journal of Psychiatry*, **148**, 1647–58.

Siever, L.J., Keefe, R., Bernstein, D.P. *et al.* (1990*a*). Eye tracking impairment in clinically identified patients with schizotypal personality disorder. *American Journal of Psychiatry*, **147**, 740–5.

Siever, L.J., Silverman, J.M., Horvath, T.B. *et al.* (1990*b*). Increased morbid risk for schizophrenia-related disorders in relatives of schizotypal personality disordered patients. *Archives of General Psychiatry*, **47**, 634–40.

Silver, D. (1985). Psychodynamics and psychotherapeutic management of the self-destructive character-disordered patient. *Psychiatric Clinics of North America*, **8**, 357–75.

Silverman, J.M., Siever, L.J., Horvath, T.B. *et al.* (1993). Schizophrenia-related and affective personality disorder traits in relatives of probands with schizophrenia and personality disorders. *American Journal of Psychiatry*, **150**, 435–42.

Simeon, D., Stanley, B., Frances, A. *et al.* (1992). Self-mutilation in personality disorders: psychological and biological correlates. *American Journal of Psychiatry*, **149**, 221–6.

Simpson, D.M. & Foster, D. (1986). Improvement in organically disturbed behaviour with trazodine treatment. *Journal of Clinical Psychiatry*, **47**, 191–3.

Sims, A.C.P. (1992). Neuroses and personality disorders. *Current Opinion in Psychiatry*, **5**, 187–9.

Skodol, A.E., Rosnick, L., Kellman, D. *et al.* (1988). Validating structured DSM-III-R personality disorder assessments with longitudinal data. *American Journal of Psychiatry*, **145**, 1297–9.

Skodol, A.E., Rosnick, L., Kellman, D. *et al.* (1990). Developments of a procedure for validating structured assessments of Axis II. In: *Personality Disorders: New Perspectives in Diagnostic Validity*, ed. J.M. Oldham, pp. 41–70. Washington DC: American Psychiatric Press Inc.

Small, I.F., Small, J.G., Alig, V.B & Moore, D.F. (1970). Passive-aggressive personality disorder: a search for a syndrome. *American Journal of Psychiatry*, **126**, 973–83.

Smith, D. (ed.) (1979). *Life Sentenced Prisoners*. Home Office Research Study No. 51. London: HMSO.

Smith, M.L., Glass, G.V. & Miller, T.I. (1980). *The Benefits of Psychotherapy*. Baltimore: The John Hopkins University Press.

Sohlberg, S. (1990). Personality, life stress and the course of eating disorders. *Acta Psychiatrica Scandinavica*, Suppl. 361, **82**, 29–33.

Sohlberg, S., Norring, C., Holmgren, S. & Rosmark, B. (1989). Impulsivity and long-term prognosis of psychiatric patients with anorexia nervosa/bulimia nervosa. *Journal of Nervous and Mental Disease*, **177**, 249–58.

Soloff, P.H. (1987). Neuroleptic treatment in the borderline patient: advantages and techniques. *Journal of Clinical Psychiatry*, **48** (8 Suppl.), 26–30.

Soloff, P.H. (1993). Pharmacological therapies in borderline personality disorder. In: *Borderline Personality Disorder*, ed. J. Paris, pp. 319–48. Washington DC: American Psychiatric Press Inc.

Soloff, P.H., Cornelius, J., George, A. *et al.* (1993). Efficacy of phenelzine and haloperidol in borderline personality disorder. *Archives of General Psychiatry*, **50**, 377–85.

Soloff, P.H., George, A. & Nathan, R.S. (1986). Progress in pharmacotherapy of borderline disorders: a double blind study of amitriptyline, haloperidol and placebo. *Archives of General Psychiatry*, **43**, 691–9.

Solomon, M.I. & Murphy, G.E. (1984). Cohort studies in suicide. In: *Suicide in the Young*, ed. H.S. Sudak, A.B. Ford & N.B. Rushford. Boston: John Wright/PSG.

Southwick, S.M., Yehuda, R. & Giller, E.L. (1993). Personality disorders in treatment-seeking combat veterans with posttraumatic stress disorder. *American Journal of Psychiatry*, **150**, 1020–3.

Southwick, S.M., Yehuda, R., Giller, E.L. & Perry, B.D. (1990). Altered platelet α_2 adrenergic receptor binding sites in borderline personality disorder. *American Journal of Psychiatry*, **147**, 1014–7.

Spitzer, R.L. (1983). Psychiatric diagnosis: are clinicians still necessary? *Comprehensive Psychiatry*, **24**, 399–411.

Spitzer, R.L., Endicott, J. & Woodruff, R.A. (1977). Classification of mood disorders. In: *Depression: Clinical, Biological and Psychological Perspectives*, ed. G. Usdin. New York: Brunner/Mazel.

Spitzer, R.L., Feister, S., Gay, M. & Pfohl, B. (1991). Results of a survey of forensic psychiatrists on the validity of the sadistic personality disorder diagnosis. *American Journal of Psychiatry*, **148**, 875–9.

Spitzer, R., Williams, J.B.W. & Gibbon, M. (1987). *Structured Interview for DSM-III-R Personality Disorders*. New York: Biometrics Research Department, New York State Psychiatric Institute.

Spitzer, R.L., Williams, J.B.W., Kass, F. & Davies, M. (1989). National field trial of the DSM-III-R diagnostic criteria for self-defeating personality disorder. *American Journal of Psychiatry*, **146**, 1561–7.

Sprock, J., Blashfield, R.K. & Smith, B. (1990). Gender weighting of DSM-III-R personality disorder criteria. *American Journal of Psychiatry*, **147**, 586–90.

Squires-Wheeler, E., Skodol, A.E., Bassett, A. & Erlenmeyer-Kimling, L. (1989). DSM-III-R schizotypal personality traits in offspring of schizophrenic disorder, affective disorder, and normal control patients. *Journal of Psychiatric Research*, **23**, 229–39.

Srole, L., Langer, T., Michael, S. *et al.* (1962). *Mental Health in the Metropolis*. New York: McGraw Hill.

Standage, K. (1989). Structured interviews and the diagnosis of personality disorders. *Canadian Journal of Psychiatry*, **34**, 906–12.

Stangl, D., Pfohl, B., Zimmerman, M. *et al.* (1985). A structured interview for the DSM-III personality disorders. *Archives of General Psychiatry*, **42**, 591–6.

Stankovic, S.R., Libb, J.W., Freeman, H.M. & Roseman, J.M. (1992). Post treatment stability of the MCMI-II personality scales in depressed outpatients. *Journal of Personality Disorders*, **6**, 82–9.

Stanley, M.A., Turner, S.M. & Borden, J.W. (1990). Schizotypal features in obsessive-compulsive disorder. *Comprehensive Psychiatry*, **31**, 511–8.

Stein, G. (1993). Drug treatment of the personality disorders. In: *Personality Disorder Reviewed*, ed. P. Pyrer & G. Stein, pp. 262–304. London: Gaskell.

Steiner, M., Links, P.S. & Korzekwa, M. (1988). Biological markers in borderline personality disorders: an overview. *Canadian Journal of Psychiatry*, **33**, 350–5.

Stern, A. (1938). Psychoanalytic investigation of and therapy in the borderline group of neuroses. *Psychoanalytic Quarterly*, **7**, 467–89.

Stern, J., Murphy, M. & Bass, L. (1993). Personality disorders in patients with somatisation disorder. *British Journal of Psychiatry*, **163**, 785–9.

Sternbach, S.E., Judd, P.H., Sabo, A.N. *et al.* (1992). Cognitive and perceptual distortions in borderline personality disorder and schizotypal personality disorder in a vignette sample. *Comprehensive Psychiatry*, **33**, 186–9.

Stevenson, J. & Meares, R. (1992). An outcome study of psychotherapy in borderline personality disorder. *American Journal of Psychiatry*, **149**, 358–62.

Stone, J.L., McDaniel, K.D., Hughes, J.R. & Hermann, B.P. (1986). Episodic dyscontrol disorder and paroxysmal EEG abnormalities: successful treatment with carbamazepine. *Biological Psychiatry*, **21**, 208–12.

Stone, M.H. (1990). *The Fate of Borderline Patients*. New York: Guilford Press.

Stone, M.H. (1992). Borderline personality disorder: course of illness. In: *Borderline Personality Disorder*, ed. J.F. Clarkin, E. Marziali & H. Munroe-Blum, pp. 67–85. New York: Guilford Press.

Stone, M.H. (1993). Long-term outcome in personality disorders. *British Journal of Psychiatry*, **162**, 299–313.

Stone, M.H., Stone, D.K. & Hurt, S.W. (1987). Natural history of borderline patients treated by intensive hospitalization. *Psychiatric Clinics of North America*, **10**, 185–206.

Stravynski, A., Lesage, A., Marcouiller, M. & Edie, R. (1989). A test of the therapeutic mechanism in social skills training with avoidant personality disorders. *Journal of Nervous and Mental Disease*, **177**, 739–44.

Stravynski, A., Marks, I. & Yule, W. (1982). Social skills problems in neurotic outpatients: social skills training with and without cognitive modification. *Archives of General Psychiatry*, **39**, 1378–85.

Streiner, D.L. & Norman, G.R. (1989). Selecting the items. In: *Health Measurement Scales*, pp. 44–6. Oxford, UK: Oxford University Press.

Strelau, J. (1983). *Temperament, Personality and Arousal*. London: Academic Press.

Stringer, A.Y. & Josef, N.C. (1983). Methylphenidate in the treatment of aggression in two patients with antisocial personality disorder. *American Journal of Psychiatry*, **140**, 1365–6.

Stuart, S., Simons, A.D., Thase, M.E. & Pilkonis, P. (1992). Are personality assessments valid in acute major depression? *Journal of Affective Disorders*, **24**, 281–90.

Suedfeld, P. & Landon, P.B. (1978). Approaches to treatment. In: *Psychopathic Behaviour: Approaches to Research*, ed. R.D. Hare & D. Schalling, pp. 347–76. New York: Wiley.

Suomi, S.J. (1983). Social development in rhesus monkey: considerations of individual differences. In: *The Behavior of Human Infants*, ed. A Oliverio & M. Zappella. New York and London: Plenum Press.

Svartberg, M. & Styles, T.C. (1991). Comparative effects of short-term psychodynamic psychotherapy: a meta-analysis. *Journal of Consulting and Clinical Psychology*, **59**, 704–14.

Svrakic, D.M., Przybeck, T.R. & Cloninger, C.R. (1992). Mood states and personality traits. *Journal of Affective Disorders*, **24**, 217–26.

Swanson, M.C.J., Bland, R.C. & Newman, S.C. (1994). Antisocial personality disorders. *Acta Psychiatrica Scandinavica*, suppl. 376, 63–70.

Szatmari, P., Bartolucci, G.& Bremner,R. (1989). A follow-up study of high-functioning autistic children. *Journal of Autism and Developmental Disorders*, **19**, 213–25.

Tantam, D. (1988). Lifelong eccentricity and social isolation. *British Journal of*

Psychiatry, **153**, 783–91.

Tantam, D. & Whittaker, J. (1992). Personality disorder and self-wounding. *British Journal of Psychiatry*, **161**, 451–64.

Tarnopolsky, A. & Berelowitz, M. (1987). Borderline personality. A review of recent research. *British Journal of Psychiatry*, **151**, 724–34.

Taylor, P.J. (1986). Psychiatric disorder in London's life sentenced offenders. *British Journal of Criminology*, **26**, 63–78.

Teicher, M.H., Glod, C.A. & Cole, J.D. (1990). Emergence of intensive suicidal preoccupation during fluoxetine treatment. *American Journal of Psychiatry*, **147**, 207–10.

Tellegen, A., Lykken, D.T., Bouchard, T.J. *et al.* (1988). Personality similarity in twins reared apart and together. *Journal of Personality and Social Psychology*, **54**, 1031–9.

Templeman, T.L. & Wollersheim, J.P. (1979). A cognitive-behavioral approach to the treatment of psychopathy. *Psychotherapy: Theory, Research and Practice*, **16**, 132–9.

Thaker, G., Adami, H., Moran, M. *et al.* (1993). Psychiatric illness in families of subjects with schizophrenia-spectrum personality disorders. *American Journal of Psychiatry*, **150**, 66–71.

Tiihonen, J. & Eronen, M. (1993). Criminality associated with mental disorders and intellectual deficiency. *Acta Psychiatrica Scandinavica*, **50**, 917–8.

Tiihonen, J. & Hakola, P. (1994). Psychiatric disorders and homicide recidivism. *American Journal of Psychiatry*, **151**, 436–8.

Tong, J.E. & McKay, G.W.(1959). A statistical follow-up of mental defectives of dangerous and violent propensities. *British Journal of Delinquency*, **9**, 276–84.

Torgerson, S. (1984). Genetic and nosological aspects of schizotypal and borderline personality disorders. *Archives of General Psychiatry*, **41**, 546–54.

Torgerson, S., Onstad, S., Skre, I., Edvardsen, J. & Kringlen, E. (1993). 'True' schizotypal personality disorder: a study of co-twins and relatives of schizophrenic probands. *American Journal of Psychiatry*, **150**, 1661–7.

Torgerson, S. & Psychol, C. (1980). The oral, obsessive, and hysterical personality syndromes: a study of hereditary and environmental factors by means of the twin method. *Archives of General Psychiatry*, **144**, 767–72.

Trower, P., Yardley, K., Bryant, B.M. & Shaw, P. (1978). The treatment of social failure: a comparison of anxiety-reduction and skills-acquisition procedures on two social problems. *Behavior Modification*, **2**, 41–60.

Trull, T.J., Widiger, T.A. & Frances, A. (1987). Co-variation of criteria sets for avoidant, schizoid and dependent personality disorder. *American Journal of Psychiatry*, **144**, 767–72.

Tupin, J.P., Smith, D.B. & Clanon, T.C. (1973). The long term use of lithium, in aggressive prisoners. *Comprehensive Psychiatry*, **14**, 311–7.

Turkat, I.D. (1990). *The Personality Disorders. A Psychological Approach to Clinical Management*. New York: Pergamon Press.

Turner, S.H., Beidel, D.C., Dancee, C.V. & Keys, D.J. (1986). Psychopathology of social phobia and comparison to avoidant personality disorder. *Journal of Abnormal Psychology*, **95**, 389–94.

Tyrer, P. (1989). Clinical importance of personality disorder. *Current Opinion in Psychiatry*, **2**, 240–3.

Tyrer, P. & Alexander, M.S. (1979). Classification of personality disorder. *British Journal of Psychiatry*, **135**, 163–7.

Tyrer, P. & Alexander, J. (1988). Personality assessment schedule. In: *Personality Disorders: Diagnosis, Management and Course*, pp. 43–62. London: Wright.

Tyrer, P., Casey, P. & Gall, J. (1983). Relationship between neurosis and personality disorder. *British Journal of Psychiatry*, 142, 404–8.

Tyrer, P. & Ferguson, B. (1988). Development of the concept of abnormal personality. In: *Personality Disorders: Diagnosis, Management and Course*, ed. P. Tyrer, pp. 1–11. London: Wright.

Tyrer, P. & Seivewright, N. (1988a). Pharmacological treatment of personality disorders. *Clinical Neuropharmacology*, 11, 493–9.

Tyrer, P. & Seivewright, N. (1988b). Studies of outcome. In: *Personality Disorders; Diagnosis, Management and Course*, ed. P. Tyrer, pp. 119–36. London: Wright.

Tyrer, P., Seivewright, N., Ferguson, B. *et al.* (1990). The Nottingham study of neurotic disorder: relationship between personality status and symptoms. *Psychological Medicine*, 20, 423–31.

Tyrer, P., Seivewright, N., Ferguson, B. *et al.* (1993). The Nottingham study of neurotic disorder. *British Journal of Psychiatry*, 162, 219–26.

Tyrer, P., Seivewright, N., Ferguson, B. & Tyer, J. (1992). The general neurotic syndrome: a coaxial diagnosis of anxiety, depression and personality disorder. *Acta Psychiatrica Scandinavica*, 85, 201–6.

Vaglum, S. & Vaglum, P. (1989). Comorbidity for borderline schizotypal personality disorders. *Journal of Nervous and Mental Disease*, 177, 279–84.

Vaillant, G.E. (1975). Sociopathy as a human process: a viewpoint. *Archives of General Psychiatry*, 32, 178–83.

Van der Kolk, B.A., Perry, J.C. & Herman, J.L. (1991). Childhood origins of self-destructive behavior. *American Journal of Psychiatry*, 148, 1665–71.

van Manen, J. & van Veelen, C.W.M. (1988). Experience in psycho-surgery in the Netherlands. *Acta Neurochirurgica*, Suppl. 44, 167–9.

Virkkunen, M., De Jong, J., Bartko, J. *et al.* (1989). Relationship of psychobiological variables to recidivism in violent offenders and impulsive fire setters. *Archives of General Psychiatry*, 46, 600–3.

Virkunnen, M., Nuutila, A., Goodwin, F.K. & Linnoila, M. (1987). Cerebrospinal fluid monoamine metabolite levels in male arsonists. *Archives of General Psychiatry*, 44, 241–7.

Von Knorring, L., Almay, B.G.L. & Johansson, F. (1987). Personality traits in patients with idiopathic pain disorder. *Acta Psychiatrica Scandinavica*, 76, 490–8.

Wagner, A.W. & Linehan, M.M. (1994). Relationship between childhood sexual abuse and topography of parasuicide among women with borderline personality disorder. *Journal of Personality Disorders*, 8, 1–9.

Waldinger, R. & Gunderson, J. (1984). Completed psychotherapies with borderline patients. *American Journal of Psychotherapy*, 38, 190–202.

Walker, N. & McCabe, S. (1973). *Crime and Insanity in England*, vol. 2. Edinburgh: Edinburgh University Press.

Wallerstein, R. (1986). *Forty-two Lives in Treatment: A Study of Psychoanalysis and Psychotherapy*. New York: The Guilford Press.

Walton, H.J. (1973). Abnormal personality. In: *Companion to Psychiatric Studies*, vol. II, pp. 15–37. Edinburgh: Churchill Livingstone.

Walton, H.J. & Presly, A.S. (1973). Use of a category system in the diagnosis of abnormal personality. *British Journal of Psychiatry*, 122, 259–68.

Weinryb, R.M., Gustavsson, J.P., Åsberg, M. & Rössel, R.J. (1992). Stability over time of character assessment using a psychodynamic instrument and personality inventories. *Acta Psychiatrica Scandinavica*, **86**, 179–84.

Weiss, G. (1985). Hyperactivity. Overview and new directions. *Psychiatric Clinics of North America*, **8**, 737–53.

Weiss, G., Hechtman, L., Perlman, T. *et al.* (1979). Hyperactives as young adults. *Archives of General Psychiatry*, **36**, 675–81.

Weiss, R.D. & Mirin, S.M. (1986). Subtypes of cocaine abusers. *Psychiatric Clinics of North America*, **9**, 491–501.

Weissman, M.M. (1993). The epidemiology of personality disorders: a 1990 update. *Journal of Personality Disorders*, Spring suppl., 44–62.

Weissman, M.M., Klerman, G.L. & Prusoff, B. (1981). Depressed outpatients one year after treatment with drugs and/or psychotherapy. *Archives of General Psychiatry*, **38**, 51–5.

Weissman, M.M., Myers, J.K. & Harding, P.S. (1978). Psychiatric disorder in a US urban community. *American Journal of Psychiatry*, **135**, 459–62.

Welch, L.W. & Bear, D. (1990). Organic disorders of personality. In: *Treating Personality Disorders*, ed. D.H. Adler. San Francisco: Jossey-Bass Inc., Publishers.

Wells, J.E., Bushnell, J.A., Hornblow, A.R. *et al.* (1989). Christchurch Psychiatric Epidemiology Study. Part I: Methodology and lifetime prevalence for specific psychiatric disorders. *Australian and New Zealand Journal of Psychiatry*, **23**, 315–26.

Wender, P.H., Reimherr, R.W., Wood, D. & Ward, M. (1985). A controlled study of methylphenidate in the treatment of attention deficit disorder, residual type, in adults. *American Journal of Psychiatry*, **142**, 547–52.

Wender, P.H., Wood, D. & Reimherr, F. (1984). Studies in attention deficit disorder, residual type (minimal brain dysfunction in adults). *Psychopharmacology Bulletin*, **20**, 18–20.

Werner, E.E. (1985). Stress and protective factors in children's lives. In: *Longitudinal Studies in Child Psychology and Psychiatry*, ed. A.R. Nicol. Chichester: Wiley.

West, D.J. (1983). The childhood origins of delinquency and antisocial behaviour. In: *Handbook of Psychiatry, vol. 4, The Neuroses and Personality Disorders*, ed. G.F.M. Russell & L. Hersov. Cambridge, UK: Cambridge University Press.

West, D.J. & Farrington, D.P. (1977). *The Delinquent Way of Life*. London: Heinemann Educational Books.

Westen, D., Ludolph, P., Misle, B. *et al.* (1990). Physical and sexual abuse in adolescent girls with borderline personality disorder. *American Journal of Orthopsychiatry*, **60**, 55–66.

Weston, S.C. & Siever, L.J. (1993). Biologic correlates of personality disorders. *Journal of Personality Disorders*, Spring Suppl., 129–48.

Whitehorn, J.C. (1952). Basic psychiatry in medical practice. *Journal of the American Medical Association*, **148**, 329–32.

Whiteley, J.S. (1970). The response of psychopaths to a therapeutic community. *British Journal of Psychiatry*, **116**, 517–29.

Whitman, R.M., Trosman, H. & Koenig, R. (1954). Clinical assessment of passive-aggressive personality. *Archives of Neurology and Psychiatry*, **72**, 540–9.

Widiger, T.A. (1987). *Personality Interview Questions II (PIQ-II)*. University of Kentucky, Lexington, KY 40506, USA.

Widiger, T.A. (1989). The categorical distinction between personality and affective disorders. *Journal of Personality Disorders*, **3**, 77–91.

Widiger, T.A. (1992). Categorical versus dimensional classification: implications from and for research. *Journal of Personality Disorders*, **6**, 287–300.

Widiger, T.A. & Frances, A. (1985*a*). The DSM-III personality disorders. *Archives of General Psychiatry*, **42**, 615–23.

Widiger, T.A. & Frances, A. (1985*b*). Axis II personality disorders: diagnostic and treatment issues. *Hospital and Community Psychiatry*, **36**, 619–27.

Widiger, T.A. & Frances, A. (1987). Interviews and inventories for the measurement of personality disorders. *Clinical Psychology Review*, **7**, 49–75.

Widiger, T.A., Frances, A., Spitzer, R.L. & Williams, J.B.W. (1988). The DSM-III-R personality disorders: an overview. *American Journal of Psychiatry*, **145**, 786–95.

Widiger, T.A. & Shea, T. (1991). Differentiation of Axis I and Axis II disorders. *Journal of Abnormal Psychology*, **100**, 399–406.

Williams, J.B.W. & Spitzer, R.L. (1982). Idiopathic pain disorder: a critique of pain-prone disorder and a proposal for a revision of the DSM-III category psychogenic pain disorder. *Journal of Nervous and Mental Disease*, **8**, 415–9.

Wimer, R.E. & Wimer, C.C. (1985). Animal behavior genetics: a search for the biological foundations of behavior. *Annual Review of Psychology*, **36**, 171–218.

Wink, P. & Gough, H.G. (1990). New narcissism scales for the California Psychological Inventory and MMPI. *Journal of Personality Assessment*, **54**, 446–62.

Winnicott, D.W. (1949). Hate in the countertransference. *International Journal of Psychoanalysis*, **30**, 69–75.

Winokur, G., Black, D.W. & Nasrallah, A. (1988). Depressions secondary to other psychiatric disorders and medical illnesses. *American Journal of Psychiatry*, **145**, 233–7.

Winston, A., Laikin, M., Pollack, J. *et al.* (1994). Short-term psychotherapy of personality disorders. *American Journal of Psychiatry*, **151**, 190–4.

Winston, A., Pollack, J., McCullough, L. *et al.* (1991). Brief psychotherapy of personality disorders. *Journal of Nervous and Mental Disease*, **179**, 188–93.

Wise, T.N., Mann, L.S. & Shay, L. (1992). Alexithymia and the five-factor model of personality. *Comprehensive Psychiatry*, **33**, 147–51.

Woerner, P.I. & Guze, S.B. (1968). A family and marital study of hysteria. *British Journal of Psychiatry*, **114**, 161–8.

Wolf, A. & Schwartz, E.K. (1962). *Psychoanalysis in Groups*. New York: Grune & Stratton.

Wolff, S. (1983). The impact of sociopathic and inadequate parents on their children (including child abuse). In: *Handbook of Psychiatry, Vol. 4. The Neuroses and Personality Disorders*, ed. G.F.M. Russell & L. Hersov, pp. 410–4. Cambridge: Cambridge University Press.

Wolff, S. (1991). 'Schizoid' personality in childhood and adult life, I, II, III. *British Journal of Psychiatry*, **159**, 615–35.

Wolff, S. & Chick, J. (1980). Schizoid personality in childhood: a controlled follow-up study. *Psychological Medicine*, **10**, 85–100.

Wolfgang, M., Figlio, R.F. & Sellin, T. (1972). *Delinquency in a Birth Cohort*. Chicago: University of Chicago Press.

Wolkind, S.N. & Rutter, M. (1985). Separation, loss and family relationships. In: *Child and Adolescent Psychiatry: Modern Approaches*, 2nd edn, ed. M.

Rutter & C. Hersov. Oxford: Blackwell Scientific.

Wonderlich, S.A., Fullerton, D., Swift, W.J. & Klein, M.H. (1994). Five-year outcome from eating disorders: relevance of personality disorders. *International Journal of Eating Disorders*, **15**, 233–43.

Wong, N. (1980). Combined group and individual treatment of borderline and narcissistic patients: heterogeneous vs. homogeneous groups. *International Journal of Group Psychotherapy*, **30**, 389–404.

Wood, D., Reimherr, R.W., Wender, P. & Johnson, G.E. (1976). Diagnosis and treatment of minimal brain dysfunction in adults. *Archives of General Psychiatry*, **33**, 1453–60.

Woody, G.E., McLellan, A.T., Luborsky, L. & O'Brien, C.B. (1985). Sociopathy and psychotherapy outcome. *Archives of General Psychiatry*, **42**, 1081–6.

Woollcott, P. (1985). Prognostic indicators in the psychotherapy of borderline patients. *American Journal of Psychotherapy*, **39**, 17–29.

World Health Organization (1978). *International Classification of Diseases*, 9th rev. (ICD-9). Geneva: World Health Organization.

World Health Organization (1992). *The ICD-10 Classification of Mental and Behavioural Disorders*. Geneva: World Health Organization.

World Health Organization (1993). *The ICD-10 Classification of Mental and Behavioural Disorders. Diagnostic Criteria for Research*. Geneva: World Health Organization.

Wrobel, T. & Lachar, D. (1982). Validity of the Weiner subtle and obvious scales for the MMPI: another example of the importance of inventory-item content. *Journal of Consulting and Clinical Psychology*, **50**, 469–70.

Yalom, I.D. (1966). Problems of neophyte group therapists. *International Journal of Social Psychiatry*, **12**, 52–7.

Yalom, I.D. (1975). *The Theory and Practice of Group Psychotherapy*. New York: Basic Books.

Yalom, I.D., Bond, G., Block, S. *et al.* (1977). The impact of a weekend group experience on individual therapy. *Archives of General Psychiatry*, **34**, 399–403.

Yalom, I.D., Brown, S. & Bloch, S. (1975). The written summary as a group psychotherapy technique. *Archives of General Psychiatry*, **32**, 605–11.

Yalom, I.D., Houts, P.S., Newell, G. & Rand, K.H. (1967). Preparation of patients for group therapy. A controlled study. *Archives of General Psychiatry*, **17**, 416–21.

Yates, W.R., Bowers, W.H., Carney, C.P. & Fulton, A.I. (1990). Is bulimia nervosa related to alcohol abuse? A personality analysis. *Annals of Clinical Psychiatry*, **2**, 23–7.

Yates, W.R., Noyes, R., Petty, F. *et al.* (1987). Factors associated with motor vehicle accidents among male alcoholics. *Journal of Studies in Alcohol*, **48**, 586–90.

Yates, W.R., Petty, F. & Brown, K. (1988). Alcoholism in males with antisocial personality disorder. *International Journal of Addictions*, **23**, 999–1010.

Yeung, A.S., Lyons, M.J., Waternaux, C.M. *et al.* (1993). Empirical determination of thresholds for case identification: validation of the Personality Diagnostic Questionnaire – Revised. *Comprehensive Psychiatry*, **34**, 384–91.

Young, M.A., Sheftner, W.A., Klerman, G.L. *et al.* (1986). The endogenous subtype of depression: a study of its internal construct validity. *British Journal of Psychiatry*, **148**, 257–67.

Yudofsky, S.C., Silver, J.M. & Jackson, W. (1986). The Overt Aggression Scale for the objective rating of verbal and physical aggression. *American Journal of Psychiatry*, **143**, 35–9.

Zanarini, M., Frankenburg, F., Chauncey, D. & Gunderson, J.G. (1987). The diagnostic interview for personality disorders: interrater and test-retest reliability. *Comprehensive Psychiatry*, **28**, 467–80.

Zanarini, M.C., Gunderson, J.G. & Frankenburg, F.R. (1990). Cognitive features of borderline personality disorder. *American Journal of Psychiatry*, **147**, 57–63.

Zanarini, M.C., Gunderson, J.G., Frankenburg, R.F. *et al.* (1991). The face validity of the DSM-III and DSM-III-R criteria sets for borderline personality disorder. *American Journal of Psychiatry*, **148**, 870–74.

Zanarini, M.C., Gunderson, J.G., Marino, M.F. *et al.* (1989). Childhood experiences of borderlines. *Comprehensive Psychiatry*, **30**, 18–25.

Zeitlyn, B.B. (1967). The therapeutic community – fact or fantasy. *British Journal of Psychiatry*, **113**, 1083–7.

Zilber, N., Schufman, N. & Lerner, Y. (1989). Mortality among psychiatric patients – the groups at risk. *Acta Psychiatrica Scandinavica*, **79**, 248–56.

Zimmerman, M. (1994). Diagnosing personality disorders. *Archives of General Psychiatry*, **51**, 225–45.

Zimmerman, M. & Coryell, W. (1989). DSM-III personality disorder diagnoses in a non patient sample. *Archives of General Psychiatry*, **46**, 682–9.

Zimmerman, M. & Coryell, W. (1990). Diagnosing personality disorders in the community. A comparison of self-report and interview measures. *Archives of General Psychiatry*, **47**, 527–31.

Zimmerman, M., Coryell, W. & Pfohl, B. (1986). ECT response in depressed patients with and without a DSM-III personality disorder. *American Journal of Psychiatry*, **143**, 1030–2.

Zimmerman, M., Pfohl, B., Coryell, W. *et al.* (1988). Diagnosing personality disorder in depressed patients. *Archives of General Psychiatry*, **45**, 733–7.

Zivich, J.M. (1981). Alcoholic subtypes and treatment effectiveness. *Journal of Consulting and Clinical Psychology*, **49**, 72–80.

Zoccolillo, M. & Rogers, K. (1991). Characteristics and outcome of hospitalized adolescent girls with conduct disorders. *Journal of American Academy of Child and Adolescent Psychiatry*, **30**, 973–81.

Zuckerman, M. (1991) Basic dimensions of personality and consistency of personality. In: *Psychology of Personality*, pp. 1–88. Cambridge, UK: Cambridge University Press.

Zuroff, D. & Mongrain, M. (1987). Dependency and self-criticism: vulnerability factors for depressive affective states. *Journal of Abnormal Psychology*, **96**, 14–22.

Index

Page numbers for tables are in italics

386